# Sleep Disorders in Children and Adolescents

*Editors*

ARGELINDA BARONI
JESSICA R. LUNSFORD-AVERY

# PSYCHIATRIC CLINICS OF NORTH AMERICA

www.psych.theclinics.com

*Consulting Editor*
HARSH K. TRIVEDI

March 2024 • Volume 47 • Number 1

**ELSEVIER**

1600 John F. Kennedy Boulevard ● Suite 1800 ● Philadelphia, Pennsylvania, 19103-2899

http://www.theclinics.com

**PSYCHIATRIC CLINICS OF NORTH AMERICA Volume 47, Number 1**
**March 2024 ISSN 0193-953X, ISBN-13: 978-0-443-24698-2**

Editor: Megan Ashdown
Developmental Editor: Varun Gopal

*Psychiatric Clinics of North America* (ISSN 0193-953X) is published quarterly by Elsevier Inc., 360 Park Avenue South, New York, NY 10010-1710. Months of issue are March, June, September, and December. Business and Editorial Offices: 1600 John F. Kennedy Blvd., Suite 1800, Philadelphia, PA 19103-2899. Periodicals postage paid at New York, NY and additional mailing offices. Subscription prices are $362.00 per year (US individuals), $100.00 per year (US students/residents), $422.00 per year (Canadian individuals), $535.00 per year (international individuals), and $220.00 per year (international students/residents), $100.00 per year (Canadian & students/residents). For institutional access pricing please contact Customer Service via the contact information below. Foreign air speed delivery is included in all *Clinics'* subscription prices. All prices are subject to change without notice. **POSTMASTER:** Send address changes to *Psychiatric Clinics of North America*, Elsevier Health Sciences Division, Subscription Customer Service, 3251 Riverport Lane, Maryland Heights, MO 63043. **Customer Service: 1-800-654-2452 (US). From outside the United States, call 1-314-447-8871. Fax: 1-314-447-8029. E-mail: journalscustomerservice-usa@elsevier.com (for print support) and journalsonlinesupport-usa@elsevier.com (for online support).**

*Reprints.* For copies of 100 or more, of articles in this publication, please contact the Commercial Reprints Department, Elsevier Inc., 360 Park Avenue South, New York, New York 10010-1710. Tel.: 212-633-3874, Fax: 212-633-3820, E-mail: reprints@elsevier.com.

*Psychiatric Clinics of North America* is covered in *MEDLINE/PubMed (Index Medicus), Current Contents/Social and Behavioral Sciences, Social Science Citation Index, Embase/Excerpta Medica,* and PsycINFO.

# Contributors

## CONSULTING EDITOR

**HARSH K. TRIVEDI, MD, MBA**
President and Chief Executive Officer, Sheppard Pratt, Clinical Professor of Psychiatry, University of Maryland School of Medicine, Baltimore, Maryland

## EDITORS

**ARGELINDA BARONI, MD**
Clinical Associate Professor, Department of Child and Adolescent Psychiatry, NYU Grossman School of Medicine, New York, New York, USA

**JESSICA R. LUNSFORD-AVERY, PhD**
Associate Professor, Department of Psychiatry, Duke University School of Medicine, Durham, North Carlina, USA

## AUTHORS

**ALEX AGOSTINI, BPsych(Hons), PhD**
Sleep and Chronobiology Laboratory, University of South Australia, Adelaide, South Australia, Australia

**LAUREN D. ASARNOW, PhD**
Assistant Professor, University of California, San Francisco, Department of Psychiatry and Behavioral Sciences, San Francisco, California, USA

**SUMAN K.R. BADDAM, MD**
Assistant Professor of Clinical Child Psychiatry, Yale Child Study Center, Yale School of Medicine, New Haven, Connecticut, USA

**ARGELINDA BARONI, MD**
Clinical Associate Professor, Department of Child and Adolescent Psychiatry, NYU Grossman School of Medicine, New York, New York, USA

**TATYANA BIDOPIA, BS**
Department of Psychology, Fordham University, Bronx, New York, USA

**OLIVIERO BRUNI, MD**
Department of Developmental and Social Psychology, Sapienza University, Rome, Italy

**CRAIG A. CANAPARI, MD**
Associate Professor of Pediatrics, Division of Pulmonary Medicine, Department of Pediatrics, Yale School of Medicine, New Haven, Connecticut, USA

**STEPHANIE CENTOFANTI, BPsych(Hons), PhD**
UniSA Online, University of South Australia, University of South Australia Online, Adelaide, South Australia, Australia

**KATHERINE CROWE, PhD**
Clinical Assistant Professor, Department of Child and Adolescent Psychiatry, Hassenfeld Children's Hospital at NYU Langone, New York, New York, USA

**MICHAEL J. CROWLEY, PhD**
Associate Professor, Yale Child Study Center, Yale School of Medicine, New Haven, Connecticut, USA

**LOURDES M. DELROSSO, MD, MEd**
Department of Internal Medicine, University of California San Francisco, Fresno, California, USA

**JENNY DIMAKOS, BSc**
Faculty of Medicine, McGill University, Montréal, Quebec, Canada

**VIJAYABHARATHI EKAMBARAM, MD, MPH**
Professor, Department of Psychiatry, University of Central Florida, HCA Florida Healthcare Program, Pensacola, Florida, USA

**MICHAEL A. FEDER, PhD**
Clinical Assistant Professor, Department of Child and Adolescent Psychiatry, Hassenfeld Children's Hospital at NYU Langone, NYC H1H/Bellevue, Child Study Center, New York, New York, USA

**VERONICA FELLMAN, DO**
Clinical Assistant Professor, Department of Child and Adolescent Psychiatry, NYU Grossman School of Medicine, Child Study Center, New York, New York, USA

**SARA N. FERNANDES, MA**
Clinical Research Assistant, New York State Psychiatric Institute, Columbia University Irving Medical Center, New York, New York, USA

**RAFFAELE FERRI, MD**
Department of Neurology I.C., Sleep Research Centre, Oasi Institute for Research on Mental Retardation and Brain Aging (IRCCS), Troina, Italy

**GABRIELLE GAUTHIER-GAGNÉ, BA**
Attention, Behaviour and Sleep Lab, Douglas Mental Health University Institute, Montréal, Quebec, Canada

**REUT GRUBER, PhD**
Director, Attention Behavior and Sleep Lab, Douglas Mental Health University Institute, Department of Psychiatry, Faculty of Medicine, McGill University, Montréal, Quebec, Canada

**PATRICK J. HEPPELL, Psy.D**
Clinical Assistant Professor, Department of Child and Adolescent Psychiatry, NYU Grossman School of Medicine, Child Study Center, New York City, New York, USA

**MADELINE HIMELFARB, BFA**
Department of Child and Adolescent Psychiatry, New York University, New York, New York, USA

**ANNA IVANENKO, MD, PhD**
Profession of Clinical Psychiatry and Behavioral Sciences, Feinberg School of Medicine, Northwestern University, Division of Child and Adolescent Psychiatry, Ann and Robert H. Lurie Children's Hospital of Chicago, Chicago, Illinois, USA

**LEAH JACKSON, MS**
Department of OB/GYN, Duke University, Durham, North Carolina, USA

**KYLE P. JOHNSON, MD**
Professor, Division of Child and Adolescent Psychiatry, Oregon Health & Science University, Portland, Oregon, USA

**LANYI LIN, BSc**
Attention, Behaviour and Sleep Lab, Douglas Mental Health University Institute, Montréal, Quebec, Canada

**JESSICA R. LUNSFORD-AVERY, PhD**
Associate Professor, Department of Psychiatry, Duke University School of Medicine, Durham, North Carolina, USA

**CHRISTOPHER MCGIRR, APRN**
Instructor in Child Psychiatry, Yale Child Study Center, Yale School of Medicine, New Haven, Connecticut, USA

**MARIA GRAZIA MELEGARI, MD**
Department of Developmental and Social Psychology, Sapienza University, Rome, Italy

**REGINA MIRANDA, PhD**
Professor, Department of Psychology, Hunter College and The Graduate Center, City University of New York, New York, New York, USA

**RIYA MIRCHANDANEY, BA**
Research Coordinator, University of California, San Francisco, Department of Psychiatry and Behavioral Sciences, San Francisco, California, USA

**MARIA PAOLA MOGAVERO, MD**
Vita-Salute San Raffaele University, San Raffaele Scientific Institute, Division of Neuroscience, Sleep Disorders Center, Milan, Italy

**ALEXANDRA Y. NASSER, DPT**
Midstate Medical Center, Meriden, Connecticut, USA

**AMY I. NATHANSON, PhD**
Professor, School of Communication, Ohio State University, Columbus, Ohio, USA

**JUDITH OWENS, MD, MPH**
Professor, Department of Neurology, Boston Children's Hospital, Harvard Medical School, Boston, Massachusetts, USA

**SUCHET RAO, MD**
Medical Director, Psychiatry and Behavioral Health, NYC Administration for Children's Services, New York, New York, USA

**SAMANTHA SCHOLES, BA**
Attention, Behaviour and Sleep Lab, Douglas Mental Health University Institute, Department of Educational and Counselling Psychology, McGill University, Montréal, Quebec, Canada

**JESS P. SHATKIN, MD, MPH**
Professor of Child and Adolescent Psychiatry and Pediatrics, Department of Child and Adolescent Psychiatry, New York University, New York, New York, USA

**JESSICA SOLIS SLOAN, PhD**
HRC Behavioral Health & Psychiatry, PA, Chapel Hill, North Carolina, USA

**CAROLYN SPIRO-LEVITT, PhD**
Clinical Psychologist, Home for Anxiety, Repetitive Behaviors, OCD, and Related Disorders (HARBOR), Philadelphia, Pennsylvania, USA

**KAREN SPRUYT, PhD**
Université Paris Cité, INSERM - NeuroDiderot, Paris, France

**IRINA TROSMAN, MD**
Division of Pulmonary and Sleep Medicine, Ann and Robert H. Lurie Children's Hospital of Chicago, Chicago, Illinois, USA

**JENNA VAN DE GRIFT, BS**
Yale Child Study Center, Yale School of Medicine, New Haven, Connecticut, USA

**PARIA ZARRINNEGAR, MD**
Assistant Professor, Division of Child and Adolescent Psychiatry, Oregon Health & Science University, Portland, Oregon, USA

**EMILY ZUCKERMAN, BA**
Research Associate, Department of Child and Adolescent Psychiatry, NYU Langone Health, New York, New York, USA

# Contents

Adequate sleep is essential for healthy development in childhood and adolescence. Healthy sleep contributes to good physical health, immune function, mental health, and academic performance. The regulation and architecture of sleep change greatly across childhood and adolescence, and the ability to obtain sufficient sleep is impacted by a range of factors that change with maturation. This article describes normal sleep across childhood and adolescence and discusses some of the most common barriers to adequate sleep, including early school start times, technology use, and changes to circadian rhythms, and sleep homeostasis across puberty.

Research suggests that technology use is associated with poorer sleep outcomes among children less than 6 years of age. These associations are evident regardless of the type of technology studied, although evening exposure may have the greatest impact compared with technology use during other parts of the day. More work is needed, particularly given that technology use is relatively high among young children. Clinicians should assess patients' technology exposure, including before bedtime, to assess whether sleep issues stem from children's technology use. Moreover, clinicians should educate caregivers about the association between technology use and sleep problems among young children.

A main childhood task is learning. In this task, the role of sleep is increasingly demonstrated. Although most literature examining this role focuses on preadolescence and middle adolescence, some studies apply napping designs in preschoolers. Studies overall conclude that without proper sleep a child's cognitive abilities suffer, but questions on how and to what extent linger. Observational studies show the hazards of potential confounders such as an individual's resilience to poor sleep as well as developmental risk factors (eg, disorders, stressors). A better understanding of cognitive sleep neuroscience may have a big impact on pediatric sleep research and clinical applications.

Sleep disturbances are common in children and adolescents but still remain unrecognized and undertreated. Several classification systems of
sleep disorders are available, which include recent attempts to develop
more specific nosologic categories that reflect developmental aspects of
sleep. The prevalence of sleep disorders has been studied across various
samples of healthy, typically developing children and those with special
medical, psychiatric, and neurodevelopmental needs. Sleep disorders
are highly prevalent in children and adolescents with psychiatric disorders,
making it important for mental health professionals to be aware of sleep
problems and to address them in the context of psychiatric comorbidities.

Sleep disturbances and sleep disorders are prevalent in children/adoles-
cents and have a bidirectional relationship with pediatric medical and mental health disorders. Screening tools and mechanisms for the evaluation
and treatment of sleep disturbances and sleep disorders in the pediatric
mental health clinic are less well-known; hence, sleep disturbances and
disorders are under-recognized in the pediatric clinics. We present specific, validated screening and evaluation tools to identify sleep disturbances and sleep disorders in children/adolescents. We offer guidance
related to the use of consumer wearables for sleep assessments and
use of sleep telemedicine in pediatric mental health and primary care
clinics.

Pediatric insomnia can affect physical and mental health and cause cognitive deficits, social deficits and decrease quality of life. There are no
Food and Drug Administration approved medications approved for pediatric insomnia. Pharmacologic interventions derive mostly from adult data
or pediatric case reports. This review focuses on Food and Drug Administration approved prescription drugs (in adults), over-the-counter drugs,
and off-label pediatric insomnia drugs. This review helps the clinician learn
general principles, practice guidelines, and pharmacologic considerations
for medication selection in the pediatric population. Pharmacologic management should be considered in combination with behavior therapy,
which is proven to have long-lasting outcomes.

Insomnia and related sleep disturbances are prevalent among youth and
are associated with adverse consequences, including poorer psychiatric
functioning. Behavioral sleep interventions, ranging from brief educational

interventions to behavioral therapies (cognitive behavior therapy–insomnia), are associated with positive outcomes for pediatric sleep health. In addition, sleep interventions may improve psychiatric health for children and adolescents with neurodevelopmental and internalizing disorders. Additional research is necessary to clarify the efficacy of these interventions over the long-term and across demographic groups; however, evidence suggests incorporating behavioral sleep strategies may prove beneficial to pediatric patients with sleep disturbances and related psychiatric complaints.

Insomnia is the most common sleep disorder among all ages; unfortunately, however, child and adolescent insomnia is infrequently addressed. Given the importance of adequate sleep for proper brain development, pediatric populations are particularly vulnerable to the negative effects of insomnia. Therefore, proper clinical assessment and treatment of pediatric insomnia is crucial. This article is the result of a comprehensive literature review and serves as a guide to the disorder and how it presents differently across child development.

Parasomnias usually present in childhood and resolve spontaneously. The diagnosis of non–rapid eye movement–related parasomnias is mainly based on clinical descriptors and can be challenging. Rapid eye movement–related parasomnias may index an underlying psychiatric disorder. Even if benign, parasomnias can affect quality of life. Pediatricians and psychiatrists should be familiarized with these sleep disorders and suggest adequate sleep hygiene, avoidance of sleep deprivation, and regular bedtimes even on weekends as the first step in management of these disorders. Clinicians should pursue the opportunity for tailoring treatments and consider referral to a sleep expert when indicated.

Children with psychiatric comorbidities frequently are referred for evaluation of sleep complaints. Common sleep symptoms can include difficulty falling asleep, frequent nocturnal awakening, restless sleep, and symptoms of restless legs syndrome (RLS). The understanding of the sleep condition in relation to the psychiatric comorbidity often is a challenge to the physician and often sleep disorders remain undiagnosed, untreated, or undertreated. Restless legs syndrome has been associated with psychiatric comorbidities and with certain medications, such as antidepressants, antihistamines, and antipsychotics. This article reviews the presentation of RLS and restless sleep, the association with psychiatric comorbidities, and treatment options.

Traumatic experiences and sleep disturbances are both common in children and adolescents. Because of the reciprocal relationship between sleep complaints and trauma, a mental health evaluation should include not only an assessment of posttraumatic stress disorder and other trauma symptoms but also a specific evaluation of sleep-related complaints. Similarly, if a history of both trauma and sleep complaints is identified, an effective trauma-informed intervention, whether psychological, psychopharmacologic, or a combination of the two, should directly address sleep issues.

This article reviews the literature on mood disorders and sleep disorders among children and adolescents. Research suggests that sleep plays an important role in the development, progression, and maintenance of mood disorder symptoms among children and adolescents. Sleep problems as early as maternal perinatal insomnia may predict and predate depression among youth. Children and adolescents who develop comorbid mood disorders and sleep problems represent a particularly high-risk group with more severe mood episode symptoms, higher rates of self-harm and suicidality, and less responsivity to treatment. Treatment research supports the idea that sleep problems can be improved through behavioral interventions.

Sleep disturbances have been linked to suicidal ideation and behaviors in adolescents. Specifically, insomnia and nightmares are associated with current suicide risk and predict future ideation. Associations between hypersomnia, sleep apnea, and suicide remain inconclusive. Potential biological mechanisms underlying these relationships include executive functioning deficits and hyperarousal. Related psychological factors may include thwarted belongingness, perceived burdensomeness, and negative appraisals. Assessing suicide risk in patients with sleep disturbances, and vice versa, is needed. Therapeutic interventions such as cognitive behavior therapy for insomnia and imagery rehearsal treatment, as well as pharmacologic treatments, show promise in treating sleep disorders and suicidal behavior.

# PSYCHIATRIC CLINICS OF NORTH AMERICA

## FORTHCOMING ISSUES

*September 2024*
**Cognitive Behavioral Therapy**
Stefan G. Hofmann, Jasper A.J. Smits, and Rianne de Kleine, *Editors*

*September 2024*
**Crisis Services**
Margie Balfour and Matthew Goldman, *Editors*

*December 2024*
**Anxiety Disorders**
Jordan Stiede and Eric Storch, *Editors*

## RECENT ISSUES

*December 2023*
**Adolescent Cannabis Use**
Paula Riggs, Jesse D. Hinckley and Jessica Megan Ross, *Editors*

*September 2023*
**Women's Mental Health**
Susan G. Kornstein and Anita H. Clayton, *Editors*

*June 2023*
**Treatment Resistant Depression**
Manish K. Jha and Madhukar H. Trivedi, *Editors*

## SERIES OF RELATED INTEREST

*Child and Adolescent Psychiatric Clinics of North America*
*https://www.childpsych.theclinics.com/*

*Neurologic Clinics*
*https://www.neurologic.theclinics.com/*

*Advances in Psychiatry and Behavioral Health*
*https://www.advancesinpsychiatryandbehavioralhealth.com/*

# Preface

# Pediatric Sleep as the Foundation for Healthy Sleep Across the Life Span

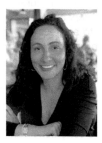
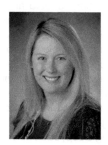

Argelinda Baroni, MD          Jessica R. Lunsford-Avery, PhD
*Editors*

Poets and philosophers acclaimed the importance of sleep long before clinicians recognized its essential role in health across the life span. Despite these long-term, widespread exhortations from both medical and nonmedical communities, sleep disorders remain common and understudied. In this issue, we focus on sleep and its disturbances in children and adolescents. Addressing sleep in youth is crucial, as sleep disturbances negatively affect children's cognitive and emotional functioning. Furthermore, childhood sleep problems often signal risk of negative patterns that persist into adult life. By intervening early, we may prevent acute detrimental effects of poor or insufficient sleep and possibly support healthier sleep and its benefits across the life course.

In this issue, Alex Agostini and Stephanie Centofanti set the stage by delineating normal sleep patterns across childhood and adolescence. They discuss developmental changes and common environmental barriers to healthy sleep, including early school start times and technology use. Amy Nathanson focuses on the impact of screens on the sleep of preschool children and the importance of facilitating long-term prevention by empowering parents. Karen Spruyt tackles the complex questions regarding neuro-cognitive effects of disrupted sleep among youth. She also provides an excellent summary of hypotheses regarding the role of sleep in cognitive function and highlights the key research questions, derived from these hypotheses, which still need to be answered.

We then turn to specific sleep disorders with Irina Trosman and Anna Ivanenko, who present the sleep disorders classification and prevalence in the general population and highlight the comorbidity between sleep and psychiatric disorders. Suman Baddam and colleagues provide an exhaustive review of screening tools to detect sleep

Psychiatr Clin N Am 47 (2024) xiii–xv
https://doi.org/10.1016/j.psc.2023.10.001
0193-953X/24/© 2023 Published by Elsevier Inc.

psych.theclinics.com

problems in the clinic, including the proliferation of wearables that provide objective indices of sleep while limiting inconvenience to the family. They also provide guidance for how to conduct a comprehensive sleep evaluation.

Although the Food and Drug Administration has not approved any medications for the treatment of pediatric insomnia, clinicians are often pressed to prescribe medications for sleep disturbances. Vijayabharathi Ekamabaram and Judith Owens review the medications that are most frequently used off-label for insomnia in children, including medications approved for use in insomnia in adults, as well as over-the-counter and other prescription drugs that are used off-label for pediatric patients. They emphasize that medications should always be adjunctive to behavioral treatments, which are the focus of the review by Jessica Lunsford-Avery and colleagues. They provide an extensive summary of behavioral techniques to address insomnia. They also show that, although multiple questions remain on how to best implement behavioral treatments, evidence for their efficacy and effectiveness is already compelling. Pediatric insomnia is also the focus of the comprehensive review by Madeline Himelfarb and Jess Shatkin, who remark that insomnia is both the most common and the most undertreated sleep disorder across the life span.

Oliviero Bruni and colleagues survey the parasomnias, which manifest as abnormal behaviors or emotions during sleep, such as sleepwalking. These conditions may herald an underlying psychiatric disorder and negatively affect quality of life of children. Recommendations are provided for the first phase of treatment, which will be sufficient for most, as well as how to proceed for those who need referrals to specialists and personalized treatments.

Lourdes DelRosso and colleagues cover the often-puzzling condition of restless legs syndrome, which can be an index of psychiatric comorbidities but can also be provoked or unmasked by certain psychotropic medications. The authors also discuss the recently introduced restless sleep disorder.

Delayed sleep phase disorder is reviewed by Michael Feder and Argelinda Baroni, who note that its prevalence in adolescents is high, and it is a frequent comorbidity with other psychiatric disorders. Fortunately, when recognized, appropriate treatments can be instituted, which combine behavioral approaches, appropriately timed light exposure, gradual shifts in sleep-wake times, and low-dose melatonin.

The complex interrelationships among sleep disorders and psychopathology are the focus of the remaining contributions, beginning with the review by Jenny Dimakos, Reut Gruber, and colleagues of the bidirectional associations between sleep and internalizing and externalizing symptoms of attention-deficit/hyperactivity disorder. They conclude that clinicians must assess and address both sleep problems and the associated clinical conditions for optimal outcomes.

Autistic youth are particularly prone to experience disturbed sleep, particularly insomnia, and this is often a major stressor for children and caregivers. Accordingly, specific recommendations, including how to modify behavioral interventions, essentials of parent education, and the judicious use of low-dose melatonin and other prescription medications, are discussed in depth by Kyle Johnson and Paria Zarrinnegar.

Katherine Crowe and Carolyn Spiro-Levitt examine the bidirectional relationship between anxiety disorders, the most prevalent form of psychopathology in youth, and sleep-related problems. The extant literature is reviewed to support the application of behavioral interventions, including the use of a transitional object for the youngest children, as well as exposure and response prevention, positive reinforcement, and cognitive self-instruction for school-aged children and adolescents.

Among the core symptoms of posttraumatic stress disorder are disturbances of sleep, including nightmares. These are reviewed by Veronica Fellman, Patrick Heppell, and

Suchet Rao, who note the importance of assessing for both trauma history and disturbances of sleep when either domain is implicated.

The greatest continuity between sleep problems in youth and in adulthood is found in the tight linkages between sleep and mood disorders, which are covered by Lauren Asornow and Riya Mirchandaney. They note that maternal perinatal insomnia can predict depression in the offspring, and that youth with cooccurring sleep problems and mood disorders are at risk of the worst long-term psychiatric outcomes. Fortunately, addressing the sleep problems may often ameliorate the cooccurring mood disturbances.

Among the worst outcomes of complex psychopathology is suicide, which is the focus of the closing contribution by Sara Fernandes and colleagues. They note that insomnia and nightmares are associated with current suicide risk, and that assessing suicide risk in patients with sleep disturbances, and vice versa, is imperative. Promising interventions include cognitive behavior therapy, including both insomnia-targeting strategies and imagery rehearsal treatment.

We thank our contributing colleagues, who include the leading experts on sleep and its disturbances in youth, and the *Psychiatric Clinics of North America* editorial staff. We hope these efforts will spur further advances in the assessment and management of sleep problems across the life span.

Argelinda Baroni, MD
Department of Child and Adolescent Psychiatry
NYU Grossman School of Medicine
One Park Avenue, 7th Floor
New York, NY 10016, USA

Jessica R. Lunsford-Avery, PhD
Department of Psychiatry
Duke University School of Medicine
2400 Pratt Street, 7th Floor
Durham, NC 27705, USA

*E-mail addresses:*
Argelinda.Baroni@nyulangone.org (A. Baroni)
Jessica.R.Avery@duke.edu (J.R. Lunsford-Avery)

# Normal Sleep in Children and Adolescence

Alex Agostini, PhD[a],*, Stephanie Centofanti, PhD[b]

## KEYWORDS

- Sleep • Mental health • Physical health • Barriers to healthy sleep • Technology
- Children • Adolescents

## KEY POINTS

- Sleep plays an integral role in the health and well-being of children and adolescence, including physical health, immune function, mental health, and academic performance.
- Sleep duration, architecture, and timing change significantly over the course of child development.
- Several biological and psychosocial factors combine to result in a preference for later bedtimes across adolescence.
- It is imperative that sleep is considered in the treatment of mental health concerns in children and adolescence.

## INTRODUCTION

Sleep is critical for the healthy development of children and teenagers. Compared with adulthood, childhood and adolescence are times of peak creativity, optimism,[1] and growth[2]; increased opportunities for extracurricular activities; and greater social support.[3] Adolescence also has been referred to, however, as "the great and terrifying transition from childhood to adulthood"[4] and is an extremely important and complex period of development. A multitude of changes occur during adolescence, including puberty, hormonal changes, and social changes, such as forging independence from parents and greater reliance on peers for social support.[5,6] It is a vulnerable period for mood disorders, such as anxiety and depression[7,8] and is also a time during

This article originally appeared in *Child and Adolescent Psychiatric Clinics*, Volume 30 Issue 1, January 2021.
[a] Sleep and Chronobiology Laboratory, University of South Australia, Adelaide, Australia; [b] UniSA Online, University of South Australia, University of South Australia Online, L4, Catherine Helen Spence Building, City West Campus, Adelaide, South Australia 5000, Australia
* Corresponding author. Sleep and Chronobiology Laboratory, University of South Australia, Magill Campus, C Building, Level 1, Room C1-82, St Bernards Road, Magill, South Australia 5072, Australia,
*E-mail address:* alex.agostini@unisa.edu.au
Twitter: @alexagostini3 (A.A.)

Psychiatr Clin N Am 47 (2024) 1–14
https://doi.org/10.1016/j.psc.2023.06.001
0193-953X/24/© 2023 Elsevier Inc. All rights reserved.

which children are likely to experience emotional pressure or bullying.[9] The teenage years are important for physical health, especially weight status,[10] but also growth.[2] During adolescence, risk taking increases as does the importance of school performance.[11] These factors all are intricately linked to sleep, which means it is imperative that health care practitioners are aware of the impact that sleep has on the physical and mental health of children and teenagers.

## IMPACT OF SLEEP ON YOUTH HEALTH AND WELL BEING
### Insufficient Sleep May Result in Poorer School Performance and Impaired Safety

Sleep is imperative for several functions, including sustained attention, learning, and academic achievement.[12–14] Being able to sustain attention and learn is extremely important during childhood and adolescence for many reasons, including school achievement.

Many studies have found relationships between sleep duration and school achievement. Obtaining less than 8 hours sleep per night has been associated with a decrease in mathematics and language skills.[15] Wolfson and Carskadon[16] also found that those receiving C, D, or F grades at school reported on average obtaining 25 minutes less sleep on school nights and going to bed 40 minutes later than those getting A or B grades. Although studies suggest a direct relationship between sleep and academic achievement, there may be indirect influences too. For example, previous research has suggested that eveningness preference (ie, a preference for later bedtimes and rise times),[17,18] lower learning motivation,[18,19] and lower socioeconomic status[20] may lower socioeconomic status may impact the relationship between sleep duration and academic performance, and many studies do not take these potential effects into account. Regardless, most studies suggest that sleep restriction likely is associated with poorer school performance.[21]

Sleep is also important from a safety perspective, because adolescence is a time at which many learn to drive. When learning to drive, adolescents are at increased risk of accidents due to their relative inexperience with driving,[22] which, when teamed with attentional lapses related to sleep loss, may result in an even greater risk of accidents.[23]

### Sleep May be Related to Physical Health

Studies in both humans and animals suggest that the sleep-wake system and the immune system are linked,[24] with sleep helping to restore immune system functioning.[25] Perhaps unsurprisingly, insufficient sleep may result in decreased immune system function, including a weakened response to vaccinations and increased infection.[26] Dickstein and Moldofsky,[27] in their review, concluded that sleep deprivation may result in changes in the levels of hormones necessary for healthy immune function.

Although there is a paucity of research conducted on the associations between health outcomes and sleep duration in healthy child populations, a few studies have investigated the immediate or possible long-term associations between short sleep and physical health. For example, Orzech and colleagues[28] found that adolescents who obtained more sleep reported fewer illnesses than those who obtained less sleep across a 16-week period. Matthews and colleagues[29] found that there also may be longer-term consequences, with shorter sleepers having higher levels of insulin resistance, which is associated with increased risk of cardiovascular disease[30] and diabetes.[31] Similarly, Klingenberg and colleagues[32] found a reduction in insulin sensitivity, which has been linked to increased risk of type 2 diabetes mellitus, in healthy adolescent boys after only 3 nights of sleep restriction. Furthermore, sleeping less than 8 hours per night has been associated with decreased physical activity,[33] which is important for several reasons, from increasing resting metabolic rate to improving blood glucose levels and protecting against chronic illnesses.[34]

Further, insufficient sleep has been associated with greater risk of injuries and increased sedentary behavior. In a study of adolescent athletes, Milewski and colleagues[35] found that insufficient sleep increases the risk of sports injuries. Together, these results suggest that poor sleep in childhood and adolescence could be associated with increased risk of both acute and chronic illness. A large-scale study, however, of sleep and health in children and adolescents is yet to be conducted.

### Poor Sleep Is Associated with Mental Health Concerns

Childhood, in particular adolescence is a vulnerable time for mental health disorders.[7,8] Early intervention for sleep problems is key, with evidence showing that sleep problems as a toddler can predict anxiety and depression in adolescence.[36] Several environmental changes occur during adolescence, as teens forge independence from their parents and rely more on social interaction with their peers.[5] This greater reliance on social interactions may make teens vulnerable to the impact of bullying,[9] which can affect an adolescent's mood and sleep.[37,38] This is a time of life when there is increased pressure to perform well at school, be involved in many extracurricular and social activities, and gain employment,[39] which can lead to increased risk of mental disorders, as can changes in hormonal levels during adolescence.[7,40]

Sleep is a factor that has been consistently related to mood and mental health in adolescence. Several studies have found associations between short sleep and depressed mood. Ojio and colleagues[41] found that the lowest risk of depression and anxiety was in boys who slept 8.5 hours or more and in girls who slept 7.5 hours or more on school nights. In a longitudinal study assessing sleep and mental health, Fredriksen and colleagues[42] found that adolescents who slept less had higher levels of depressive symptoms. Similarly, positive correlations have been found between sleep problems and depressive mood and anxiety.[43] Insufficient sleep also has been found to influence adolescents' ability to deal with stressors such as bullying, having a further impact on mental health.[38]

Studies have also found associations between sleep duration and suicidal thoughts and self-harm behaviors.[44] McKnight-Eily and colleagues[33] found that obtaining less than 8 hours of sleep per night was associated with greater odds of feeling sad or hopeless and seriously considering attempting suicide. Similarly, voluntary sleep curtailment has been correlated with increased suicidality, even after controlling for depression scores.[45] Further, poor sleep quality and duration have been related to emotional and peer-related problems, anxiety, conduct issues, and suicide ideation.[46] Using sleep extension and restriction protocols, experimental studies have supported the findings of these naturalistic studies, showing that adolescents suffer from lower mood and greater emotion regulation problems during periods of sleep restriction.[47,48]

Insufficient sleep can also have an impact on physical and mental health indirectly, via behavioral factors. A study by Owens and colleagues[49] found that decreasing amounts of sleep were associated with increasing odds of risky behaviors, such as antisocial behaviors, drug use, and gang involvement. Furthermore, Weaver and colleagues[50] found that, compared with adolescents who obtained more than 8 hours of sleep, those who obtained less than 6 hours of sleep were approximately twice as likely to engage in risky driving; marijuana, alcohol, and tobacco use; risky sexual behavior; and aggressive behaviors. Alarmingly, this likelihood increased to more than 3 times for considering or attempting suicide and/or making a suicide attempt plan and more than 4 times for an attempted suicide that required treatment. These findings suggest that both direct and indirect impacts of poor sleep may have negative consequences for the mental health of children and adolescents.

In sum, the existing research strongly suggests that sleep is crucial for academic performance and physical and mental health. The following section describes what can be considered normal sleep, how this differs across childhood and adolescence, and the common barriers to healthy sleep.

## SLEEP CHANGES ACROSS CHILD DEVELOPMENT
### Sleep Architecture

The structure of sleep differs with age. For the first 16 weeks of life, sleep has little to no structure, with infants sleeping around the clock.[51] From 16 weeks, sleep begins to adhere to a more diurnal, consolidated nighttime pattern but with frequent naps throughout the day.

The 2 main stages of sleep for infants are referred to as quiet sleep and active sleep. Quiet sleep is characterized by even respiration and discontinuous electroencephalography (EEG) pattern in infants and turns into non–rapid eye movement (NREM) stages of sleep as the infant matures. By 6 weeks to 9 weeks of age, NREM begins to differentiate into light sleep (stages 1 and 2) and deep (slow wave sleep [SWS]), and by 2 months to 3 months of age, the sleep spindles characteristic of stage 2 sleep appear. Active sleep is characterized by uneven respiration, muscle atonia, continuous EEG pattern, rapid eye movements (REMs), sucking movements, and twitches. This stage of sleep matures into REM sleep.

**Fig. 1** displays a typical sleep period in childhood compared with adulthood. In adulthood, a sleep cycle typically lasts 90 minutes and includes a period in each stage of sleep. During early childhood, the percentage of REM sleep often is higher than during adulthood, at approximately 30% compared with 20% to 25% in adulthood, and sleep cycles often are shorter, at approximately 60 minutes compared with 90 minutes in adulthood.[52] Furthermore, during early childhood, the amount of time spent in SWS often is longer compared with during adulthood.[52] Throughout childhood, changes in sleep staging and cycles occur, predominantly in reductions in percentages of REM sleep and SWS. This reduction of REM sleep and SWS makes way for the increase in stage 1 and stage 2 sleep characteristic of adult sleep. Some suggest that by early adolescence, sleep patterns often mirror those of mature adults.[52] Others show continuing alterations, however, in amount of time spent in SWS across development, from preadolescence through adulthood.[53,54] Higher amounts of REM sleep and SWS across childhood and adolescence may reflect higher rates of growth, development, and learning during these periods.[52]

### Sleep Duration

Sleep duration also changes across the course of childhood. In infancy, children sleep approximately 12 hours to 16 hours across the 24-hour period, including 1 nap to 2 naps per day. The daytime nap is lost for most Western children between the ages of 3 years and 5 years, which corresponds with children beginning kindergarten and school. With the loss of this nap, total sleep duration decreases, as nighttime sleep duration remains stable. During the school years and across adolescence, sleep duration continues to decline (**Table 1**).

### The 2-Process Model of Sleep: Biological and Behavioral Changes in Adolescence

Although some changes to sleep timing and duration occur from infancy to early childhood, arguably the most meaningful changes occur during puberty. The processes

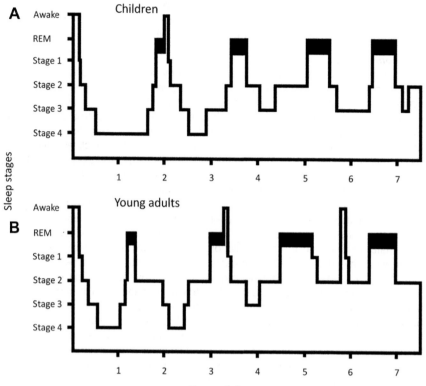

**Fig. 1.** A typical nocturnal sleep period for children (*A*) and young adults (*B*). (*Adapted from* Chokroverty S. Overview of normal sleep. In: Chokroverty S, editor. Sleep disorders medicine: Basic science, technical considerations, and clinical aspects. 2nd edition. Boston: Butterworth-Heinemann; 1999. p. 11; with permission.)

controlling sleep regulation change drastically in adolescence. The 2-process model suggests that sleep is regulated by both homeostatic sleep and circadian factors. The circadian rhythm interacts with homeostatic sleep pressure to regulate the sleep/wake cycle in humans.[55] Although homeostatic sleep pressure increases

| Table 1 |  |
|---|---|
| **Sleep duration recommendations** |  |
| **Age** | **Recommendation per 24 Hours** |
| Infants (4–12 mo) | 12–16 h |
| 1–2 y | 11–14 h |
| 3–5 y | 10–13 h |
| 6–12 y | 9–12 h |
| 13–18 y | 8–10 h |

*Data from* Paruthi S, Brooks LJ, D'Ambrosio C, et al. Recommended amount of sleep for pediatric populations: a consensus statement of the American Academy of Sleep Medicine. J Clin Sleep Med. 2016;12(6):785–6.

throughout the day (with increased time awake), the circadian rhythm works to keep humans active and alert until the night, helping them maintain optimal sleep/wake alignment with the environmental patterns of dark/light.[55]

### Sleep homeostasis

Homeostasis refers to an organism's tendency to maintain stability and equilibrium.[56] Sleep homeostasis—or the drive for sleep—is dependent on sleep/wake processes, as homeostatic sleep pressure rises during wake and declines during sleep.[55] This pressure increases the propensity for sleep, increasing the likelihood that a person falls asleep.[55] When sleep is delayed, there is a continued increase in the propensity for sleep until sleep occurs, at which point the homeostatic sleep pressure declines until waking. When deprived of sleep, the subsequent sleep often is longer and deeper than typical in order to dissipate sleep propensity.[57] SWS (ie, deep sleep) is considered a measure of homeostatic sleep pressure, because SWS declines throughout a sleep period, regardless of the timing of sleep onset,[58] suggesting a homeostatic, rather than circadian, process. SWS also increases during recovery sleep after periods of sleep deprivation.[59]

Several cross-sectional studies have shown that there is a decline in SWS as teenagers mature[60] and that the accumulation of sleep drive across the day becomes slower with maturation.[61,62] This suggests that more mature adolescents may take longer to accumulate a sufficient sleep drive over the day than younger adolescents, meaning that older adolescents are less likely to want or need to fall asleep until later in the evening. The reduction in the rate of build-up of sleep drive across the day may encourage later bedtimes in more mature teens.[62] Although the later drive for sleep can have an impact on bedtimes, the dissipation of this drive across the sleep period remains stable across adolescence.[63] This suggests that although adolescent sleep is pushed later, the amount of sleep needed is unchanged. It is not only the changing homeostat that promotes later bedtimes during adolescence, however, as the primary factor that pushes bedtimes later is the changing circadian system.

### Circadian rhythms

Many of the body's biological processes, including sleep and wakefulness, body temperature, and hormone levels, fluctuate according to a circadian rhythm,[64] that is, over the course of an approximately 24 hour period.[65] Because circadian rhythms often run on a slightly longer than 24-hour period, with adolescent studies finding them approximately 24.3 hours,[66] they need to be externally reset each day. This is achieved predominantly by exposure to light, which is a major zeitgeber, or time cue, for the body's circadian rhythms.[52] Melatonin is a hormone with a strong 24-hour rhythm and provides an indication of circadian timing. Melatonin secretion begins just prior to the onset of sleep and ceases around wake up time.[67] As such, melatonin often is considered to be a sleep promoting hormone,[68] and changes in the timing of melatonin onset are considered effective markers of circadian phase,[69,70] which is known to shift during puberty (**Fig. 2**).

Several studies have found that melatonin secretion delays across adolescence. For example, using dim light melatonin onset (DLMO) as a measure of circadian phase, Crowley and colleagues[71] found that older adolescents had a later DLMO than younger adolescents. In addition to the slower build-up of homeostatic sleep drive, this later melatonin-onset time in more mature teenagers facilitates later sleep-onset times and makes it difficult to fall asleep early in the evening and rise in the mornings.

## PSYCHOSOCIAL BARRIERS TO SLEEP ACROSS CHILDHOOD AND ADOLESCENCE

There are many psychosocial factors that may prevent good sleep among youth and lead to abnormal sleep patterns in the long-term. In younger children, the major factor

## Interaction between homeostatic and circadian processes

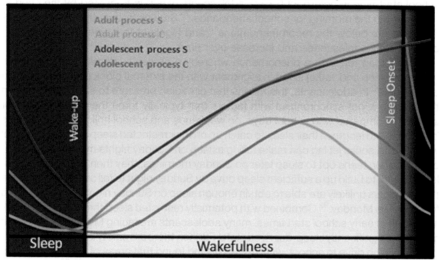

**Fig. 2.** Diagram of the 2-process model of sleep and wake. The X axis shows a 24-hour period. The blue panel displays the environmental day and the black panels display the environmental night. As process S (homeostatic drive for sleep) increases across the day with time spent awake and dissipates over the sleeping period. Process C (circadian drive for wake) fluctuates across the 24-hour period and works to keep human beings awake until the biological night. The later circadian and homeostatic processes during adolescence are displayed over the earlier processes of adults.

contributing to changes in sleep patterns is starting school. As discussed previously, the start of schooling usually results in the end of daytime napping, which can be problematic if nighttime sleep duration does not increase. Normal sleep routines may also be more difficult to achieve for children in chaotic households[72] and those whose guardians have less parental control.[73] Despite these barriers to normal sleep in children, the most significant changes and barriers to normal sleep manifest during the transition into adolescence.

### Social Barriers

In conjunction with biological changes, social factors, such as increased freedom from parents and after-school employment, also contribute to later bedtimes during adolescence.[42,74,75] Adolescents also face an increase in demands across multiple life domains. For example, after school, teenagers need to complete increasingly complex homework; and are involved in extracurricular activities,[76] spending time with friends, and potentially gaining part-time employment.[74] These factors can push bedtimes later and contribute to difficulties obtaining adequate sleep before waking early in the morning to attend school.

### School Schedules

Later bedtimes alone may not necessarily be a problem, especially given the later circadian rhythms of teens. It seems there are physiologic allowances for later bedtimes during adolescence, so later bedtimes may be beneficial rather than detrimental, especially for sleep quality.[77] Later bedtimes may become a problem, however, when considering school schedules. Particularly in the United States, when the average school start time is before 8:00 AM,[78] adolescents' sleep is truncated by the need to wake early in the morning for school attendance.[79] Studies frequently find sleep durations that are below the recommendations[16] and highlight that sleep restriction may begin in early adolescence and increase over time.

Social jet lag refers to a phenomenon whereby a person's internal clock (circadian rhythm of sleep and wake) is not in alignment with the external clock (the external light/dark cycle).[80] In adolescents, this means that circadian pressure to stay awake later in the evening is not synchronized with factors that typically force them to rise early for school.[80] Compared with school days, on weekends and school holidays, adolescents both delay and lengthen their sleep to catch up on their restricted sleep across the school week.[81] This social jet lag can make falling asleep on Sunday nights more difficult. Specifically, when teens opt to sleep later on Sunday mornings, they then are not awake for long enough to build up a sufficient sleep drive by Sunday night to fall asleep. This means that teenagers unlikely are able to obtain enough sleep on Sunday night to be well-rested for school on Monday.[82] Combined with potentially restricted sleep throughout the week as a result of early school start times, many adolescents are facing Monday mornings at school in a significantly sleep-deprived state. Further, there are safety implications for adolescents who drive to school, with studies having found that areas of the United States with earlier school start times have more teen motor vehicle accidents.[83–85]

### Technology Use

Perhaps the biggest threat to adequate sleep today is overuse of technology. Greater access to technology can result in later bedtimes, with children choosing to be in contact with friends, watch television or movies, or play computer games until later in the evening.[76] In the United States, 75% of children have at least 1 electronic device in the bedroom, and 16% report reading and/or sending messages after initially going to sleep.[86] Several studies have found that access to digital devices in the bedroom leads to significant reductions in sleep quantity and quality in children.[87–90]

Nighttime technology use disrupts sleep through 2 pathways. First, the bright, blue wavelength light emitted from mobile phones, laptops, and tablets can delay sleep onset by suppressing the release of melatonin.[91] This is especially problematic for adolescents, who already have a biological tendency toward delayed circadian rhythms.[92] Second, technology use can increase physiologic arousal.[93] When this occurs in the evening, the hormonal processes involved in the onset of sleep, for example, a decrease in cortisol and an increase in melatonin, can be altered, leading to a state of hyperarousal, which makes it difficult to wind down.[94] Social media use at night has also been related to shorter sleep duration, reduced sleep quality and mental health[95] as well as poorer academic outcomes.[96]

Setting boundaries surrounding technology use in the evening and limiting technology in the bedroom can be beneficial, with a recent study finding that children who reported having rules at home about restricting technology use at certain times were more likely to report earlier weekday bedtimes.[97] Refraining from using devices for even 1 hour before bed may improve sleep duration.[98] Further interventions targeting nighttime technology use and sleep are needed, however, to assist parents with providing clear guidelines on technology use in the evenings.

### SUMMARY

This article identifies some of the common consequences of disturbed sleep and some of the barriers to healthy sleep across childhood and adolescence. Several factors combine to influence adolescent sleep patterns. Biological changes interact with environmental and social factors to result in the facilitation of later bedtimes, while school start times force early awakenings. This truncation of sleep can result in sleep deprivation in this age group, as studies show that—although sleep duration is reduced—the need for sleep does not decrease throughout adolescence. Sleep restriction has many negative consequences for daytime functioning and health, including poorer academic performance, increased sleepiness and weight gain, and worsened mental and physical health. Further research must be conducted in younger children, especially given the increase in nighttime technology use in this age group.

## CLINICS CARE POINTS

- Psychoeducation on sleep health (eg, recommended sleep duration) is important for maintaining normal sleep across childhood, especially in the primary years.

- Sleep and mental health are intrinsically linked; greater patient care could be provided by practitioners, including questions about sleep when children and adolescents present with mental health symptoms. Improvements to sleep behaviors/patterns may result in lessened mental health concerns.

- Reduced academic outcomes and poorer mental health during adolescence may have an impact on quality of life across adulthood, so early intervention targeting sleep is imperative to improve outcomes across the lifespan.

- Technology use should be limited in the evening hours; guidelines should be set by parents to minimize technology use in the hours before bed and in the bedroom.

## DISCLOSURE

The authors have nothing to disclose.

## REFERENCES

1. Cropley AJ. Creativity in education & learning: a guide for teachers and educators. Psychology Press; 2001.
2. Malina RM. Growth. In: Mooren FC, editor. Encyclopedia of exercise medicine in health and disease. Berlin (Heidelberg): Springer Berlin Heidelberg; 2012. p. 376–8.
3. Lavoie J, Pereira L, Talwar V. Understanding healthy development in children and adolescents: themes of resilience. American Psychological Association Newsletter 2014;10.
4. Dement WC. Foreward. In: Carskadon MA, editor. Adolescent sleep patterns: biological, social, and psychological influences. Cambridge(United Kingdom): Cambridge University Press; 2002. p. ix–xi.
5. Dusek JB. Adolescent development and behavior. Prentice-Hall, IncQ; 1987.
6. World Health Organisation. Adolescent development 2020. Available at: https://www.who.int/maternal_child_adolescent/topics/adolescence/development/en/. Accessed April 24, 2020.
7. Henker B, Whalen CK, Jamner LD, et al. Anxiety, affect, and activity in teenagers: monitoring daily life with electronic diaries. J Am Acad Child Adolesc Psychiatry 2002;41(6):660–70.

8. Lewinsohn PM, Rohde P, Seeley JR. Major depressive disorder in older adolescents: prevalence, risk factors, and clinical implications. Clin Psychol Rev 1998;18(7):765–94.

9. Sourander A, Helstelä L, Helenius H, et al. Persistence of bullying from childhood to adolescence—a longitudinal 8-year follow-up study. Child Abuse Negl 2000; 24(7):873–81.

10. Arora T, Taheri S. Associations among late chronotype, body mass index and dietary behaviors in young adolescents. Int J Obes 2015;39(1):39–44.

11. Steinberg L. A social neuroscience perspective on adolescent risk-taking. Dev Rev 2008;28(1):78–106.

12. Beebe DW, Field J, Milller MM, et al. Impact of multi-night experimentally induced short sleep on adolescent performance in a simulated classroom. Sleep 2017; 40(2):zsw035.

13. Beebe DW, Rose D, Amin R. Attention, learning, and arousal of experimentally sleep-restricted adolescents in a simulated classroom. J Adolesc Health 2010; 47(5):523–5.

14. Fogel SM, Smith CT. Learning-dependent changes in sleep spindles and stage 2 sleep. J Sleep Res 2006;15(3):250–5.

15. Perkinson-Gloor N, Lemola S, Grob A. Sleep duration, positive attitude toward life, and academic achievement: the role of daytime tiredness, behavioral persistence, and school start times. J Adolesc 2013;36(2):311–8.

16. Wolfson AR, Carskadon MA. Sleep schedules and daytime functioning in adolescents. Child Dev 1998;69(4):875–87.

17. Escribano C, Díaz-Morales JF, Delgado P, et al. Morningness/eveningness and school performance among Spanish adolescents: further evidence. Learn Individ Differ 2012;22(3):409–13.

18. Roeser K, Schlarb AA, Kübler A. The chronotype-academic performance model (CAM): daytime sleepiness and learning motivation link chronotype and school performance in adolescents. Pers Individ Dif 2013;54(7):836–40.

19. Meijer AM, van den Wittenboer GL. The joint contribution of sleep, intelligence and motivation to school performance. Pers Individ Dif 2004;37(1):95–106.

20. Pagel JF, Forister N, Kwiatkowki C. Adolescent sleep disturbance and school performance: the confounding variable of socioeconomics. J Clin Sleep Med 2007; 3(01):19–23.

21. Wolfson AR, Carskadon MA. Understanding adolescents sleep patterns and school performance. Sleep Med Rev 2003;7:491–506.

22. McKnight AJ, McKnight AS. Young novice drivers: careless or clueless? Accid Anal Prev 2003;35(6):921–5.

23. National Commission Against Drunk Driving. Youth driving without impairment: report on the youth impaired driving public hearings, Atlanta, Boston, Chicago, Fort Worth, Seattle: "A community challenge". Washington, DC: National Commission Against Drunk Driving; 1988.

24. Moldofsky H. Sleep and the immune system. Int J Immunopharmacol 1995;17(8): 649–54.

25. Moldofsky H. Central nervous system and peripheral immune functions and the sleep-wake system. J Psychiatry Neurosci 1994;19(5):368.

26. Majde JA, Krueger JM. Links between the innate immune system and sleep. J Allergy Clin Immunol 2005;116(6):1188–98.

27. Dickstein JB, Moldofsky H. Sleep, cytokines and immune function. Sleep Med Rev 1999;3(3):219–28.

28. Orzech KM, Acebo C, Seifer R, et al. Sleep patterns are associated with common illness in adolescents. J Sleep Res 2014;23(2):133–42.
29. Matthews KA, Dahl RE, Owens JF, et al. Sleep duration and insulin resistance in healthy black and white adolescents. Sleep 2012;35(10):1353–8.
30. Ginsberg HN. Insulin resistance and cardiovascular disease. J Clin Invest 2000; 106(4):453–8.
31. Ceriello A, Motz E. Is oxidative stress the pathogenic mechanism underlying insulin resistance, diabetes, and cardiovascular disease? The common soil hypothesis revisited. Arterioscler Thromb Vasc Biol 2004;24(5):816–23.
32. Klingenberg L, Chaput J-P, Holmbäck U, et al. Acute sleep restriction reduces insulin sensitivity in adolescent boys. Sleep 2013;36(7):1085–90.
33. McKnight-Eily LR, Eaton DK, Lowry R, et al. Relationships between hours of sleep and health-risk behaviors in US adolescent students. Prev Med 2011;53(4–5): 271–3.
34. Miles L. Physical activity and health. Nutr Bull 2007;32(4):314–63.
35. Milewski MD, Skaggs DL, Bishop GA, et al. Chronic lack of sleep is associated with increased sports injuries in adolescent athletes. J Pediatr Orthop 2014; 34(2):129–33.
36. Becker SP, Langberg JM, Byars KC. Advancing a biopsychosocial and contextual model of sleep in adolescence: a review and introduction to the special issue. J Youth Adolesc 2015;44:239–70.
37. Williams K, Chambers M, Logan S, et al. Association of common health symptoms with bullying in primary school children. BMJ 1996;313(7048):17–9.
38. Agostini A, Lushington K, Dorrian J. Sleep, bullying, and physical and mental health in adolescence. Sleep Med 2019;64:S4.
39. Carskadon MA. Adolescent sleepiness: increased risk in a high-risk population. Alcohol Drugs Diving 1990;5(4):317–28.
40. Kessler RC, Berglund P, Demler O, et al. Lifetime prevalence and age-of-onset distributions of DSM-IV disorders in the national comorbidity survey replication. Arch Gen Psychiatry 2005;62(6):593–602.
41. Ojio Y, Nishida A, Shimodera S, et al. Sleep duration associated with the lowest risk of depression/anxiety in adolescents. Sleep 2016;39(8):1555–62.
42. Fredriksen K, Rhodes J, Reddy R, et al. Sleepless in Chicago: tracking the effects of adolescent sleep loss during the middle school years. Child Dev 2004;75(1): 84–95.
43. Giannotti F, Cortesi F. Sleep patterns and daytime function in adolescence: an epidemiological survey of an Italian high school student sample. J Sleep Res 2002;11(3):191–9.
44. Matamura M, Tochigi M, Usami S, et al. Associations between sleep habits and mental health status and suicidality in a longitudinal survey of monozygotic twin adolescents. J Sleep Res 2014;23(3):292–6.
45. Lee YJ, Cho S-J, Cho IH, et al. Insufficient sleep and suicidality in adolescents. Sleep 2012;35(4):455–60.
46. Sarchiapone M, Mandelli L, Carli V, et al. Hours of sleep in adolescents and its association with anxiety, emotional concerns, and suicidal ideation. Sleep Med 2014;15(2):248–54.
47. Baum KT, Desai A, Field J, et al. Sleep restriction worsens mood and emotion regulation in adolescents. J Child Psychol Psychiatry 2014;55(2):180–90.
48. Vriend JL, Davidson FD, Corkum PV, et al. Manipulating sleep duration alters emotional functioning and cognitive performance in children. J Pediatr Psychol 2013;38(10):1058–69.

49. Owens J, Wang G, Lewin D, et al. Association between short sleep duration and risk behavior factors in middle school students. Sleep 2017;40(1). https://doi.org/10.1093/sleep/zsw004.

50. Weaver MD, Barger LK, Malone SK, et al. Dose-dependent associations between sleep duration and unsafe behaviors among us high school students. JAMA Pediatr 2018;172(12):1187–9.

51. Kleitman N, Engelmann TG. Sleep characteristics of infants. J Appl Phys 1953; 6(5):269–82.

52. Sheldon SH, Ferber R, Kryger MH, et al. Principles and practice of pediatric sleep medicine e-book. Elsevier Health Sciences; 2014.

53. Carskadon MA, Harvey K, Duke P, et al. Pubertal changes in daytime sleepiness. Sleep 1980;2(4):453–60.

54. Paruthi S, Brooks LJ, D'Ambrosio C, et al. Recommended amount of sleep for pediatric populations: a consensus statement of the American academy of sleep medicine. J Clin Sleep Med 2016;12(06):785–6.

55. Borbély AA. A two process model of sleep regulation. Hum Neurobiol 1982;1(3): 195–204.

56. Passer MW, Smith RE. Psychology: the science of mind and behavior. 2nd edition. North Ryde (New South Wales): McGraw-Hill Education; 2015.

57. Brunner DP, Dijk D-J, Borbély AA. Repeated partial sleep deprivation progressively changes the EEG during sleep and wakefulness. Sleep 1993;16(2):100–13.

58. Åkerstedt T, Gillberg M. The circadian variation of experimentally displaced sleep. Sleep 1981;4(2):159–69.

59. Ferrara M, De Gennaro L, Bertini M. Selective slow-wave sleep (SWS) deprivation and SWS rebound: do we need a fixed SWS amount per night. Sleep Res Online 1999;2(1):15–9.

60. Carskadon MA. The second decade. In: Guilleminault C, editor. Sleeping and waking disorders: indications and techniques. Menlo Park (CA): Addison Wesley; 1982. p. 99–125.

61. Jenni OG, Achermann P, Carskadon MA. Homeostatic sleep regulation in adolescents. Sleep 2005;28(11):1446–54.

62. Taylor DJ, Jenni OG, Acebo C, et al. Sleep tendency during extended wakefulness: insights into adolescent sleep regulation and behavior. J Sleep Res 2005;14(3):239–44.

63. Tarokh L, Carskadon MA, Achermann P. Dissipation of sleep pressure is stable across adolescence. Neuroscience 2012;216:167–77.

64. Kryger MH, Roth T, Dement WC. Principles and practice of sleep medicine. 5th edition. St Louis (MI): Elsevier Saunders.; 2011.

65. Czeisler CA, Duffy JF, Shanahan TL, et al. Stability, precision, and near-24-hour period of the human circadian pacemaker. Science 1999;284(5423):2177–81.

66. Carskadon MA, Labyak SE, Acebo C, et al. Intrinsic circadian period of adolescent humans measured in conditions of forced desynchrony. Neurosci Lett 1999; 260(2):129–32.

67. Cajochen C, Kräuchi K, Wirz-Justice A. Role of melatonin in the regulation of human circadian rhythms and sleep. J Neuroendocrinol 2003;15(4):432–7.

68. Zhdanova IV, Lynch HJ, Wurtman RJ. Melatonin: a sleep-promoting hormone. Sleep 1997;20(10):899–907.

69. Lewy AJ, Sack RL. The dim light melatonin onset as a marker for orcadian phase position. Chronobiol Int 1989;6(1):93–102.

70. Voultsios A, Kennaway DJ, Dawson D. Salivary melatonin as a circadian phase marker: validation and comparison to plasma melatonin. J Biol Rhythms 1997; 12(5):457–66.
71. Crowley SJ, Acebo C, Fallone G, et al. Estimating dim light melatonin onset (DLMO) phase in adolescents using summer or school-year sleep/wake schedules. Sleep 2006;29(12):1632–41.
72. Whitesell CJ, Crosby B, Anders TF, et al. Household chaos and family sleep during infants' first year. J Fam Psychol 2018;32(5):622.
73. Pieters D, De Valck E, Vandekerckhove M, et al. Effects of pre-sleep media use on sleep/wake patterns and daytime functioning among adolescents: the moderating role of parental control. Behav Sleep Med 2014;12(6):427–43.
74. Carskadon MA. Patterns of sleep and sleepiness in adolescents. Pediatrician 1990;17(1):5–12.
75. Dahl RE, Lewin DS. Pathways to adolescent health sleep regulation and behavior. J Adolesc Health 2002;31(6):175–84.
76. O'Malley EB, O'Malley MB. School start time and its impact on learning and behavior. In: Sleep and psychiatric disorders in children and adolescents. New York: Informa Healthcare; 2008. p. 79–94.
77. Zhu L, Zee PC. Circadian rhythm sleep disorders. Neurol Clin 2012;30(4): 1167–91.
78. Edwards F. Early to rise? the effect of daily start times on academic performance. Econ Educ Rev 2012;31(6):970–83.
79. Carskadon MA, Wolfson AR, Acebo C, et al. Adolescent sleep patterns, circadian timing, and sleepiness at a transition to early school days. Sleep 1998;21(8): 871–81.
80. Wittmann M, Dinich J, Merrow M, et al. Social jetlag: misalignment of biological and social time. Chronobiol Int 2006;23(1–2):497–509.
81. Agostini A, Pignata S, Camporeale R, et al. Changes in growth and sleep across school nights, weekends and a winter holiday period in two Australian schools. Chronobiol Int 2018;35:691–704.
82. Olds T, Blunden S, Dollman J, et al. Day type and the relationship between weight status and sleep duration in children and adolescents. Aust N Z J Public Health 2010;34(2):165–71.
83. Danner F, Phillips B. Adolescent sleep, school start times, and teen motor vehicle crashes. J Clin Sleep Med 2008;4(06):533–5.
84. Vorona RD, Szklo-Coxe M, Wu A, et al. Dissimilar teen crash rates in two neighboring southeastern Virginia cities with different high school start times. J Clin Sleep Med 2011;7(02):145–51.
85. Vorona RD, Szklo-Coxe M, Lamichhane R, et al. Adolescent crash rates and school start times in two central Virginia counties, 2009-2011: a follow-up study to a southeastern Virginia study, 2007-2008. J Clin Sleep Med 2014;10(11): 1169–77.
86. National Sleep Foundation. Sleep in America poll: sleep in the modern family 2014. Arlington (VA).
87. Buxton OM, Chang A-M, Spilsbury JC, et al. Sleep in the modern family: protective family routines for child and adolescent sleep. Sleep Health 2015;1(1):15–27.
88. Cain N, Gradisar M. Electronic media use and sleep in school-aged children and adolescents: a review. Sleep Med 2010;11(8):735–42.
89. Garmy P, Nyberg P, Jakobsson U. Sleep and television and computer habits of Swedish school-age children. J Sch Nurs 2012;28(6):469–76.

90. Van den Bulck J. Television viewing, computer game playing, and Internet use and self-reported time to bed and time out of bed in secondary-school children. Sleep 2004;27(1):101–4.

91. Cajochen C, Frey S, Anders D, et al. Evening exposure to a light-emitting diodes (LED)-backlit computer screen affects circadian physiology and cognitive performance. J Appl Phys 2011;110(5):1432–8.

92. Carskadon MA. Sleep in adolescents: the perfect storm. Pediatr Clin North Am 2011;58(3):637–47.

93. Higuchi S, Motohashi Y, Liu Y, et al. Effects of playing a computer game using a bright display on presleep physiological variables, sleep latency, slow wave sleep and REM sleep. J Sleep Res 2005;14(3):267–73.

94. Bonnet MH, Arand DL. Hyperarousal and insomnia: state of the science. Sleep Med Rev 2010;14(1):9–15.

95. Woods HC, Scott H. # Sleepyteens: social media use in adolescence is associated with poor sleep quality, anxiety, depression and low self-esteem. J Adolesc 2016;51:41–9.

96. Grover K, Pecor K, Malkowski M, et al. Effects of instant messaging on school performance in adolescents. J Child Neurol 2016;31(7):850–7.

97. Bowers JM, Moyer A. Adolescent sleep and technology-use rules: results from the California health interview survey. Sleep Health 2020;6(1):19–22.

98. Bartel K, Scheeren R, Gradisar M. Altering adolescents' pre-bedtime phone use to achieve better sleep health. Health Commun 2019;34(4):456–62.

# Sleep and Technology in Early Childhood

Amy I. Nathanson, PhD

## KEYWORDS

- Early childhood • Preschoolers • Sleep • Insomnia • Technology • Television
- Media

## KEY POINTS

- Research on the impact of technology use on children less than 6 years old is relatively new and constitutes a relatively small portion of the work on technology and sleep.
- Technology use among young children is related to worse sleep outcomes, including delayed bedtimes, shorter sleep duration, and daytime sleepiness.
- Although little research has been conducted among infants and toddlers, the available evidence suggests that the negative impact of technology on sleep may be stronger among this age group.
- Technology use before bedtime may have the most harmful effect on sleep.
- It is not clear why technology use affects young children's sleep, but scholars speculate it could be due to the melatonin-suppressing blue light exposure, increased arousal, or time displacement.

## INTRODUCTION

With technology's ubiquitous presence in young children's lives, attention has turned to the potential and real outcomes of sustained exposure to electronic devices during development.[1] Although this is not an entirely new topic— indeed, scholars and the public alike have been studying or pondering the impact of media exposure on children for decades—the observed shift downward in the average age of first exposure to media combined with the increasing amount of time young children now devote to media[2–5] has raised new questions about how technology use affects young children.

Before the emergence and proliferation of mobile media, the study of technology use in early childhood was mostly focused on the impact of television. Moreover, because television content developed for young children is among the highest quality material available on television (eg, programming available on America's Public Broadcasting Station[6]), research on the educational and prosocial benefits of

This article originally appeared in *Child and Adolescent Psychiatric Clinics*, Volume 30 Issue 1, January 2021.

School of Communication, Ohio State University, Columbus, OH 43210, USA

*E-mail address:* nathanson.7@osu.edu

exposure is prevalent. But the media landscape has changed dramatically. The same high-quality material still exists, but now it is available at any time of the day through streaming services. In addition, thanks to mobile media, that content is also available in any location with an Internet connection, including the bedroom, the dining room, and outside of the house as well. Furthermore, more content has been developed with this youngest audience in mind, providing children with a plethora of entertainment and educational options, but of mixed quality. As a result, researchers studying the uses and effects of technology among young children must consider the implications of both a larger range of media platforms (eg, television, computer, tablet, smartphone) consumed in a variety of settings (eg, bedroom, living room, outside of the house) and with a wider range of content. To put it mildly, the complexity of the impact of technology on young children has increased.

Although the majority of work on technology and young children—both historically and today—focuses on the social or educational outcomes of technology use, it is important to consider the health implications of young children's media as well. In fact, health outcomes are very likely mediators in the relation between technology exposure and social and educational outcomes. A critical health outcome, particularly for young children, is sleep. With the rise of mobile media and the increased availability of media content more generally, it is important to examine if and how exposure to technology affects young children's sleep.

In this article, I review the research that has been conducted on the uses and impact of technology among young children. I will highlight some important considerations when reviewing this work. Later, I offer suggestions for future directions. It should be noted that many of the speculations offered in this article are based on knowledge that has already accrued in this area from research on older children and adolescents. Finally, I will provide guidance for clinicians who are working with families of young children about how to assess and address their patients' technology-induced sleep problems.

## DEFINITIONS

In this article, I use the term *technology* as an umbrella term encompassing a variety of media or devices (including television, video games, smartphones, tablets, and computers, either laptop or desktop) and platforms (eg, YouTube, Netflix). The reviewed research will address either the impact of technology exposure per se (eg, overall time with technology, technology use before bedtime) or the effects from exposure to specific types of technology (eg, educational technology, violent technology content).

In addition, the term *young children* will refer to children under the age of 6 years and before they have commenced formal schooling. Although the majority of research on sleep and young children focuses on children between the ages of 3 and 5 years, there are a handful of studies that have been devoted to children who are younger than 3 years. My review and recommendations will pertain to all children under the age of 6.

## RESEARCH

To date, the majority of work investigating the impact of technology on children's sleep has focused on school-aged children and adolescents (eg,[7–10]). This review focuses on the available research focusing on younger children, sometimes using insights from the work conducted among older children.

### Effects of Technology on Young Children's Sleep

There is a growing body of research showing that young children's technology use is negatively related to their sleep quality. Still the amount of research pales in comparison with the volume of work conducted among school-aged children and, in particular, adolescents.[11,12]

To date, the most work has explored the links between television viewing and sleep outcomes. In particular, the presence of a television in the bedroom has been shown to correlate with disrupted sleep among young children, such as nightmares and feeling tired in the morning.[11] This association may be particularly strong among racial/ethnic minority children, who experience a 31-minute per day decrease in sleep time when a television is present in their bedroom.[13] In addition, evening television exposure is linked with poor sleep outcomes[11,14] among 3- to 5-year-old children. For example, Brockmann and colleagues[11] found that 55% of preschool-aged children with sleep disturbances watched television in the evening compared with 33% of children without abnormal sleep patterns.

Nathanson and Beyens[15] examined the links between 3- to 5-year-old children's sleep and their use of "mobile electronic media" (including tablets, smartphones, hand-held video games, laptops, and iPods), both in the daytime and in the evening. Their cross-sectional survey of caregivers examined 3 indicators of sleep quality, derived from the Children's Sleep Habits Questionnaire.[16] They found that both daytime and evening use of technology were related to poorer sleep quality. The relations were strongest between tablet use and bedtime resistance. This finding may seem to be counterintuitive to parents who use technology to calm children and prepare them for bedtime; in fact, this work suggests that mobile device use achieves the opposite effect. It is important to note that these relations held even when traditional television viewing amounts were controlled, suggesting that mobile device use makes an independent contribution to children's sleep quality.

Most research examines the impact of technology on outcomes such as bedtime, wake time, and sleep duration. However, when it comes to young children, it is also important to examine sleep maturity as an outcome. Specifically, sleep consolidation reflects the proportion of total sleep that occurs at night and represents a mature sleep pattern.[17] Children's sleep becomes more consolidated as they age and shifts away from daytime napping and they experience the majority of their sleep during the nighttime. Sleep consolidation is linked with enhanced cognitive function[17,18] and its achievement is considered a developmental milestone.[19]

Beyens and Nathanson[20] found that multiple forms of technology use (ie, television, tablets, smartphones) were related to less sleep consolidation among 3- to 5-year-old children. Relatedly, television viewing was associated with more daytime napping. It is possible that parents use mid-day television viewing as a means of promoting napping behavior among their young children. Overall, this study suggested that technology use was associated with less mature sleep patterns among young children. Sleep consolidation and napping behaviors are seldom investigated in connection with technology use, however, so more work is needed before drawing any conclusions.

The majority of research in this area relies on parent reports of young children's sleep behaviors, such as reports of bedtimes and wake times, or responses to the Children's Sleep Habits Questionnaire.[16] However, Downing and colleagues[21] used actigraphy, an accelerometer device that estimates sleep objectively, and found a negative association between 3- to 5-year old boys' television viewing and their sleep time, lending more support to the research showing a negative association between technology use and young children's sleep.

An even smaller body of work examines the links between technology use and sleep behavior among infants and toddlers. The existing work generally supports the research conducted among older populations, regardless of whether the focus of the research is on touchscreens,[22] televisions,[23] mobile media,[24] or evening-time exposure.[25] For example, Chen and colleagues[26] found that screen viewing (either television or mobile device use) was related to shorter sleep duration among children under 2 years of age. They found that children exposed to screens in excess of 1 hour per day slept 1.5 hours less compared with infants who did not view any screen media. The associations were strongest among children who were 6 months of age or younger. According to Janssen and colleagues's[12] meta-analysis, the impact of technology use is particularly strong on infants and toddlers compared with preschoolers.

Within this small body of research on infants and toddlers, 3 longitudinal studies are particularly noteworthy. Marinelli and colleagues[27] found that television exposure at 2 years of age was associated with shorter sleep duration, as reported by parents, at age 4. In addition, children who experienced increases in television exposure (from <1.5 hours per day to >1.5 hours per day of exposure) experienced reduced sleep duration over time. Likewise, Genuneit and colleagues[28] found that electronic media use at age 2 predicted worse sleep outcomes by age 3, as measured by the Children's Sleep Habits Questionnaire. Using an even longer time period, Cespedes and colleagues[13] found that television viewing during infancy was related to shorter sleep durations concurrently and into middle childhood. These studies are helpful because they suggest that technology exposure can have long-term implications for young children's sleep.

### Sleep Quality as a Mediator

Some research has considered the role of sleep as a mediator of relations between technology use and other effects. As a result, this work examines whether the impact of technology on children's sleep has implications for other outcomes.

Nathanson and Beyens[29] found that 3- to 5-year-old children who used tablet devices in the evening hours (1) went to bed later, (2) resisted bedtime more, and (3) had shorter sleep durations compared with other children; moreover, each of the 3 sleep variables was related to worse effortful control (a form of self-regulation) among the children. Nathanson and Fries[30] found a similar indirect effect of technology use via sleep. They found that total sleep time among 3- to 5-year-old children mediated the relation between their television viewing time and their theory of mind. More specifically, television viewing time was related to fewer sleep hours at night, which, in turn, predicted weaker theory of mind performance. Finally, Sigtsma and colleagues[31] found that sleep time was a mediator in the relation between television viewing and body mass index among 3- to 4-year-old children, such that more exposure was related to a shorter sleep duration, which, in turn, predicted high body mass index. As a result, it seems that technology-induced sleep problems have concerning implications for young children's physical and cognitive outcomes.

### Sleep Quality as a Moderator

Another possibility, albeit one that has not been thoroughly investigated, is that sleep quality moderates the relation between young children's technology use and particular outcomes. That is, the quality of children's sleep could either exacerbate or mitigate the impact of technology. There is evidence from other bodies of literature that sleep plays this type of role; for example, the impact of high-quality maternal communication is stronger among children who receive adequate sleep.[32]

In support of this finding, Nathanson and Beyens[29] found there was a negative relation between 3- to 5-year-old children's tablet use and their effortful control (a form of self-regulation), but only among children with shorter nighttime sleep durations (less than about 11 hours of sleep per night). In contrast, there was a positive relation between using hand-held video-game players (such as a Nintendo DS) and effortful control, but only among children experiencing longer nighttime sleep durations (more than about 10.5 hours of sleep per night). Golshevsky and colleagues[33] also found that sleep was a moderator of the impact of television on the body mass index of 4 to 17-year-old children, such that negative associations were only found among children who were getting less sleep. These findings suggest that the impact of technology on young children may depend on how well children are sleeping.

Because these studies were correlational, however, alternative explanations exist. For example, it is possible that parents are more likely to provide tablets to children who are sleep deprived and with poor effortful control, perhaps as a means of occupying them throughout the day. Likewise, perhaps parents of children who get enough sleep and have stronger effortful control recognize that their children can benefit from interactive games and therefore provide them more readily. Longitudinal research is needed to understand these relations more.

## CONSIDERATIONS AND CONTROVERSIES

To understand the impact of technology on children, it is necessary to consider several factors that play mitigating or exacerbating roles. First, technology exposure may have effects owing to the particular content that is viewed or because of the timing or duration or exposure. For example, children's sleep may suffer more after exposure to a scary movie compared with a light-hearted family movie. Or, children may have a harder time falling asleep after playing an intense, competition-based video game compared with listening to soothing music on the radio. At the same time, the overall duration of technology exposure—regardless of the content—may play a role in affecting children's sleep. Longer exposures to technology emitting short-wave, blue light, particularly close to bedtime, may inhibit sleep transitions more than shorter exposures and those occurring earlier in the day.[14] Or, longer exposure to technology may displace activities that facilitate healthy sleep patterns, such as physical exercise, more than shorter daily exposures to technology.[7]

A second consideration when examining the impact of technology on young children is where exposure occurs. In particular, technology use that occurs in a child's bedroom may have unique effects compared with use that occurs either in other parts of the house or outside of the house. Research shows that children with bedroom television sets have worse outcomes (eg, on sleep, academic performance) compared with children without bedroom televisions.[34,35] With the increase of mobile media, this issue has become even more important; today's children can use both mobile and stationary forms of technology in their bedrooms. And yet, it is important to note that the location of exposure could be a proxy for another important variable—such as technology use before bedtime, increased exposure hours, or lack of parental supervision of technology use. Where the location of exposure becomes meaningful in and of itself is when it refers to the relative quiet of the environment. For example, technology use in the bedroom could theoretically be conducive to learning if the room is quiet and the child is able to concentrate on the content. In contrast, technology use that occurs in a public space, whether that is a loud living room or a noisy restaurant, may leave children feeling overwhelmed and unable to focus on the material at hand. Perhaps the overstimulation caused by mobile technology use will ultimately affect children's ability to transition to sleep. The possibility that technology exposure's impact will vary according to the location in which it is used has not been empirically examined to date, but is worth considering in synthesizing the extant work.

Finally, it is important to consider the reasons why technology use and sleep are associated. One hypothesis is that exposure to short wavelength blue light from self-illuminating screens, such as televisions, computers, and smartphones disrupts sleep.[36] This explanation is biological in nature and suggests that technology exposure interferes with the body's natural circadian rhythm. Specifically, blue light exposure results in delayed onset in the timing of melatonin secretion, among both adults and children,[37,38] which then delays the onset of sleep.[39] Although there is not yet consensus regarding the impact of short wavelength light from electronic screens on sleep quality (eg, see the research by Higuchi and colleagues[40] on a small sample of adults), many experts recommend that screen time should not occur in the hours before bed.

Another hypothesis predicts that exposure to specific content prevents children from settling down and successfully transitioning to sleep.[9] Certain types of content may be seen as particularly effective in arousing either positive (excitement, joy) or negative (fear, sadness) emotions. For example, some speculate the video games are particularly arousing compared with other media forms, although Yland and colleagues[41] found that exposure to television and computers was more disruptive to 9-year-olds' sleep than was video game playing. With young children in particular, it may be difficult to engage in sufficient self-regulation to manage these strong emotions and prepare for sleep. Relatedly, certain types of content may be disturbing or upsetting enough to interfere with sleep. For example, young children are exposed to upsetting media content (eg, the news, horror films) either intentionally or accidently.[42] It is not uncommon for such exposure to result in sleep disruptions among children, either in the form of nightmares, fear of being alone in the bedroom, or difficulty falling asleep. Moreover, the effects of this type of exposure can last for days, weeks, months, and in rarer cases, years.[42]

## FUTURE DIRECTIONS

Much of the work to date has relied on less-than-ideal measures of both children's technology use and sleep, such as parent reports, which are subject to bias and error. Media diaries are believed to constitute the best possible approach to assessing children's media use and should be considered in future work. Likewise, parent reports are frequently used to gather information about children's sleep. More objective measures of sleep, such as actigraphy, should be considered as well, even though this approach is not flawless.[43]

Relatedly, researchers should consider other types of sleep outcomes as potentially vulnerable to technology use, such as napping and sleep consolidation. To date, scholars have mostly focused on nighttime sleep duration and sleep disturbances as key indicators of sleep quality. However, when it comes to children—and young children in particular—napping and sleep consolidation are important markers of sleep development.

More longitudinal research is needed to understand whether technology use affects sleep or whether a reverse chain of events explains the connections. For example, it is possible that caregivers are more likely to provide technology devices to young children who have trouble sleeping. Because sleep has a negative effect on children's behavior (and children's sleep disturbances affect parents' sleep quality as well), technology devices may be viewed by parents as palatable solutions to keeping young children entertained, because parents may observe that their children become calm when using technology.[44] In addition, because technology can provide "easy" entertainment, sleep-deprived children may prefer them over more demanding activities. Moreover, it is possible that there is a cyclical relation between technology use and sleep among children, such that use disrupts sleep, which then encourages more technology use to cope with sleep deprivation, and so on. This type of relation has been observed in prior work focused on television, computers, and sleep.[45]

One understudied factor in this area of research concerns the physical distance between the child and the screen. There is speculation that devices that are held close to the face can heighten the negative impact of technology use on sleep.[46] Theoretically, the intensity of blue light decays over greater distances, thereby diminishing the impact of exposure on sleep from devices viewed at a distance but intensifying the impact from devices held close to the face. So far the research is mixed concerning whether television or mobile devices have the strongest impact on young children's sleep; nevertheless, future research should consider the distance between the screen and the user in considering technology's potential impact.

In addition, more work is needed to understand whether there are developmental differences in blue-light sensitivity. Some research shows that, compared with adults and older adolescents, children and younger adolescents are more sensitive to blue light.[47,48] One reason may be because of younger children's relatively larger pupil sizes compared with older individuals.[48] Given the relative scarcity of research on the impact of technology on young children, scholars may apply guidelines designed for adolescents or adults to younger children. However, if indeed younger children are more at risk for experiencing negative effects of blue light compared with older individuals, then distinct guidelines need to be developed with this unique population in mind. As a result, the relative vulnerability of younger children to the impact of technology needs to be studied more extensively, including this group's potential heightened vulnerability to blue light.

## CLINICAL ASPECTS OF TECHNOLOGY USE AND SLEEP

Clinicians addressing sleep issues among young children should evaluate the extent to which children's technology use may be contributing to poor sleep hygiene and shortened sleep duration (defined as not meeting the American Academy of Sleep Medicine's[49] recommended total daily sleep time hours: 10–13 hours, 11–14 hours, and 12–16 hours for preschoolers, toddlers, and infants, respectively). During interviews with caregivers or via questionnaires, clinicians should obtain a record of the child's access to and use of technology on both typical weekdays and weekends. This should include information about the types of devices that children use (eg, television, mobile media), the locations that devices are used (eg, bedrooms), the overall duration of exposure throughout the day (and especially the duration of exposure in the evening and before bedtime), and the nature of the content that is viewed (eg, violent content, potentially upsetting content). Clinicians should be aware of the American Academy of Pediatrics screen time recommendations (eg, keeping bedrooms as tech-free zones, limiting screen time to no more than 1 hour per day of high-quality programming for children over 2 years[50]) and should understand that the majority of parents (particularly those from backgrounds of a lower socioeconomic status) are not aware of these guidelines.[3] Clinicians should also conduct formal assessments of their clients' sleep patterns (see the Suman K.R. Baddam's article, "Screening and Evaluation of Sleep Disturbances and Sleep Disorders in Children and

Adolescents," in this issue for recommended tools) and consider the potential association between technology usage habits and sleep behaviors.

If evening technology use is present, clinicians should obtain a detailed understanding of the nature of young children's bedtime rituals, including whether screen time plays a role. Clinicians should help parents to develop healthy bedtime rituals for their children that include setting a consistent bedtime and engaging in quiet activities before bedtime. In addition, parents should be encouraged to remove technology devices from children's bedrooms and to decrease their reliance on technology as part of the child's bedtime ritual. If children have become habituated to consuming media before bedtime, parents can be instructed to gradually decrease the amount of time devoted to technology and to work toward a goal of no screen time in the 1 to 2 hours before bedtime. Caregivers should be instructed to replace electronic screen time with calm activities, such as reading, coloring, or listening to quiet music (with no accompanying visuals, such as with music videos). If this type of goal is not achievable for caregivers, they should be encouraged to instead focus on the type of content their child consumes before bedtime and to select content that is free of violence or other potentially frightening content as well as material that is slower paced. Clinicians can direct caregivers to Common Sense Media's website (commonsensemedia.org), which provides detailed descriptions of media content and research-backed recommendations about the appropriateness of media content for different age groups. When screen time is perceived to be needed in a bedtime ritual, caregivers should be advised to select specific programs with clear beginnings and endings (rather than permitting open-ended searching through a series of unrelated videos, such as on YouTube) to ease the transition from screen time to bedtime. In addition, caregivers should be encouraged to coview the material with their young children, if possible, a practice that not only assists parents in monitoring media content but also provides a sense of warmth and connection for the child.

## SUMMARY

Although the body of work is relatively small, research suggests that most technology use is associated with poorer sleep outcomes among children less than 6 years of age (some types of technology have not yet been extensively studied in relation to sleep, such as video-calling platforms). The limited longitudinal work further suggests that technology use causes sleep disturbances in this population. These associations are evident regardless of the type of technology that has been studied, although evening exposure seems to have the worst impact compared with technology use during other parts of the day. The range of sleep outcomes studied include sleep duration, bedtime, frequency of nightmares, bedtime resistance, daytime sleepiness, napping frequency, and sleep consolidation. Sleep quality can be studied as a mediator or moderator of effects or as an outcome in and of itself. More work is needed with this population, particularly given that technology use is relatively high among young children. Researchers should expand the types of measures used to study both technology use and sleep outcomes, and consider other ways of conceptualizing sleep behaviors, such as considering them as mediators and moderators of other types of outcomes, like physical and emotional health. Because caregivers are often unaware of the detrimental impact of technology—coupled with a tendency among parents to use media as a sleep aid for children—clinicians should assess patients' exposure to technology in general and especially before bedtime to determine whether sleep issues may stem from children's technology use. Moreover, clinicians should educate caregivers about the association between technology use and sleep problems among young children.

## CLINICS CARE POINTS

- Because parental concern over the impact of technology on children's sleep is low,[51] clinicians should educate caregivers on the disruptive qualities of technology for sleep.

- During parent interviews or in parent questionnaires, clinicians should assess children's technology habits when determining the source of young children's sleep problems. In particular, clinicians should ask parents to (1) estimate the amount of time their child spends with media (during the day, in the evening, and before bedtime); (2) indicate the type of technology content the child uses, especially in the evening (eg, frightening content, highly arousing content); and (3) provide information about the presence of media devices in the child's bedroom.

- During parent interviews or in parent questionnaires, clinicians should determine whether parents contribute to their children's technology use by (1) using technology as a sleep aid; and/or (2) providing technology to occupy children who are sleep-deprived or because of the parent's own sleep deprivation.

- Clinicians should make specific recommendations to caregivers concerning the use of technology for children, including recommending that bedrooms are free of technology and that exposure is prohibited or limited in the hours preceding bedtime.

- Clinicians should encourage parents to shield their young child from scary media content, such as violent programming and games.

- Clinicians should advise parents to consult Common Sense Media for guidance and recommendations for age-appropriate media content.

- Clinicians should work with parents to develop screen-free (or screen-limited) bedtime rituals for their young children.

- Clinicians should encourage parents to co-use media with their children to both monitor content and to build and strengthen parent–child relationships.

## DISCLOSURE

The author has nothing to disclose.

## REFERENCES

1. Radesky JS, Schumacher J, Zuckerman B. Mobile and interactive media use by young children: the good, the bad, and the unknown. Pediatrics 2014;135(1):1–3.
2. Chassiakos YL, Radesky J, Christakis D, et al. Children and adolescents and digital media. Pediatrics 2016;138(5):e20162593.
3. Rideout V. The common sense consensus: media use by kids ages zero to eight. San Francisco (CA): Common Sense Media; 2017.
4. Cristia A, Seidl A. Parental reports on touch screen use in early childhood. PLoS One 2015;10(5):e0128338.
5. Kabali H, Irigoyen MM, Nunez-Davis R, et al. Exposure and use of mobile media devices by young children. Pediatrics 2015;136:1044–50.
6. Woodward EH. The 1999 State of children's television report. Programming for children over broadcast and cable television. Philadelphia: Annenberg Public Policy Center; 1999. Available at: https://cdn.annenbergpublicpolicycenter.org/

Downloads/Media_and_Developing_Child/Childrens_Programming/19990628_State_of_Children/childrensTVreport1999.pdf.

7. Cain N, Gradisar M. Electronic media use and sleep in school-aged children and adolescents: a review. Sleep Med 2010;11:735–42.

8. Carter B, Rees P, Hale L, et al. A meta-analysis of the effect of media devices on sleep outcomes. JAMA Pediatr 2016;170(12):1202–8.

9. Hale L, Guan S. Screen time and sleep among school-aged children and adolescents: a systematic literature review. Sleep Med Rev 2015;21:50–8.

10. LeBorgeois ML, Hale L, Chang A-M, et al. Digital media and sleep in childhood and adolescence. Pediatrics 2017;140:s92–6.

11. Brockmann PE, Diaz B, Damiani F, et al. Impact of television on the quality of sleep in preschool children. Sleep Med 2016;20:140–4.

12. Janssen X, Martin A, Hughes AR, et al. Associations of screen time, sedentary time and physical activity with sleep in under 5s: a systematic review and meta-analysis. Sleep Med Rev 2020;49:101226.

13. Cespedes EM, Gilman MW, Kleinman K, et al. Television viewing, bedroom television, and sleep duration from infancy to mid-childhood. Pediatrics 2014;133(5): e1163–71.

14. Garrison MM, Liekweg K, Christakis DA. Media use and child sleep: the impact of timing, content, and environment. Pediatrics 2011;128(1):29–35.

15. Nathanson AI, Beyens I. The relation between use of mobile electronic devices and bedtime resistance, sleep duration, and daytime sleepiness among preschoolers. Behav Sleep Med 2018;16:202–19.

16. Owens JA, Spirito A, McGuinn M. The children's sleep habit questionnaire (CSHQ): psychometric properties of a survey instrument for school-aged children. Sleep 2000;23(8):1–9.

17. Bernier A, Beauchamp MH, Bouvette-Tourcot, et al. Sleep and cognition in preschool years: specific links to executive functioning. Child Dev 2013;84(5): 1542–53.

18. Dionne G, Touchette E, Forget-Dubois N, et al. Associations between sleep-wake consolidation and language development in early childhood: a longitudinal twin study. Sleep 2011;34(8):987–95.

19. Sadeh A, De Marcas G, Guri Y, et al. Infant sleep predicts attention regulation and behavior problems at 3-4 years of age. Dev Neuropsychol 2015;40(3):122–37.

20. Beyens I, Nathanson AI. Electronic media use and sleep among preschoolers: evidence for time-shifted and less consolidated sleep. Health Commun 2019; 34:537–44.

21. Downing KL, Hinkley T, Salmon J, et al. Do the correlates of screen time and sedentary time differ in preschool children? BMC Public Health 2017;17:285.

22. Cheung CHM, Bedford R, Saez De Urabain I, et al. Daily touchscreen use in infants and toddlers is associated with reduced sleep and delayed sleep onset. Sci Rep 2017;7:46104.

23. Thompson DA, Christakis DA. The association between television viewing and irregular sleep schedules among children less than 3 years of age. Pediatrics 2005;116(4):851–6.

24. Chindano S, Buja A, DeBattisti E, et al. Sleep and new media usage in toddlers. Eur J Pediatr 2019;178:483–90.

25. Vijakkhana N, Wilaisakditipakorn T, Ruedeekhajorn K, et al. Evening media exposure reduces night-time sleep. Acta Paediatr 2014;104(3):306–12.

26. Chen B, van Dam RM, Seng Tang C, et al. Screen viewing behavior and sleep duration among children aged 2 and below. BMC Public Health 2019;19:59.

27. Marinelli M, Sunyer J, Alvarez-Pedrerol M, et al. Hours of television viewing and sleep duration in children: a multicenter birth cohort study. JAMA Pediatr 2014; 168(5):458–64.
28. Genuneit J, Brockmann PE, Schlarb AS, et al. Media consumption and sleep quality in early childhood: results from the Ulm SPATZ Study. Sleep Med 2018; 45:7–10.
29. Nathanson AI, Beyens I. The role of sleep in the relation between children's mobile media use and effortful control. Br J Dev Psychol 2018;36:1–21.
30. Nathanson AI, Fries P. Television exposure, sleep time, and neuropsychological function among preschoolers. Media Psychol 2014;17:237–61.
31. Sigtsma A, Koller M, Sauer PJJ, et al. Television, sleep, outdoor play and BMI in young children: the GECKO Drenthe cohort. Eur J Pediatr 2015;174:631–9.
32. Bernier A, Belanger M-E, Tarabulsy GM, et al. My mother is sensitive, but I am too tired to know: infant sleep as a moderator of prospective relations between maternal sensitivity and infant outcomes. Infant Behav Dev 2014;37:682–94.
33. Golshevsky DM, Magnussen C, Juonala M, et al. Time spent watching television impacts body mass index in youth with obesity, but only in those with shortest sleep duration. J Pediatr Child Health 2019. https://doi.org/10.1111/jpc.14711.
34. Barr-Anderson DJ, van den Berg P, Neumark-Sztainer D, et al. Characteristics associated with older adolescents who have a television in their bedrooms. Pediatrics 2008;121(4):718–24.
35. Wethington H, Pan L, Sherry B. The association of screen time, television in the bedroom, and obesity among school-aged youth: 2007 National Survey of Children's Health. J Sch Health 2013;83(8):573–81.
36. Wood B, Rea MS, Plitnick B, et al. Light level and duration of exposure determine the impact of self-luminous tablets on melatonin suppression. Appl Ergon 2013; 44:237–40.
37. Salti R, Tarquini R, Sagi S, et al. Age-dependent association of exposure to television screen and children's urinary melatonin secretion. Neuroendocrinology Letter 2006;27:73–80.
38. Wood B, Rea MS, Plitnick B, et al. Light level and duration of exposure determine the impact of self-luminous tablets on melatonin suppression. Applied Ergonomics 2013;44:237–40.
39. Chang A-M, Aeschbach D, Duff JF, et al. Evening use of light-emitting eReaders negatively affects sleep, circadian timing, and next-morning alertness. Proceedings of the National Academy of Sciences 2015;112:1232–7.
40. Higuchi S, Motohashi Y, Liu Y, et al. Effects of playing a computer game using a bright display on preschool physiological variables, sleep latency, slow wave sleep and REM sleep. J. Sleep Res. 2005;14:267–73.
41. Yland J, Guan S, Emanuele E, et al. Interactive vs passive screen time and nighttime sleep duration among school-aged children. Sleep Health 2015;1(3):191–6.
42. Cantor J. "Mommy I'm Scared": How TV and movies frighten children and what we can do to protect them. New York, NY: Houghton Mifflin Harcourt; 1998.
43. Galland B, Meredith-Jones K, Terrill P, et al. Challenges and emerging technologies within the field of pediatric actigraphy. Front Psychiatry 2014;5:1–5.
44. Radesky JS, Peacock-Chambers E, Zuckerberg B. Use of mobile technology to calm upset children: associations with social-emotional development. JAMA Pediatr 2016;170:397–9.
45. Magee CA, Kyu Lee J, Vella SA. Bidirectional relationships between sleep duration and screen time in early childhood. JAMA Pediatr 2014;168(5):465–70.

46. Calamaro CJ, Mason TBA, Ratcliffe SJ. Adolescents living the 24/7 lifestyle: effects of caffeine and technology on sleep duration and daytime functioning. Pediatrics 2009;123:e1005–10.

47. Crowley SJ, Cain SW, Burns AC, et al. Increased sensitivity of the circadian system to light in early/mid-puberty. J Clin Endocrinol Metab 2015;100:4067–73.

48. Higuchi S, Nagafuchi Y, Lee S, et al. Influence of light at night on melatonin suppression in children. J Clin Endocrinol Metab 2014;99(9):3298–303.

49. Paruthi S, Brooks LJ, D'Ambrosio C, et al. Recommended amount of sleep for pediatric populations: a consensus statement of the American Academy of Sleep Medicine. J Clin Sleep Med 2016;12(6):785–6.

50. AAP Council on Communications And Media. Media and young minds. Pediatrics 2016;138(5):e20162591.

51. Owens J, Maxim R, McGuinn M, et al. Television viewing habits and sleep disturbances in school children. Pediatrics 1999;104(3):e27.

# Neurocognitive Effects of Sleep Disruption in Children and Adolescents

Karen Spruyt, PhD

## KEYWORDS

- Cognition • Sleep • Child • Adolescent • Performance

## KEY POINTS

- Recently, there has been an upsurge of experimental cognitive neuroscience study designs with sleep measures, as well as observational sleep studies investigating cognition beyond memory in children and adolescents.
- Subjective sleep studies in childhood show associations with school achievements, executive function and attention; objective sleep studies seem to highlight relationships with working memory.
- The sleep–cognition interdependency is complex, and requires a developmental perspective.
- Sleep duration, timing, quality, and regulation are examined in this review, and although each play a role, their impact on cognition needs to be understood in the context of the individual child's need for sleep.

## INTRODUCTION
### Sleep and Development: The Importance Toward Neurocognition

Sleep is necessary for optimal performance both physically and mentally, promoting learning and memory.[3] The sleep macrostructure is neurophysiologically divided into non-REM (NREM) sleep and REM sleep, and is characterized in terms of behavioral, neurologic, and functional anatomy features. NREM sleep is further divided in 3 subtypes according to electroencephalographic (EEG) oscillations: NREM stage 1, with slow waves, vertex waves, or wake rhythm fragmentation; NREM stage 2, with a phasic activity as K complex and sleep spindles; and NREM stage 3, also called slow wave sleep, with slow wave activity, consisting of delta range oscillations.

Although sleep macrostructure classification seems complete, this classical approach to sleep analysis may fail to recognize EEG microstructural changes. That

This article originally appeared in *Child and Adolescent Psychiatric Clinics*, Volume 30 Issue 1, January 2021.
Université Paris Cité, INSERM - NeuroDiderot, Paris, France
*E-mail addresses:* karen.spruyt@inserm.fr; karen.spruyt@univ-lyon1.fr

Psychiatr Clin N Am 47 (2024) 27–45
https://doi.org/10.1016/j.psc.2023.06.003
0193-953X/24/© 2023 Elsevier Inc. All rights reserved.

is, during sleep the brain is switched into an activation state that is distinct from wakefulness at both microscopic (eg, spike timing, amplitude) and macroscopic (eg, neocortical EEG oscillations) levels. In sleep microstructure analysis, the microstructural cyclicity of NREM sleep and sleep spindles (ie, bursts of neural oscillatory activity) are examined and have been considered as the window onto brain maturation.

In children specifically, this role of sleep in cognition is extremely important because NREM sleep EEG synchronization changes considerably with age.[4–7] In light of such maturational changes in terms of feature number, density, duration, frequency, and regional distribution, both REM and NREM sleep cycles have defining EEG features that are increasingly investigated in relation to cognition during childhood. The current review summarizes recent findings regarding sleep and cognition to inform both research and clinical applications in the fields of psychiatry and sleep medicine.

### Sleep Is for Cognition: The Supporting Mechanisms

Animal studies have shown that sleep and sleep disruption influence brain plasticity[8–10] and, specifically, learning and memory.[11,12] This has led to at least one widespread hypothesis known as the synaptic homeostasis hypothesis.[9,10] Other studies speculated that sleep promotes hippocampal structural plasticity[13,14] such as dendritic spine density.[15] In other words, sleep promotes synaptic activity.[11,16] Converging evidence, from the molecular to the clinical, leaves little doubt that sleep is involved in development—be it maturation and/or learning. The "how" is a vigorously studied question.[3,17] The synaptic homeostasis hypothesis has pushed a vast majority of human studies toward investigating the role of slow-wave sleep (0.5–4.0 Hz), and especially the less than 1 Hz slow oscillations, in our learning aptitude. This phenomenon may have overshadowed the early interest in REM sleep, an interest driven by its abundant presence in early childhood.[18] Recent animal studies,[19,20] however, (re)support the critical role of REM for neuronal circuit development and learning.

Regarding cognitive functioning specifically, several sleep hypotheses have been published, including the sleep-dependent memory consolidation,[21] the active system consolidation,[16,22,23] the role of neural replay in memory formation,[24–26] and the dual process hypothesis[27] (**Table 1**). Based on these findings, progressively more studies in adults confirm that sleep provides optimal conditions for consolidation, stabilization, and transformation of memories and their subsequent integration into "cognitive functioning".[23,28] Hence, publications of studies in childhood showing slow oscillations, spindle oscillations, sharp-wave ripples (ie, rapid bursts of synchronized neuronal activity elicited by the hippocampus), and REM sleep linked to (optimal) sleep conditions and performance are increasing.

### CURRENT EVIDENCE ON SLEEP MACROSTRUCTURE DISRUPTION AND COGNITION

Maturation is presumably the indispensable component in determining our sleep,[29] yet in childhood sleep evolves in complex ways. In fact, worldwide normative, age-appropriate sleep needs (ie, the amount of sleep required for optimal functioning) remain poorly characterized. Notwithstanding, several types of reviews on cognitive outcomes of poor sleep have been published lately. With Spruyt (**Fig. 1**),[1] recent reviews reported on sleep restriction,[30,31] weekend-to-weekday sleep differences,[32] napping,[33] sleep in general,[34,35] and with a focus on adolescence specifically.[31,36] Each of them concludes that, without optimal sleep, a child's cognitive abilities suffer.

More specifically, the narrative review by Lo and Chee[31] proposes that multiple successive nights of restricted sleep impairs multiple cognitive functions, with limited benefits gained by weekend recovery sleep. Davidson and colleagues[30] had a slightly

| Table 1 | |
|---|---|
| **Sleep hypotheses regarding cognitive functioning** | |
| **Hypothesis** | **Synopsis** |
| The sleep-dependent memory consolidation[21] | This hypothesis supposes an improvement in recall after an interval with sleep relative to an interval with wake. |
| The active system consolidation[16,22,23] | In the systems consolidation approach, the redistribution of the "to be memorized information" between different brain systems led researchers to explore the dialogue between neocortex and hippocampus in particular. In the synaptic consolidation approach, the local changes in synaptic connections in neuronal circuits, or scrutinizing the neurobiology of the concept "consolidation" has been the topic of research. |
| The role of neural replay in memory formation[24–26] | Sleep primes certain memories to be preferentially replayed or a sleep-associated memory consolidation process is in play. The sleep-dependent generalization[67] counteracts the abundance in declarative memory (ie, explicit recognition or recall of facts and events) studies and sets stage for studies investigating cognitive flexibility or creativity. Or the idea that memory traces become unstable to facilitate their interaction and extraction of common features. |
| The dual process hypothesis[27] | This hypothesis proposes that slow wave sleep plays its role in declarative memories, whereas REM sleep might play a role in the consolidation of nondeclarative (or implicit), procedural and emotional memories. |

broader scope with a main interest in children with attention deficit hyperactivity disorder (ADHD). The authors concluded that too few experimental sleep manipulation research studies exist in children, with either typical or atypical development, to stipulate causal relationships with specific cognitive and emotion regulation domains. Because predominantly attention has been studied, particularly children with ADHD compared with others have been investigated. Results are variable, but the scarce correlational and subjective studies in children with ADHD suggest poorer academic competence, more variable reaction times, and difficulties across executive function tasks.[30]

Up to 2018, 20 observational studies quantified the adverse impact of week-to-weekend sleep differences on academic performance (see **Fig. 1**).[32] Only 6 studies published data on a broad range of cognitive performances, with mixed results likely to be ascribed to methodologic challenges.[32] The narrative review by Horváth and Plunkett[33] concluded that for preschoolers daytime napping is crucial for early memory development (ie, possibly for generalization and retention abilities). We may additionally conclude that the napping paradigm in children less than 5 years of age is popular for investigating the sleep–cognition relationship in this age group (note, daytime sleep is not readily generalizable to nighttime sleep). In the 39 studies systematically meta-reviewed by Matricciani and colleagues,[34] only 3 had a focus on cognition, and 5 had a broader scope, including cognitive or academic performance, among other outcomes. Findings[1,32,34] concur that, in the case of sleep macrostructure disruption, the bulk of research investigated health-related outcomes, and firm conclusions on cognitive performance are difficult.

Nearly all of these reviews captured studies until 2017, and show that poor sleep affects cognition in complex ways. Our auxiliary systematic literature search conducted for this review adds a total of 29 original papers (**Table 2**). Most were subjective

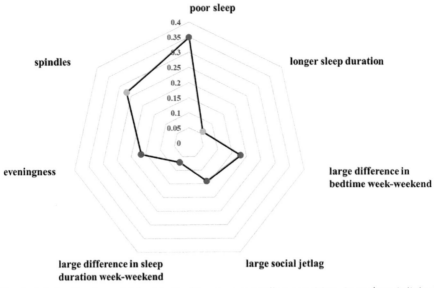

**Fig. 1.** Point estimates published in the literature regarding cognition. Poor sleep is linked to poor cognitive performance by Spruyt[1]; longer sleep duration associated with better cognition[56]; large differences in bedtime, midpoint of sleep (social jetlag), and sleep duration between week–weekend are associated with poor academic performance by Sun and colleagues[32]; eveningness associated with worse academic performance by Tonetti and colleagues[60]; and there was a positive correlation between spindles and cognition by Reynolds and colleagues.[53]

reports on sleep (predominantly sleep duration), with 2 applying standard polysomnography parameters and 5 using actigraphy. Chiefly school-aged children (37.9%) and adolescents (31%; in particular 15–17 year olds) have been participants. Most of these individual studies do not have an experimental design, a few had a(n) (surrogate) approach to a sleep-dependent memory consolidation design,[37,38] and one investigated the dual process hypothesis.[39] An equal interest in memory (20.7%), cognitive development/abilities (20.7%), academic performance (20.7%), and mixed cognitive outcomes (20.7%) (ie, several cognitive tests, or combined cognitive and behavioral outcomes) is seen. One study tested whether training the working memory of children would improve their sleep,[40] which was unsuccessful.

Looking at **Table 2**, it becomes clear that firm conclusions are challenged by how the sleep measures and concepts were defined, which cognitive assessments have been applied, and the type of design used (ie, observational, experimental, and what kind of experiment). In addition, studies are plagued by inconsistent controlling for potential confounders such as age, sex,[41,42] fatigue,[41,43] stress, familial factors,[44–49] and (co)morbidities (eg, prematurity[50]). Roughly, we may infer the following across childhood regarding sleep macrostructure disruptions. Before the age of 5 years, sleep continuity (ie, sleep uninterrupted by night wakings) and the regularity of sleep patterns promote overall development and memory. At school age, sleep quality relates to verbal performance, achievement, and executive functioning, whereas adequate sleep duration may prevent forgetting and improve executive control. Morningness (ie, circadian preference for early wake time/bedtimes) in adolescence, likely interlinked with increased sleep duration, nurtures enhanced scholastic

**Table 2**
**Recent findings on sleep macrostructure disruptions and cognition**

| Author, Year | Age (y), Mean ± SD; Range | Sleep Aim | Sleep Variables | Cognitive Variables |
| --- | --- | --- | --- | --- |
| Smithson et al,[68] 2018 | Birth cohort | Sleep duration | Sleep duration, sleep disordered breathing | At 2 y Bayley Scale of Infant Development |
| Trajectory analysis identified 4 total sleep durations phenotypes: short sleepers, decline to short sleepers, intermediate sleepers and long sleepers; compared with children with intermediate sleep durations, short sleepers had a 5.2-point lower cognitive development score at 2 y of age; nocturnal sleep duration, compared with daytime sleep duration, had the greatest effect on cognitive development | | | | |
| Sun et al,[69] 2018 | 2–30 mo | Sleep | Sleep duration, night waking | Bayley Scales of Infant Development |
| Frequent nighttime awakenings are associated with poor cognitive functions in toddlers | | | | |
| Spanò et al,[37] 2018 | 33.4 ± 5.1 mo | Nap time | Natural, in-home naps | Word learning |
| Naps benefitted memory performance; these beneficial effects of napping persisted 24 h later; memory retention for object–label associations correlated positively with percent of time in REM sleep | | | | |
| Schlieber et al,[70] 2018 | 3–4 | Sleeping patterns | Parent interviews | Peabody Picture Vocabulary Test-IV, the Expressive One-Word Picture Vocabulary Test, and Subtests of the Woodcock Johnson III) in addition to teacher report |
| Sleeping through the night and having a consistent bedtime were found to be predictive of many areas of cognitive and behavioral development | | | | |

(continued on next page)

**Table 2**
*(continued)*

| Author, Year | Age (y), Mean ± SD; Range | Sleep Aim | Sleep Variables | Cognitive Variables |
|---|---|---|---|---|
| McCann et al,[65] 2018 | 6–7 (born very preterm) | Parent-reported sleep | Snoring, nighttime sleep quality, and daytime sleepiness | A verbal working memory task, measures of processing speed and verbal storage capacity; a direct measure of executive functioning |
| | Poor sleep has an impact on the executive component of working memory; problematic sleeping adversely impacted executive functioning in the very preterm group | | | |
| Xing et al,[71] 2018 | 6.3 ± 0.4 | Sleep | Total daily sleep duration, ratio of nighttime sleep to total daily sleep, sleep compensation over the weekend | Executive function |
| | Longer night time sleep = ↑ executive function; initial ratio of nighttime sleep predicts subsequent executive function; ↑ sleep compensation = ↑ executive function | | | |
| Quach et al,[40] 2018 | 6.9 ± 0.4 | Sleep | Parent-reported sleep | CogMed program |
| | Adaptive working memory training during the school day cannot improve children's sleep (6 mo later), regardless of the time of day training is delivered | | | |
| Blunden et al,[72] 2018 | 7–9 | Sleep | Sleep duration, bedtimes, wake times, variability in bedtimes from weekdays to weekends | National Assessment Program–Literacy and Numeracy |
| | Short sleep was associated with poorer school performance, with this performance worsening over time for some performance indicators | | | |

| | | | | |
|---|---|---|---|---|
| Prehn-Kristensen et al,[38] 2018 | 7–11 | Sleep | Sleep; encoding session in the evening + fixed retention interval of 12 h, the retrieval session in next morning; in the wake condition, the time schedule was the same but reversed | Learn the location of 18 object pairs; one-half of the object locations were allocated to a high-rewarded condition and the other half to a low-rewarded condition |
| Results show that 12 h of wakefulness can deteriorate the memory performance for highly rewarded representations, whereas sleep can prevent the forgetting of these rewarded representations | | | | |
| Zinke et al,[73] 2018 | 10–12 | Sleep | Between the training sessions, participants first spent a full night sleeping + a normal day awake (evening groups) or vice versa (morning groups) | Trained on 3 sessions of an n-back task comprising 3 runs of blocks (6 blocks with 20 responses each) |
| Sleep after training facilitates cognitive procedures related to executive control | | | | |
| Cusick et al,[62] 2018 | 12–14 | Previous night's sleep | Sleep quality, sleep duration, and number of night waking | Standardized tests of processing speed and working memory, as well as word reading, numerical operations, math fluency academic achievement |
| Participants reporting $\geq$2 night wakings the previous night had slightly more than one-half of a standard deviation lower scores on average compared with participants reporting 0 night wakings | | | | |
| Arrona-Palacios et al,[42] 2018 | 13.9 $\pm$ 0.7 | Afternoon school shift | Morningness–Eveningness Scale for Children (MESC) + sleep habits survey | Test of academic performance, inductive reasoning subtest of the Primary Mental Abilities battery |
| Female sex, sleep length, inductive reasoning, and morningness were associated with academic performance in the morning shift | | | | |

(continued on next page)

**Table 2**
*(continued)*

| Author, Year | Age (y), Mean ± SD; Range | Sleep Aim | Sleep Variables | Cognitive Variables |
|---|---|---|---|---|
| Tashjian et al,[74] 2018 | 14–18 | Sleep | Actigraphy over 14 d | Resting state functional connectivity |
| | Variation in sleep quality, but not duration, was related to weaker intrinsic default mode network connectivity, such that those with worse quality sleep evinced weaker intranetwork connectivity at rest | | | |
| Fuligni, et al,[75] 2018 | 15.03 | Daily variability in sleep duration | Reported nightly sleep times for 2 wk; ~80% repeated the same protocol 1 y later | A composite grade point average; California Standards Test in mathematics and English from school records; attendance; Child Behavior Checklist |
| | ↑ Daily variability = ↑ symptomatology and mixed academic outcomes | | | |
| Cohen-Zion et al,[41] 2018 | 15–18 | Sleep | Survey on sleep, phase preference | Academic performance, executive functions |
| | Female sex, grade status, sleepiness, and evening chronotype accounted for approximately 25%–30% of the variance in daily executive ability; sleep duration was a weak predictor of executive skills; lower school grades were associated with increased sleepiness, evening preference and poorer executive skills | | | |
| Cousins et al,[76] 2018 | 15–18 | Partial sleep restriction (5 consecutive nights of 5 h time in bed) | Time in bed | A picture-encoding task |
| | Memory encoding is impaired after multiple nights of partial sleep restriction; this impairment was not correlated with a decrease in vigilance | | | |
| Estevan et al,[49] 2018 | 16.6 ± 1.1 | Sleep | School start times: morning or afternoon shifts | Mean midterm teachers' ratings of students' performance and the number of absences |
| | Eveningness influence on school performance is contingent on the temporal arrangement of scholar activities | | | |

| Study | Age | Type | Measure | Outcome |
|---|---|---|---|---|
| Pisch et al,[77] 2019 | Within 2 wk of 4, 6, 8, and 10 mo since their date of birth | Sleep | Sleep (1 wk actigraphy) + sleep questionnaire) | Eye tracking; remember the location of a toy previously linked to a sound |
| | Night wake time can serve as a marker for different cognitive trajectories | | | |
| Hoyniak et al,[46] 2019 | 30, 36, and 42 mo | Sleep | Various sleep problems, using actigraphy | Standardized test of cognitive abilities |
| | ↑ Delayed sleep schedules on average = ↓ cognitive abilities; delayed sleep explains part of the association between family socioeconomic context and child cognitive abilities | | | |
| Franco et al,[78] 2019 | | Sleep | Standard sleep parameters from birth | Intelligence quotient |
| | Night sleep fragmentation or longer naps could be associated with impaired cognitive function at 3 y of age | | | |
| Nieto et al,[45] 2019 | 3–6 | Sleep | Parental self-report | Autobiographical memory |
| | Time slept during the night or the day positively correlated with autobiographical memory specificity, regardless of memory valence | | | |
| Smith et al,[47] 2019 | 49–72 mo | Napping behaviors | Those who nap (nappers), sometimes nap (transitioners), do not nap (resters), and neither nap, nor lie still (problem nappers) | Woodcock Johnson III; Brief Intellectual Ability Scale |
| | Nappers had significantly shorter duration of nighttime sleep, were younger, and had lower cognitive functioning scores | | | |
| El-Sheikh et al,[44] 2019 | 9.4 ± 0.7 | Sleep | Actigraphy sleep parameters (7 consecutive nights) + sleep self-report | Cognitive performance tests; academic achievement data through school |
| | Nonlinear associations were detected between both actigraphy-derived and subjective reports of sleep quality and multiple developmental domains including academic functioning; the best functioning corresponded with the highest levels of sleep quality | | | |

(continued on next page)

**Table 2**
*(continued)*

| Author, Year | Age (y), Mean ± SD; Range | Sleep Aim | Sleep Variables | Cognitive Variables |
|---|---|---|---|---|
| Adelantado-Renau et al,[79] 2019 | 13.9 ± 0.3 | Sleep | Self-reported sleep + accelerometry | Spanish version of the SRA Test of Educational Ability |
| | ↓Objective sleep duration = ↓ verbal ability; ↑self-reported sleep quality = ↑ academic performance; no associations between self-reported sleep duration and objective sleep quality with academic and cognitive performance | | | |
| Wetter et al,[48] 2019 | Young children | Sleep | Sleep | Executive functioning |
| | Sleep is a protective mechanism for executive functioning in children from low-income homes | | | |
| Stormark et al,[80] 2019 | 7–9; at 11–13 | Difficulties initiating and maintaining sleep | Concurrent, transitory and persistent difficulties | Academic performance |
| | Sleep problems in children are associated with impaired academic performance; sleep problems may not increase the risk of poor academic performance unless they persist over time | | | |
| Möhring et al,[39] 2019 | 7–12 (preterm/full-term born) | Sleep | Ambulatory polysomnography | Dual-task situations; simultaneously perform different cognitive tasks |
| | ↑ Disrupted sleep = ↓ dual-task performance; REM sleep seems more related to performance in procedural tasks whereas slow wave sleep seems more related to performance in declarative tasks | | | |
| Cheng et al,[81] 2020 | 9–11 | Sleep | Sleep Disturbance Scale for Children | Structural magnetic resonance imaging |
| | Volume of the orbitofrontal cortex, prefrontal and temporal cortex, precuneus, and supramarginal gyrus correlated with longer sleep duration; higher cognitive scores were associated with higher volume of the prefrontal cortex, temporal cortex, and medial orbitofrontal cortex | | | |
| Preckel et al,[82] 2020 | 14.98 | Circadian preference | A quadrant-based typology of circadian preference | Academic performance |
| | Types did not differ in sleep duration; lower academic performance related to having an evening preference | | | |

achievements. Stable, good quality sleep in adolescents seems to promote optimal brain connectivity as seen in executive control tasks.

Despite the limited experimental studies investigating the impact of sleep macrostructure disruptions, a vast amount of sleep studies in general,[1] and in children with various disorders such as ADHD,[51] sleep-disordered breathing[52] or other sleep disorders, or for instance examining shifted school start times, support the following clinical implications: (1) sleepiness and sleep duration affect executive functions, complex cognitive tasks, and school grades, (2) primarily subjective reports of poor sleep have been associated with deficits in attention, memory performance, or problem solving tasks, and (3) decreased sleep time seems to affect vigilance, whereas increased sleep time seems to improve working memory.

## CURRENT EVIDENCE OF SLEEP MICROSTRUCTURE DISRUPTION AND COGNITION

Because sleep duration, quality, and timing of sleep are interrelated, it is difficult to abstract the specific, related cognitive dysfunction when studies do not apply polysomnography. Defining the measurement of a phenomenon, or its operationalization, is much clearer when studying sleep microstructure. Especially here, the influx of cognitive neuroscientists is visible in the sleep literature.

Despite a boom in original research papers, few have recently reviewed the cognitive outcomes of sleep microstructure disruptions. Moreover, studies have primarily focused on adolescents,[36,53] whereas in preschoolers[33] 4 studies were described. Reynolds and colleagues[53] concluded a positive relationship between spindles (ie, bursts of neural oscillatory activity believed to mediate many sleep-related functions, from memory consolidation to cortical development) and cognition (see **Fig. 1**). Similar to other investigators,[1,54–56] they highlighted that the impact or relationship may vary according to the functional domain (eg, attention, speed, and memory), age of the participant, and specific study design. Such multifariousness is also hampering firm conclusions with respect to imaging results.[57] Namely, developing brain functions and structures tend to be sensitive to sleep, yet again to date we cannot be much more specific.

In analogy with our approach to sleep macrostructure disruption, we searched the literature (**Table 3**). Seven original papers were retrieved, applying in primarily school-aged children and (pre/early) adolescents sleep studies toward microstructural analysis. The majority of them (n = 3) examine memory and learning. Findings indicate small but significant associations between sleep microstructural changes and cognition. Roughly, we could summarize from these preliminary reports the following: (1) across childhood both NREM and REM features foster development and (2) in early infancy, the oscillatory changes link to developmental changes, whereas during the school-age period and adolescence spindle activity relates to memory performance.

## DISCUSSING THE CLINICAL RELEVANCE

The notions on the role of sleep in cognitive functioning[16,22,58] provide us improved insights that sleep is for cognition, we just do not know exactly how. In this blooming period of cognitive sleep neurosciences,[17] however, 3 aspects need to be highlighted. First, brain development is a nonlinear process both structurally and functionally, and continues throughout childhood and adolescence. Although gray matter growth peaks in the first 2 decades of life, which virtually goes hand in hand with cerebral blood flow changes, white matter follows a more gradual growth. Findings on the sleep–cognition relationship, therefore, need to incorporate developmental influences on brain maturation (eg, the faster growth pace of white matter volume in girls vs boys during

**Table 3**
Recent findings on sleep microstructure disruptions and cognition

| Author, Year | Age (y) Mean ± SD; Range | Sleep Aim | Sleep Variables | Cognitive Variables |
|---|---|---|---|---|
| Page et al,[63] 2019 | 20 ± 5.2 mo | Sleep network dynamics of NREM sleep | Sleep topography with high-density electroencephalography | Motor, language, and social skills by Mullen Early Scales of Learning and the Vineland Adaptive Behavior Scales—2nd Edition |
| | | | Delta, theta, and beta oscillations and sleep spindles exhibited clear developmental changes; low delta and high theta oscillations correlated with motor, language, and social skills, independent of age | |
| Hahn et al,[83] 2019 | 8–11; at 14–18 | Sleep | Ambulatory polysomnography 2 nights (baseline and experimental) | Wechsler Intelligence Scale |
| | | | Mature fast spindles play crucial role in sleep-dependent memory consolidation; slow spindle changes across adolescence were related to general cognitive abilities | |
| Bestmann et al,[61] 2019 | 9–12 ↑Sigma power = ↑ reaction times | Sleep | Sigma power | Reaction times |
| Vermeulen et al,[84] 2019 | 10.7 ± 0.8 | Sleep | Sleep stages and microstructural sleep characteristics | Repeated assessments of the Tower of Hanoi task (planning and problem-solving skills) |
| | | | Stronger performance improvement across wake in children with more stage NREM stage 2 sleep and less slow-wave sleep; stronger improvements across sleep were present in children in whom slow spindles were more dense, and in children in whom fast spindles were less dense, of shorter duration and had less power | |

| Study | Age | Domain | Measure | Description |
|---|---|---|---|---|
| Bothe et al,[85] 2019 | 11–14 | Sleep | Sleep stages, microstructural sleep characteristics | A complex gross motor adaptation task by using a bicycle with an inverse steering device; training in morning/evening + a 9-hr retention interval |
| | | | | Overnight gains in accuracy were associated with an increase in left hemispheric NREM stage 2 slow sleep spindle activity from control to learning night; decreases in REM and tonic REM duration were related to higher overnight improvements in accuracy; regarding speed, an increase in REM and tonic REM duration was favorable for higher overnight gains in riding time |
| Kuula et al,[86] 2019 | 16.9 ± 0.1 | Spindles | Sleep spindle activity | Deese, Roediger & McDermott (DRM) false memory procedure |
| | | | | Higher sleep spindle activity is associated with fewer false memories; no association between slow-wave sleep and false memory recollection |
| Wilhelm et al,[87] 2020 | 11–13 | Sleep | REM sleep | Targeted memory reactivation during sleep; half of the words were presented via loudspeakers during postlearning periods of NREM sleep |
| | | | | Improvement on the oscillatory level (not behavioral), that is, successful reactivation during sleep resulted in the characteristic increase in theta power over frontal brain regions |

puberty). Second, the bulk of research investigated hippocampus-dependent memories, yet an early decrease in hippocampal neurogenesis has been postulated.[59] This finding may question the usability of adult models to address pediatric questions. Indeed few of these scientific sleep–cognition heuristics (see **Table 1**; eg, sleep-dependent memory consolidation) are completely established on pediatric research, or a developing brain. And last, particularly in children, creativity, problem solving, and cognitive flexibility are cardinal in their cognitive functioning, yet these functions have received little attention.

In Spruyt,[1] we reported a pooled estimate (0.35) for cognition, based on 19 reviews investigating poor sleep (eg, duration, quality) published in the last 5 years. Other pooled estimates have been published,[32,53,56,60] as shown in **Fig. 1**. Only sleep restriction/extension studies (ie, studies in which sleep is experimentally shortened or lengthened)[54,55] lack a pooled estimate; nonetheless, the current data indicate that sleep is clearly implicated in cognitive functioning, particularly, attention, executive functioning, and memory. Despite methodologic challenges, pediatric sleep research, therefore, has an important task ahead. Progressively more studies echo that, beyond sleep duration, other aspects of sleep, including quality, timing, and regulation, each have their role in cognition. At the moment, this might not be directly detectable on the behavioral level per the subjective reports on sleep and its macrostructure, but more so might be rippling at the microscopic level (eg, microstructure disruptions early in life impacting later developmental performance).

Optimal sleep is important for supporting development. Studies in children with developmental disabilities or sleep disorders (eg, ADHD,[30,61,62] autism,[63] Down syndrome,[37] and sleep-disordered breathing) bring pieces to the puzzle in terms of sleep macrostructural and microstructural findings. Taken together, they support that sleep is important in the cognitive processing of different abilities. However, they also suggest an increased vulnerability toward outcomes of poor sleep (eg, in Down syndrome, comorbid severe sleep-disordered breathing was accompanied by greater difficulties with executive function and verbal intelligence).[2,64–66] Alternatively, in typically developing children, studies suggest that sleep is an active brain process; regretfully one in which the individual child's need for sleep[1] has been systematically overlooked.

Converging evidence in the literature at large underpins that "what fires together, wires together." Although in the early years primarily the role of REM sleep in neural circuitry was speculated and (still) pedantically investigated, nowadays studies progressively more show that, during sleep, neural oscillations contribute to synapse formation, neuronal differentiation and migration, apoptosis, and the refinement of topographic mapping. Therefore, sleep is to forget (downscaling) and to remember (replay/generalize), so without a doubt to learn.

To conclude, the evidence linking sleep and cognition remains scattered, likely because there is more than one type of cognition, but also because sleep is not a homogenous state (eg, its macro/microstructure) and—foremost—children develop. Likely, their interdependence needs examination that is more comprehensive.

### Critical Points for Future Research

1. To radically understand the role of sleep on cognition, we need to (dis)entangle its components. "Sleep" is a multidimensional concept. Aside from sleep macrostructure/microstructure characteristics, it involves several parameters that are interrelated: bedtime/rise time and how long it takes to fall asleep/to wake up; sleep duration and quality; alertness following awakening; timing(s) of sleep within the 24-hour rhythm; variability of each of these parameters; sleepiness/sleeplessness;

and several biomarkers such as endogenous melatonin production during dim light conditions. Intertwined, yet each will contribute to cognitive performance.
2. A publication bias may exist because some functions are more readily investigated in cross-sectional studies or via questionnaires. Cognition has often been investigated in terms of attention, executive function, memory, and more globally as development or intellectual performance. Replication studies are needed.

## CLINICS CARE POINTS

---

- Despite the caveats in current research: sleep is for cognition. Accordingly, improving sleep (or any of its components) will improve cognition (whichever subfunction/domain) across childhood. Moreover, studies gradually accumulate evidence that poor sleep early in life may have adverse developmental outcomes later in childhood.

- For clinical practice, it remains pertinent to promote optimal sleep in the absence of more science pinpointing the specific gains. Too few studies have investigated the impact of sleep disruptions on cognition in children with atypical development to specify well-founded conclusions. Generally, one may speculate that their characteristic sleep disruption may have a selective impact on a sensitive cognitive domain. However, more research is needed to better understand the potential of such (a) risk/protective marker(s).

- Key players toward optimal sleep are age-appropriate sleep schedules; regularity in time, behavior, and environment; and appropriate sleep hygiene behaviors (eg, limited screen times, proper exercise and diet, sleep-promoting circumstances).

---

## DISCLOSURE

The author has nothing to disclose.

## REFERENCES

1. Spruyt K. A review of developmental consequences of poor sleep in childhood. Sleep Med 2019;60:3–12.
2. Spruyt K. Impact of sleep in children. In: Accardo JA, editor. Sleep in children with neurodevelopmental disabilities: an evidence-based guide. Cham (Switzerland): Springer International Publishing; 2019. p. 3–16.
3. Tononi G, Cirelli C. Sleep and the price of plasticity: from synaptic and cellular homeostasis to memory consolidation and integration. Neuron 2014;81(1):12–34.
4. Bruni O, Ferri R, Miano S, et al. Sleep cyclic alternating pattern in normal school-age children. Clin Neurophysiol 2002;113(11):1806–14.
5. Bruni O, Novelli L, Finotti E, et al. All-night EEG power spectral analysis of the cyclic alternating pattern at different ages. Clin Neurophysiol 2009;120(2):248–56.
6. Dan B, Boyd SG. A neurophysiological perspective on sleep and its maturation. Dev Med child Neurol 2006;48(9):773–9.
7. Shinomiya S, Nagata K, Takahashi K, et al. Development of sleep spindles in young children and adolescents. Clin Electroencephalogr 1999;30(2):39–43.
8. Del Rio-Bermudez C, Kim J, Sokoloff G, et al. Active sleep promotes coherent oscillatory activity in the cortico-hippocampal system of infant rats. Cereb Cortex 2020;30(4):2070–82.
9. Raven F, Van der Zee EA, Meerlo P, et al. The role of sleep in regulating structural plasticity and synaptic strength: implications for memory and cognitive function. Sleep Med Rev 2018;39:3–11.

10. Tononi G, Cirelli C. Sleep and synaptic homeostasis: a hypothesis. Brain Res Bull 2003;62(2):143–50.
11. Born J, Feld GB. Sleep to upscale, sleep to downscale: balancing homeostasis and plasticity. Neuron 2012;75(6):933–5.
12. Raven F, Meerlo P, Van der Zee EA, et al. A brief period of sleep deprivation causes spine loss in the dentate gyrus of mice. Neurobiol Learn Mem 2019; 160:83–90.
13. Chauvette S, Seigneur J, Timofeev I. Sleep oscillations in the thalamocortical system induce long-term neuronal plasticity. Neuron 2012;75(6):1105–13.
14. Durkin J, Aton SJ. Sleep-dependent potentiation in the visual system is at odds with the synaptic homeostasis hypothesis. Sleep 2016;39(1):155–9.
15. Aton SJ, Suresh A, Broussard C, et al. Sleep promotes cortical response potentiation following visual experience. Sleep 2014;37(7):1163–70.
16. Dudai Y. The neurobiology of consolidations, or, how stable is the engram? Annu Rev Psychol 2004;55:51–86.
17. Hobson JA, Pace-Schott EF. The cognitive neuroscience of sleep: neuronal systems, consciousness and learning. Nat Rev Neurosci 2002;3(9):679–93.
18. Kleitman N, Engelmann TG. Sleep characteristics of infants. J Appl Phys 1953; 6(5):269–82.
19. Del Rio-Bermudez C, Blumberg MS. Active sleep promotes functional connectivity in developing sensorimotor networks. BioEssays 2018;40(4):e1700234.
20. Li W, Ma L, Yang G, et al. REM sleep selectively prunes and maintains new synapses in development and learning. Nat Neurosci 2017;20(3):427–37.
21. Stickgold R. Sleep-dependent memory consolidation. Nature 2005;437(7063): 1272–8.
22. Klinzing JG, Niethard N, Born J. Mechanisms of systems memory consolidation during sleep. Nat Neurosci 2019;22(10):1598–610.
23. Dudai Y, Karni A, Born J. The consolidation and transformation of memory. Neuron 2015;88(1):20–32.
24. Born J, Rasch B, Gais S. Sleep to remember. Neuroscientist 2006;12(5):410–24.
25. Jegou A, Schabus M, Gosseries O, et al. Cortical reactivations during sleep spindles following declarative learning. NeuroImage 2019;195:104–12.
26. Wilhelm I, Diekelmann S, Molzow I, et al. Sleep selectively enhances memory expected to be of future relevance. J Neurosci 2011;31(5):1563.
27. Ackermann S, Rasch B. Differential effects of non-REM and REM sleep on memory consolidation? Curr Neurol Neurosci Rep 2014;14(2):430.
28. Chambers AM. The role of sleep in cognitive processing: focusing on memory consolidation. Wiley Interdiscip Rev Cogn Sci 2017;8(3). https://doi.org/10.1002/wcs.1433.
29. Roffwarg HP, Muzio JN, Dement WC. Ontogenetic development of the human sleep-dream cycle. Science 1966;152(3722):604–19.
30. Davidson F, Rusak B, Chambers C, et al. The impact of sleep restriction on daytime functioning in school-age children with and without ADHD: a narrative review of the literature. Can J Sch Psychol 2019;34(3):188–214.
31. Lo JC, Chee MW. Cognitive effects of multi-night adolescent sleep restriction: current data and future possibilities. Curr Opin Behav Sci 2020;33:34–41.
32. Sun W, Ling J, Zhu X, et al. Associations of weekday-to-weekend sleep differences with academic performance and health-related outcomes in school-age children and youths. Sleep Med Rev 2019;46:27–53.
33. Horváth K, Plunkett K. Spotlight on daytime napping during early childhood. Nat Sci Sleep 2018;10:97–104.

34. Matricciani L, Paquet C, Galland B, et al. Children's sleep and health: a meta-review. Sleep Med Rev 2019;46:136–50.
35. Göder R, Prehn-Kristensen A. Sleep and cognition in children and adolescents. Z Kinder Jugendpsychiatr Psychother 2018;46(5):405–22.
36. Galvan A. The need for sleep in the adolescent brain. Trends Cogn Sci 2020; 24(1):79–89.
37. Spanò G, Gómez RL, Demara BI, et al. REM sleep in naps differentially relates to memory consolidation in typical preschoolers and children with Down syndrome. Proc Natl Acad Sci U S A 2018;115(46):11844–9.
38. Prehn-Kristensen A, Böhmig A, Schult J, et al. Does sleep help prevent forgetting rewarded memory representations in children and adults? Front Psychol 2018; 9:9.
39. Möhring W, Urfer-Maurer N, Brand S, et al. The association between sleep and dual-task performance in preterm and full-term children: an exploratory study. Sleep Med 2019;55:100–8.
40. Quach J, Spencer-Smith M, Anderson PJ, et al. Can working memory training improve children's sleep? Sleep Med 2018;47:113–6.
41. Cohen-Zion M, Shiloh E. Evening chronotype and sleepiness predict impairment in executive abilities and academic performance of adolescents. Chronobiol Int 2018;35(1):137–45.
42. Arrona-Palacios A, Diaz-Morales JF. Morningness-eveningness is not associated with academic performance in the afternoon school shift: preliminary findings. Br J Educ Psychol 2018;88(3):480–98.
43. Gais S, Lucas B, Born J. Sleep after learning aids memory recall. Learn Mem 2006;13(3):259–62.
44. El-Sheikh M, Philbrook LE, Kelly RJ, et al. What does a good night's sleep mean? Nonlinear relations between sleep and children's cognitive functioning and mental health. Sleep 2019;42(6):zsz078.
45. Nieto M, Ricarte JJ, Griffith JW, et al. Sleep and cognitive development in preschoolers: stress and autobiographical performance associations. J Appl Dev Psychol 2019;63:16–22.
46. Hoyniak CP, Bates JE, Staples AD, et al. Child sleep and socioeconomic context in the development of cognitive abilities in early childhood. Child Development 2019;90(5):1718–37.
47. Smith SS, Edmed SL, Staton SL, et al. Correlates of naptime behaviors in preschool aged children. Nat Sci Sleep 2019;11:27–34.
48. Wetter SE, Fuhs M, Goodnight JA. Examining sleep as a protective mechanism for executive functioning in children from low-income homes. Early Child Dev Care 2019;189:1–12.
49. Estevan I, Silva A, Tassino B. School start times matter, eveningness does not. Chronobiol Int 2018;35(12):1753–7.
50. Bennet L, Walker DW, Horne RSC. Waking up too early – the consequences of preterm birth on sleep development. J Physiol 2018;596(23):5687–708.
51. Spruyt K, Gozal D. Sleep disturbances in children with attention-deficit/hyperactivity disorder. Expert Rev Neurother 2011;11(4):565–77.
52. Galland B, Spruyt K, Dawes P, et al. Sleep disordered breathing and academic performance: a meta-analysis. Pediatrics 2015;136(4):e934–46.
53. Reynolds CM, Short MA, Gradisar M. Sleep spindles and cognitive performance across adolescence: a meta-analytic review. J Adolesc 2018;66:55–70.
54. Lowe CJ, Safati A, Hall PA. The neurocognitive consequences of sleep restriction: a meta-analytic review. Neurosci biobehavioral Rev 2017;80:586–604.

55. de Bruin EJ, van Run C, Staaks J, et al. Effects of sleep manipulation on cognitive functioning of adolescents: a systematic review. Sleep Med Rev 2017;32:45–57.

56. Short MA, Blunden S, Rigney G, et al. Cognition and objectively measured sleep duration in children: a systematic review and meta-analysis. Sleep health 2018; 4(3):292–300.

57. Dutil C, Walsh JJ, Featherstone RB, et al. Influence of sleep on developing brain functions and structures in children and adolescents: a systematic review. Sleep Med Rev 2018;42:184–201.

58. Stickgold R, Walker MP. Sleep-dependent memory consolidation and reconsolidation. Sleep Med 2007;8(4):331–43.

59. Sorrells SF, Paredes MF, Cebrian-Silla A, et al. Human hippocampal neurogenesis drops sharply in children to undetectable levels in adults. Nature 2018;555(7696): 377–81.

60. Tonetti L, Natale V, Randler C. Association between circadian preference and academic achievement: a systematic review and meta-analysis. Chronobiol Int 2015;32(6):792–801.

61. Bestmann A, Conzelmann A, Baving L, et al. Associations between cognitive performance and sigma power during sleep in children with attention-deficit/hyperactivity disorder, healthy children, and healthy adults. PloS one 2019; 14(10):e0224166.

62. Cusick CN, Isaacson PA, Langberg JM, et al. Last night's sleep in relation to academic achievement and neurocognitive testing performance in adolescents with and without ADHD. Sleep Med 2018;52:75–9.

63. Page JM. Characterizing early development and NREM sleep in infants and toddlers and risk for autism spectrum disorder [D.E.]. The University of North Carolina at Chapel Hill; 2019.

64. Spruyt K, Gozal D. A mediation model linking body weight, cognition, and sleep-disordered breathing. Am J Respir Crit Care Med 2012;185(2):199–205.

65. McCann M, Bayliss DM, Anderson M, et al. The relationship between sleep problems and working memory in children born very preterm. Child Neuropsychol 2018;24(1):124–44.

66. Sanchez E, El-Khatib H, Arbour C, et al. Brain white matter damage and its association with neuronal synchrony during sleep. Brain 2019;142(3):674–87.

67. Stickgold R, Walker MP. Sleep-dependent memory triage: evolving generalization through selective processing. Nat Neurosci 2013;16(2):139–45.

68. Smithson L, Baird T, Tamana SK, et al. Shorter sleep duration is associated with reduced cognitive development at two years of age. Sleep Med 2018;48:131–9.

69. Sun W, Li SX, Jiang Y, et al. A community-based study of sleep and cognitive development in infants and toddlers. J Clin Sleep Med 2018;14(6):977–84.

70. Schlieber M, Han J. The sleeping patterns of head start children and the influence on developmental outcomes. Child Care Health Dev 2018;44(3):462–9.

71. Xing S, Li Q, Gao X, et al. Differential influence of sleep time parameters on preschoolers' executive function. Acta Psychologica Sinica 2018;50(11):1269–81.

72. Blunden S, Magee C, Attard K, et al. Sleep schedules and school performance in Indigenous Australian children. Sleep health 2018;4(2):135–40.

73. Zinke K, Noack H, Born J. Sleep augments training-induced improvement in working memory in children and adults. Neurobiol Learn Mem 2018;147:46–53.

74. Tashjian SM, Goldenberg D, Monti MM, et al. Sleep quality and adolescent default mode network connectivity. Soc Cogn Affect Neurosci 2018;13(3):290–9.

75. Fuligni AJ, Arruda EH, Krull JL, et al. Adolescent sleep duration, variability, and peak levels of achievement and mental health. Child Development 2018;89(2): e18–28.
76. Cousins JN, Sasmita K, Chee MWL. Memory encoding is impaired after multiple nights of partial sleep restriction. J Sleep Res 2018;27(1):138–45.
77. Pisch M, Wiesemann F, Karmiloff-Smith A. Infant wake after sleep onset serves as a marker for different trajectories in cognitive development. J Child Psychol Psychiatry 2019;60(2):189–98.
78. Franco P, Guyon A, Stagnara C, et al. Early polysomnographic characteristics associated with neurocognitive development at 36 months of age. Sleep Med 2019;60:13–9.
79. Adelantado-Renau M, Diez-Fernandez A, Beltran-Valls MR, et al. The effect of sleep quality on academic performance is mediated by Internet use time: DA-DOS study. J Pediatr (Rio J) 2019;95(4):410–8.
80. Stormark KM, Fosse HE, Pallesen S, et al. The association between sleep problems and academic performance in primary school-aged children: findings from a Norwegian longitudinal population-based study. PloS one 2019;14(11): e0224139.
81. Cheng W, Rolls E, Gong W, et al. Sleep duration, brain structure, and psychiatric and cognitive problems in children. Mol Psychiatry 2020. https://doi.org/10.1038/s41380-020-0663-2.
82. Preckel F, Fischbach A, Scherrer V, et al. Circadian preference as a typology: latent-class analysis of adolescents' morningness/eveningness, relation with sleep behavior, and with academic outcomes. Learn Individ Differ 2020;78.
83. Hahn M, Joechner AK, Roell J, et al. Developmental changes of sleep spindles and their impact on sleep-dependent memory consolidation and general cognitive abilities: a longitudinal approach. Dev Sci 2019;22(1):e12706.
84. Vermeulen MCM, Van der Heijden KB, Swaab H, et al. Sleep spindle characteristics and sleep architecture are associated with learning of executive functions in school-age children. J Sleep Res 2019;28(1):e12779.
85. Bothe K, Hirschauer F, Wiesinger H-P, et al. The impact of sleep on complex gross-motor adaptation in adolescents. J Sleep Res 2019;28(4):1–11.
86. Kuula L, Tamminen J, Makkonen T, et al. Higher sleep spindle activity is associated with fewer false memories in adolescent girls. Neurobiol Learn Mem 2019; 157:96–105.
87. Wilhelm I, Schreiner T, Beck J, et al. No effect of targeted memory reactivation during sleep on retention of vocabulary in adolescents. Sci Rep 2020;10(1):4255.

# Classification and Epidemiology of Sleep Disorders in Children and Adolescents

Irina Trosman, MD[a], Anna Ivanenko, MD, PhD[b],*

## KEYWORDS

- Sleep disorders • Classification • Prevalence • Children • Adolescents

## KEY POINTS

- Sleep disorders are included in several major classifications systems such as the *International Classification for Sleep Disorders*, 3rd Edition (ICSD-3), the *Diagnostic and Statistical Manual of Mental Disorders*, 5th Edition (DSM-5), and the *International Classification of Diseases*, 10th Edition, the Clinical Modification (ICD-10-CM).
- Sleep disorders are highly prevalent in children of all ages.
- Higher prevalence of sleep disorders is documented in pediatric patients with special medical, neurologic, and psychiatric conditions.
- Associations between sleep problems and depression, anxiety, and suicidality have been demonstrated.

Sleep disturbances are common in children and adolescents but still remain unrecognized and undertreated. There are several classification systems of sleep disorders available, some of which include recent attempts to develop more specific nosologic categories that reflect developmental aspects of sleep. The purpose of this review is to provide an overview of currently available classification systems of sleep disorders and their prevalence in pediatric patients.

## CLASSIFICATION SYSTEMS FOR SLEEP DISORDERS

The *International Classification for Sleep Disorders*, 3rd Edition (ICSD-3)[1] is a comprehensive classification system that includes several nosologic categories, such as

This article originally appeared in *Child and Adolescent Psychiatric Clinics*, Volume 30 Issue 1, January 2021.
[a] Division of Pulmonary and Sleep Medicine, Ann and Robert H. Lurie Children's Hospital of Chicago, 225 East Chicago Avenue Box 43, Chicago, IL 60611-2991, USA; [b] Division of Child and Adolescent Psychiatry, Ann and Robert H. Lurie Children's Hospital of Chicago, Chicago, IL, USA
* Corresponding author. 800 Biesterfield Road, Suite 510, Elk Grove Village, IL 60007.
*E-mail address:* a-ivanenko@northwestern.edu

insomnias, parasomnias, hypersomnias, sleep-related breathing disorders, circadian-rhythm disorders, sleep-related movement disorders, and other sleep disorders. Behavioral insomnia of childhood is a distinct subtype of insomnia to emphasize its pathophysiology in children. Other ICSD-3 insomnia subtypes include psychophysiologic, idiopathic, and paradoxical insomnias, and inadequate sleep hygiene.

There are several classification systems available for sleep disorders, including the International Classification for Sleep Disorders, 3rd Edition (ICSD-3), the Diagnostic and Statistical Manual of Mental Disorders-5 (DSM-5-TR), the International Classification of Diseases, 10th Edition, the Clinical Modification (ICD-10-CM), and the Diagnostic Classification, Zero to Three (DC: 0-5)[1–4]. The *Diagnostic and Statistical Manual of Mental Disorders*, 5th Edition (DSM-5)[2] is a multiaxial classification system that divides sleep-wake disorders into insomnia disorder, hypersomnolence disorder, narcolepsy, breathing-related sleep disorders, circadian-rhythm sleep-wake disorders, parasomnias, restless legs syndrome (RLS), rapid eye movement (REM) sleep behavior disorder, other specified and unspecified insomnia disorder, other specified and unspecified hypersomnolence disorder, and other specified and unspecified sleep-wake disorder. The DSM-5 no longer divides insomnia disorder into "primary insomnia" and "insomnia related to another mental/medical condition" but defines a single diagnostic entity with a specification for "coexisting with other mental or medical comorbidities and/or sleep disorders." Of note, DSM-5 fails to recognize sleep disorders seen in younger children, especially infants and toddlers.

The *Diagnostic Classification, Zero to Three* (DC:0–5)[4] is a less frequently used multiaxial classification system that categorizes behavioral and emotional disorders in infants and toddlers. Axis I sleep disorder is called "sleep behavior disorder" and can be paired with other axis I disorders (eg, regulatory disorder, adjustment disorder).

## EPIDEMIOLOGY OF SLEEP DISORDERS
### Insomnia Disorder

Pediatric insomnia is generally defined as "a repeated difficulty with sleep initiation, duration, consolidation, or quality that occurs despite age-appropriate time and opportunity for sleep and results in daytime functional impairment for the child and/or family."[5] It is common in young children, with both bedtime difficulties and frequent night waking reported in 20% to 30% of children younger than 3 years[6,7] and 25% to 50% of preschool-aged children.[7–10] One study reported nighttime awakenings in 23% of children at 1 year, 24% at 18 months, and 14% at 3 years.[11] According to parents' reports, 69% of children have problems falling and staying asleep a few times a week, and 51% of adolescents report difficulties initiating sleep at least once a week.[12,13]

According to the ICSD-3, behavioral insomnia is defined by sleep-onset association, limit setting, or combined types, and reflects maladaptive associations developed by the child or attributable to poor parental limit setting, which results in an inability to fall asleep in the absence of behavioral associations (eg, rocking, watching television, falling asleep in the parents' bed, holding a favorite stuffed animal). Most children suffering from behavioral insomnia also have difficulty returning to sleep after normal nocturnal awakenings, leading to sleep loss. Both sleep-onset association type and limit-setting type occur in 10% to 30% of children. Infants and toddlers are commonly at higher risk.[14] The problems tend to diminish as the children grow older, especially after age 4 years. Sleep complaints, such as bedtime resistance, refusal to sleep alone, increased nighttime fears, and nightmares, are also common in children who have experienced traumatic events, including physical and sexual abuse.[15]

Psychophysiologic insomnia is typically experienced by older children and adolescents. It is characterized by increased arousal and learned negative sleep associations that prevent sleep onset. Insomnia is the most prevalent sleep disorder in adolescence, with a 10.7% lifetime and a 9.4% current prevalence among 13- to 16-year-olds.[16] Up to 35% of adolescents report insomnia at least several times a month.[16–18] There is strong female prevalence that occurs after puberty.[16] Rates of adolescent insomnia in other studies range from 4% to 39%, with differences in prevalence rates related to the diagnostic criteria used, characteristics of the sample, and study design. Recently, a prevalence rate of 18.5% (23.6% in girls and 12.5% in boys) was reported for DSM-5 insomnia in older adolescents (16–18 years).[18]

Prevalence data for idiopathic insomnia, defined by long-standing sleep difficulties that arise in early childhood and persist over time, are limited, although it seems to be unrelated to specific life events, psychological trauma, or medical disorders during childhood.[1]

Growing evidence suggests that insomnia is a risk factor for the development of psychiatric conditions, particularly depression and anxiety later in life.[19,20] For example, sleep disturbances in depressed adolescents increase the risk of suicidal ideation and suicide attempts,[21] even after controlling for depression.[22]

### Hypersomnias of Central Origin

#### Narcolepsy

Narcolepsy is a rare disorder attributed to dysfunction of the hypocretin (orexin) brain system and characterized by sudden sleep attacks, hypnagogic hallucination, cataplexy, and sleep paralysis. Onset of narcolepsy typically occurs during adolescence, with rare cases of childhood onset. Genetic and environmental factors have been suggested as possible causes.[23] Narcolepsy is difficult to diagnose in younger children because of the inconsistency of cataplexy and other REM-related phenomena.

DSM-5 uses modifiers for narcolepsy that include narcolepsy without cataplexy, with cataplexy, and secondary to another medical condition.[2] ICSD-3 classifies narcolepsy as type 1 (NT1) and type 2 (NT2). NT1 is defined by excessive sleepiness and either cerebrospinal fluid (CSF) hypocretin (orexin) deficiency or the combination of cataplexy and specific polysomnographic (PSG)/multiple sleep latency test (MSLT) findings. MSLT mean sleep latency (MSLT-SL) should be 8 minutes or less with at least 2 sleep-onset REM periods (SOREMs) between PSG and MSLT recordings.[1] For a diagnosis of NT2, individuals must have an MSLT-SL less than 8 minutes and at least 2 SOREMs, but cannot have cataplexy, hypocretin deficiency, or other conditions that may explain the symptoms. It is estimated that about 1 in 2000 individuals of all ages are affected by narcolepsy. However, up to 50% of individuals may remain undiagnosed, and current prevalence is underestimated.[24]

**Narcolepsy with cataplexy.** Narcolepsy with cataplexy has a prevalence of 0.02% to 0.18% in the United States and western European nations and 0.16% to 0.18% in Japan. Males seem to be more commonly affected than females. Human leukocyte antigen (HLA) subtypes DR2/DRB1*1501 and DQB1*0602 are associated with the disorder in whites and Asians, while DQB1*0602 alone is associated with the disorder in African Americans. Some HLA subtypes are protective against narcolepsy in the presence of DQB1*0602, such as DQB*0501 and DQB1*0601, while DQB1*0301 increases susceptibility. A previous study in monozygotic twins showed a concordance rate of

29% for narcolepsy with cataplexy. Environmental triggers include head trauma, viral illness, an abrupt change in sleep-wake patterns, or sustained sleep deprivation. First-degree relatives of patients with narcolepsy with cataplexy have a 10- to 50-fold increased risk of developing the disorder.[23,25]

**Narcolepsy without cataplexy.** Narcolepsy without cataplexy is thought to represent about 15% to 36% of narcoleptic patients; however, the exact prevalence remains unknown.[1] Both males and females are affected at any age, although it seems to more commonly onset in adolescence. A small percentage of patients demonstrate CSF hypocretin deficiency. Possible environmental triggers include head trauma and viral illnesses. A recent review showed associations between central disorders of hypersomnolence and psychiatric symptoms, including anxiety, depression, and/or other emotionally based problems in children. Depression is particularly associated with hypersomnolence.[26,27]

### Kleine-Levin syndrome
Kleine-Levin syndrome (KLS) is a rare, ICSD-3 defined, relapsing-remitting disorder characterized by severe hypersomnolence episodes (median 10 days) associated with neurologic and neuropsychiatric symptoms, including confusion, slowness, amnesia, derealization, apathy, increased appetite, hypersexuality, anxiety, depressed mood, hallucinations, delusions, and behavioral problems.[28] KLS prevalence is estimated at around 1 to 2 cases per million, with a male-to-female ratio of 2:1 and frequent adolescent onset, although KLS cases have also been reported in younger children. An autoimmune basis was suggested because of an occasional association with HLA DQB1*02.[29] Environmental factors, such as infections, alcohol consumption, head trauma, or exposure to anesthetics, may be possible triggers.

### Hypersomnolence disorder
DSM-5 defines hypersomnolence disorder as "self-reported excessive sleepiness despite a main sleep period lasting at least 7 hours," with either recurrent periods of sleep, prolonged main sleep episode of more than 9 hours per day, or difficulty being fully awake after abrupt awakening, occurring at least three times per week for at least 3 months.[2] ICSD-3 defines idiopathic hypersomnia as "daily periods of irrepressible need to sleep or daily lapses into sleep occurring for at least 3 months".[1] Cataplexy and hypocretin deficiency must be absent. Objective confirmation includes an MSLT sleep latency ≤8 minutes but without at least 2 SOREMs, and/or at least 660 minutes (11 hours) of sleep time measured over 24 hours of PSG or wrist actigraphy and sleep logs, averaged over at least 1 week of unrestricted sleep. Children are rarely affected. It generally occurs before age 25 years and has an equal male-to-female ratio. There may be an increased predisposition to hypersomnia in psychiatric disorders, which might be genetic in nature. An autosomal dominant mode of inheritance has been suggested.

### Childhood Obstructive Sleep-Disordered Breathing

Childhood obstructive sleep-disordered breathing is a spectrum of disorders that includes primary snoring (PS), upper airway resistance syndrome, obstructive sleep apnea syndrome (OSAS), and obesity hypoventilation syndrome. Children with OSAS experience partial or complete obstruction of the upper airways during sleep, which may result in arousals and/or awakenings. OSAS, especially when associated with hypoxia and obstructive hypoventilation, is considered an extreme of the "sleep-disordered breathing" (SDB) spectrum.

### Primary snoring or habitual snoring

PS or habitual snoring is not associated with apnea, hypopnea, gas-exchange abnormalities, or architectural sleep disruption as detected by PSG.[30] Historically, PS has been considered a benign condition[31]; however, growing evidence suggests that children with PS may develop neurocognitive and behavioral problems similar to children with OSAS.[32–36] Most commonly, habitual snoring is defined as snoring more than 3 times per week. PS prevalence rates have been reported to be between 10% and 15%. However, some studies have reported prevalence as high as 35%[37,38] or as low as 3%.[39] This variation may be attributed to use of different PS definitions, reliance on parental and self-reports, individual or cultural differences in perceptions of snoring, cosleeping practices, and differences in definitions of snoring frequency and "habitual snoring."[40–46]

### Obstructive sleep apnea syndrome

OSAS affects about 2% to 3.5% of children. The first peak occurs in children from 2 to 8 years of age, with the presence of enlarged adenoid and/or tonsils. A second peak arises during adolescence in relation to weight gain. However, description of pediatric OSAS epidemiology is complicated by variances in methodology used to diagnose OSAS, child's age, progression of illness, and presence of medical and neurologic morbidities. As a result, pediatric OSAS studies are methodologically heterogeneous and inconsistent.[37,43,47–52]

Common risk factors for pediatric OSAS include Black race, obesity,[53] adenotonsillar hypertrophy, sinus problems, allergies, asthma,[50] family history of OSAS,[54] prematurity, craniofacial abnormalities, low muscle tone, and neurologic disorders impairing respiratory control (ie, meningomyelocele, Chiari malformation). Black children have a 4- to 6-fold higher risk than white children, independent of factors such as obesity, premature birth, and maternal smoking.[43,55] Asian children have more severe OSAS than white children, although the overall OSAS prevalence in Asian children is relatively low.[51] Differences in craniofacial features between Asians and whites are thought to explain these findings.[56,57] In general, soft-tissue factors may be more relevant to predicting risk in African Americans while skeletal features are more predictive in Asians.[58,59]

Obesity is one of the strongest risk factors for OSAS. The pediatric OSAS profile has changed over the last 2 decades. Earlier studies reported more frequent OSAS association with growth failure (GF).[60] In the mid-2000s, the relationship between weight and OSAS shifted along with the increase in pediatric obesity in the United States.[61,62] This change in dynamics is exemplified by a study showing that less than 15% of all symptomatic habitually snoring children were obese in the early 1990s compared with more than 50% of children in the early 2000s.[63] Subsequently, there has been a shift from the classic presentation of children with OSAS, from children with adenotonsillar hypertrophy (ATH) and GF to children with obesity with or without ATH. This epidemiologic change triggered an intense interest in exploring the relationship between OSA and weight gain, and OSAS and obesity in particular.[64]

## Circadian-Rhythm Sleep Disorders

### Delayed sleep-wake phase disorder

Delayed sleep-wake phase disorder (DSWPD)[1] is thought to be the most common circadian-rhythm sleep-wake disorder. The exact prevalence of DSWPD remains unknown. Comparison across studies is complicated by use of inconsistent diagnostic criteria and lack of objective assessments. For instance, according to DSM-5 DSP criteria, the use of sleep diaries or actigraphy is required for diagnosis. However, earlier epidemiologic studies based their estimates on assessments with screening questionnaires, sleep diaries, and clinical interviews and did not include actigraphy.[65,66] In addition, prevalence studies are unable to differentiate between "circadian" and "noncircadian" DSWPD.[67] One clinic-based study of DSWPD patients found that only 57% had a true phase delay (as measured by salivary dim light melatonin onset [DLMO] occurring after desired bedtime), and as such were designated true "circadian" DSWPD. The remaining 43% of the sample had DLMO occurring before desired bedtime and were designated "noncircadian" DSWPD.[68]

DSWPD is common in adolescents, with a reported prevalence of from 0.13% to 8%[69–72] and significant overlap with insomnia.[72] One study reported higher prevalence of DSWPD in girls than boys (3.7% vs 2.7%), whereas others demonstrated higher male-to-female ratios.[73] It is unclear whether prevalence differs as a function of geographic location or socioeconomic factors. For instance, differences in school start times (later in western Europe than in the United States) may explain reported regional prevalence variability. DSWPD has been associated with mental health problems,[74] including depression,[75–77] attention deficit-hyperactivity disorder (ADHD),[78] and autism spectrum disorder (ASD).[79]

### Advanced sleep-wake phase disorder

Advanced sleep-wake phase disorder (ASWPD) is a marked phase advance of the sleep-wake cycle accompanied by a sleep-related complaint. The prevalence of ASWPD is unknown. However, one study reported an ASWPD prevalence of 0.04% for individuals presenting with advanced sleep phase before age 30 years.[80] Familial cases have been identified with the possibility of an autosomal dominant mode of inheritance.[80]

### Non–24-hour sleep-wake rhythm disorder

Non–24-hour sleep-wake rhythm disorder (N24SWD) is characterized by an inability to entrain to the 24-hour environment. A diagnosis of N24SWD is made by monitoring an individual's sleep-wake pattern for a minimum of 14 days with sleep logs and/or actigraphy.[1] N24SWD can occur in both blind[81] and sighted individuals[82,83]; however, it is more common in blind individuals (about 50%), including children with congenital blindness. In a case series[82] of sighted individuals, the majority began to exhibit symptoms in their teens or 20s, and 28% had a premorbid psychiatric disorder. An additional 25% developed depression symptoms after N24SWD onset.

### Sleep-Related Movement Disorders

### Restless legs syndrome and periodic limb movement disorder

RLS is a common sensorimotor disorder occurring at a prevalence of 4% to 10% in adults,[84] approximately 25% to 40% of whom report symptom onset before age 20 years.[85] Despite increasing recognition of RLS in children, there is a paucity of epidemiologic data regarding RLS prevalence in this age group. Diagnostic criteria for pediatric RLS were first created in 2003[84] and have been modified over the years, making it challenging to compare epidemiologic data published over the last few decades. The ICSD-3, DSM-5, and International RLS Study Group (IRLSSG) each list separate diagnostic criteria for RLS. An updated version of pediatric RLS diagnostic criteria was published by the IRLSSG in 2013 to improve clinical practice and facilitate research.[86]

Earlier studies reported RLS prevalence as high as 17% in children in general pediatric clinics and 5.9% in children referred to sleep clinics.[87,88] The largest-ever study assessing RLS in children found a prevalence of 1.9% in 8- to 11-year-olds and 2% in 12- to 17-year olds, with no differences among boys and girls.[89] More recent epidemiologic studies demonstrated similar findings, with pediatric RLS prevalence of 2% to 4%.[90,91]

Among youth, RLS is more frequent in those with ADHD,[88] periodic limb movements (PLMS),[92,93] growing pains,[94] and renal insufficiency.[95] Comorbid psychiatric conditions including mood disorders, ADHD, anxiety, and behavioral disturbances were found in two-thirds of children younger than age 18 years with RLS.[96] RLS prevalence among children with ADHD has been reported at 10.5% to 44%.[97,98] Increased parasomnia incidence has been reported in children with RLS caused by possible PLM sleep disruption and sleep deprivation.[99] RLS appears to follow a familial pattern of inheritance, with up to 50% of patients with RLS reporting a familial association.[89,100,101] An autosomal dominant mode of inheritance has also been observed in some families.[102]

PLMS are characterized by the presence of repetitive stereotyped limb movements during sleep, generally involving extension of the big toe and dorsiflexion of the ankle, with the PLMS index of >5 per hour as detected by PSG. About 80% of the patients diagnosed with RLS also have periodic limb movement disorder (PLMD).[85] PLMS are considered a supportive diagnostic criterion for RLS. PLMS occur in a variety of sleep disorders, including RLS, narcolepsy, OSAS, and REM sleep behavior disorder, and may be induced by certain medications. PLMD diagnosis requires PSG-documented PLMS and exclusion of SDB.[86] Pediatric studies have revealed a 5% to 25% prevalence rate of PLMS in children referred for sleep studies.[103–106] One of the biggest studies found a PLMD prevalence of 14% and no age or gender differences. However, PLMD was more common in white than in Black children (49% vs 26%).[103]

PLMD may precede the onset of sensory symptoms required for diagnosing RLS in children.[93] PLMS are also associated with insomnia and sleep-related eating disorder, the latter of which is responsive to dopaminergic therapy.

### Parasomnias

Parasomnias are common during childhood[107] and include undesirable physical events (complex movements, behaviors) or experiences (emotions, perceptions, dreams) occurring during entry into sleep, within sleep, or during arousals from sleep.[1] Parasomnia is further divided into REM parasomnia (sleep paralysis, nightmare disorder, REM sleep without atonia, REM behavioral disorder) and non-REM parasomnia (confusional arousals, sleep enuresis, exploding head syndrome, sleep-related hallucinations, night terrors, sleep talking, and sleepwalking).

### Non-REM parasomnia

In a large prospective study conducted among children ages 2.5 to 6 years, 88% manifested at least one parasomnia,[108] including sleep terrors (40%), sleepwalking (15%), nocturnal enuresis (25%), nocturnal bruxism (46%), and rhythmic movement disorder (9%). Similar findings and a high resolution of parasomnia within a 5-year period have also been reported.[109] Most studies base parasomnia incidence on parental recall.[108]

Childhood parasomnias are primarily due to genetic and developmental factors.[110] Approximately 50% of school-aged children have a sleep-talking episode at least once a year, whereas less than 10% experience sleep talking every night.[111] Another study showed sleepwalking prevalence to be 16.7% in children aged 12 years.[112] Nocturnal enuresis occurs in ~30% of 4-year-olds, 10% of 6-year-olds, 5% of 10-year-olds, and 3% of 12-year-olds.[113–116] A recent study found a 12-month prevalence of enuresis of 4.45% among United States children, along with a strong association with ADHD.[117] A large survey reported a childhood history of nocturnal bruxism in 15.1% of university students.[118] Bruxism prevalence progressively decreases from childhood through preadolescence.[119]

### REM parasomnia

**Nightmares.** Nightmares are common in children, with the highest prevalence rates between ages 5 and 10 years.[119–123] Nightmares are strongly associated with sleep-walking and sleep-talking as well as a family history of sleepwalking.[119] Between 70% and 90% of young adults reported that they experienced childhood nightmares.[124] Chronic nightmares and psychopathology, such as anxiety and stress, are closely correlated.[123,125] Nightmares and sleep disturbances were also found to be more common in children with emotional problems (eg, separation anxiety, severe traumatic experience).[126–128] However, some studies did not find this relationship.[129–131] Post-trauma nightmares may occur during both REM and non-REM sleep.[132] One study found that 18.8% of adults with post-traumatic stress disorder reported nightmares as opposed to 4.2% of healthy adults.[133] Pediatric studies have documented similar, if not higher, rates of nightmares in children with a trauma history (50%-80%).[134,135]

**REM behavior disorder.** In childhood, cases of REM behavior disorder (RBD) are associated with structural brainstem lesions including neoplasms, juvenile Parkinson disease, Chiari type 1 malformation in combination with SDB, autism, narcolepsy, Tourette syndrome, use of antidepressant medications, and Smith-Magenis syndrome.[136–147] Pediatric RBD literature is sparse and composed of single case reports or small case series; thus, the incidence is unknown. RBD semiology does have some resemblance to nightmares because the child experiences a terrifying dream. Therefore, some reported childhood nightmares may be unrecognized RBD.

## PREVALENCE OF SLEEP DISTURBANCES IN CHILDREN WITH PSYCHIATRIC DISORDERS

Sleep disorders are far more frequently reported among children and adolescents with coexisting psychiatric morbidities. Only a handful of studies, however address the prevalence of sleep problems in psychiatric cohorts of children. In one of the earlier studies, sleep complaints in children evaluated at a mental health clinic were compared to sleep symptoms reported by parents of children from the general population.[148] This study found a significantly greater prevalence of nightmares and restless sleep in children with anxiety and depression, as well as a significantly higher prevalence of snoring, head banging, and nocturnal awakenings and restlessness among children with ADHD. In a more recent surveys conducted among children attending a psychiatric clinic, sleep problems were more frequently reported in children with psychiatric disorders than in children without a psychiatric history and vise versa, children and adolescents evaluated at the specialty sleep clinic for insomnia exhibited high rate of psychiatric disorders and mental health symptoms.[149,150] Among those with psychiatric disorders, a high rate of nocturnal awakenings and nightmares was documented in children with ADHD and comorbid mood and anxiety disorders and in those with mood or anxiety disorders alone. Sleep duration and sleep latency strongly correlated with aggression, hyperactivity and depression, while restless sleep highly correlated with all psychiatric symptoms.

There have been growing numbers of studies indicating a high prevalence of insomnias, parasomnias and disorders of excessive daytime sleepiness in children with ADHD, mood and anxiety disorders, and autism spectrum disorders. For example, sleep complaints have been reported by 25-50% of parents of children with ADHD.[151,152] Symptoms like bedtime resistance, delayed sleep onset, and frequent night time awakenings have been most frequently reported in patients with ADHD. Other intrinsic sleep disorders have also been associated with ADHD.[153] Sleep disordered breathing has been reported in patients with ADHD and appears to be implicated in the pathophysiology of neurocognitive and behavioral deficits seen in affected children. Recent meta-analysis suggested that ADHD symptoms are related to SDB and improve after adenotonsillectomy.[154]

Sleep disruptions are highly prevent among children and adolescents with anxiety disorders. Some clinician and parent reports found that about 85% of children and adolescents with anxiety disorders have transient sleep problems, and up to 50% have chronic sleep disturbance.[155] Recent studies demonstrated frequent problems with sleep initiation, nighttime awakenings, nightmares, and bedtime resistance among youth with anxiety disorders.[155–157]

Significant life events where children feel a loss of control (eg, divorce, separation, and relocation) may cause them to react in the form of night terrors.[158] Some studies have suggested that parasomnias, especially enuresis, are associated with socioeconomic factors, such as low social class, low parental education, and family disruption.[113,159] Children with Autism Spectrum Disorders (ASD) have a high prevalence rate of sleep problems. It has been reported that 44 – 83% of children with ASD have sleep initiation and maintenance difficulties and suffer from irregular sleep-wake patterns, early morning awakenings, and poor sleep routines.[160,161]

Early onset depression has been associated with symptoms of sleep initiation and maintenance insomnia and early morning awakenings. Earlier study of depressed children and adolescents revealed that 72.7% had sleep disturbance, 53.5% had insomnia alone, 9% had hypersomnia, and 10.1% had both insomnia and hypersomnia. Children with more severe depression had more disturbed sleep with the most severely affected ones having both insomnia and hypersomnia.[162] More recent survey conducted among adolescents demonstrated association between sleep problems and suicidality[163] with a strong association between sleep problems and suicide attempts in adolescents already engaging in non-suicidal self-injury.[164] This further emphasizes the importance of sleep evaluation in adolescents with depression.

## SUMMARY

Several classification systems of sleep disorders are currently available for use with pediatric populations. Sleep disorders are highly prevalent in children and adolescents and significantly affect their neurocognitive, emotional, and behavioral development. Children with medical, neurodevelopmental, and psychiatric disorders have a significantly higher rate of sleep-related problems that can persist over time if not properly treated. Thus, it is critical for mental health professionals to assess and address sleep problems in the context of psychiatric comorbidities.

## CLINICS CARE POINTS

- Apply ICSD-3 or DSM-5 classification systems for diagnosing older children and adolescents and DC:0–5 to diagnose infants and toddlers.

- Given the high prevalence rates of sleep disorders among children and adolescents with medical, neurodevelopmental, and psychiatric disorders, routinely assess for sleep problems in youth presenting with these concerns.

- Early identification and treatment of disrupted sleep improves daytime functioning, academic performance, and behavioral and emotional regulation.

## DISCLOSURE

The authors have nothing to disclose.

## REFERENCES

1. American Academy of Sleep Medicine. International classification of sleep disorders. 3rd edition. Westchester (IL): American Academy of Sleep Medicine; 2014.
2. American Psychiatric Association. Diagnostic and statistical manual of mental disorders. 4th edition. Washington, DC: American Psychiatric Association; 2013. text revision.
3. International classification of diseases, tenth revision, clinical modification (ICD-10-CM). Available at: http://www.cms.hhs.gov/ICD10/02m_2009_ICD_10_CM. asp#TopOfPage. Accessed September 27, 2020.
4. Zero to Three. DC:0–5: diagnostic classification of mental health and developmental disorders of infancy and early childhood. Arlington (VA): Zero to Three; 2016.
5. Mindell JA, Emslie G, Blumer J, et al. Pharmacological management of insomnia in children and adolescents: consensus statement. Pediatrics 2006;117(6): e1223–32.
6. Mindell JA, Kuhn B, Lewin DS, et al. Behavioral treatment of bedtime problems and night wakings in infants and young children. Sleep 2006;29(10):1263–76.
7. Sadeh A, Mindell JA, Luedtke K, et al. Sleep and sleep ecology in the first 3 years: a web-based study. J Sleep Res 2009;18(1):60–73.
8. Meltzer LJ, Mindell JA. Sleep and sleep disorders in children and adolescents. Psychiatr Clin North Am 2006;29:1059–76.
9. Owens J. Classification and epidemiology of childhood sleep disorders. Sleep Med Clin 2007;2(3):353–61.
10. Gaylor EE, Burnham MM, Goodlin-Jones BL, et al. A longitudinal follow-up study of young children's sleep patterns using a developmental classification system. Behav Sleep Med 2005;3(1):44–61.
11. Jenkins S, Bax MCO, Hart H. Behavior problems in preschool children. J Child Psychol Psychiatry 1980;21:5–17.
12. National Sleep Foundation. Children and sleep. Sleep in America poll. Washington (DC): SleepFoundation.org; 2004. Available at: http://www.sleepfoundation.org.
13. National Sleep Foundation. Adolescents and sleep. Sleep in America poll. Washington (DC): SleepFoundation.org; 2006. Available at: http://www. sleepfoundation.org.
14. Owens JA, Moore M. Insomnia in infants and young children. Pediatr Ann 2017; 46(9):e321–6.
15. Sadeh A. Sleep, trauma, and sleep in children. Child Adolesc Psychiatr Clin N Am 1996;5(3):685–700.
16. Johnson E, Roth T, Schultz L, et al. Epidemiology of DSM-IV insomnia in adolescence: lifetime prevalence, chronicity, and an emergent gender difference. Pediatrics 2006;117(2):e247–56.

17. Roberts RE, Roberts CR, Duong HT. Chronic insomnia and its negative consequences for health and functioning of adolescents: a 12-month prospective study. J Adolesc Health 2008;42(3):294–302.

18. Hysing M, Pallesen S, Stormark K, et al. Sleep patterns and insomnia among adolescents: a population-based study. J Sleep Res 2013;22(5):549–56.

19. Roane BM, Taylor DJ. Adolescent insomnia as a risk factor for early adult depression and substance abuse. Sleep 2008;31(10):1351–6.

20. Alvaro P, Roberts R, Harris J, et al. The direction of the relationship between symptoms of insomnia and psychiatric disorders in adolescents. J Affect Disord 2016;207:167–74.

21. Wong MM, Brower KJ, Craun EA. Insomnia symptoms and suicidality in the national comorbidity survey—adolescent supplement. J Psychiatr Res 2016; 81:1–8.

22. Wong MM, Brower KJ. The prospective relationship between sleep problems and suicidal behavior in the National Longitudinal Study of Adolescent Health. J Psychiatr Res 2012;46(7):953–9.

23. Guilleminault C, Zvonkina V, Tantrakul V, et al. Advances in narcolepsy syndrome and challenges in the pediatric population. Sleep Med Clin 2007;2(3): 397–404.

24. Dye TJ, Gurbani N, Simakajornboon N. Epidemiology and pathophysiology of childhood narcolepsy. Paediatr Respir Rev 2018;25:14–8.

25. Kotagal S. Narcolepsy and idiopathic hypersomnia in childhood. In: Ivanenko A, editor. Sleep and psychiatric disorders in children and adolescents. New York: London Informa Healthcare; 2008. p. 163–73.

26. Maski K, Steinhart E, Williams D, et al. Listening to the patient voice in narcolepsy: diagnostic delay, disease burden, and treatment efficacy. J Clin Sleep Med 2017;13(3):419–25.

27. Ludwig B, Smith S, Heussler H. Associations between neuropsychological, neurobehavioral and emotional functioning and either narcolepsy or idiopathic hypersomnia in children and adolescents. J Clin Sleep Med 2018;14(4):661–74.

28. Arnulf I, Groos E, Dodet P. Kleine-Levin syndrome: a neuropsychiatric disorder. Rev Neurol (Paris) 2018;174(4):216–27.

29. Dauvilliers Y, Mayer G, Lecendreux M, et al. Kleine-Levin syndrome: an autoimmune hypothesis based on clinical and genetic analyses. Neurology 2002; 59(11):1739–45.

30. Katz E, D'Ambrosio C. Pathophysiology of pediatric obstructive sleep apnea. Proc Am Thorac Soc 2008;5:253–62.

31. American Thoracic Society. Standards and indications for cardiopulmonary sleep studies in children. Am J Respir Crit Care Med 1996;153:866–78.

32. Blunden S, Lushington K, Kennedy D, et al. Behavior and neurocognitive performance in children aged 5-10 years who snore compared to controls. J Clin Exp Neuropsychol 2000;22:554–68.

33. Tripuraneni M, Paruthi S, Armbrecht ES, et al. Obstructive sleep apnea in children. Laryngoscope 2013;123:1289–93.

34. Beebe DW, Ris MD, Kramer ME, et al. The association between sleep disordered breathing, academic grades, and cognitive and behavioral functioning among overweight subjects during middle to late childhood. Sleep 2010;33: 1447–56.

35. Beebe D, Wells C, Jeffries J, et al. Neuropsychological effects of pediatric obstructive sleep apnea. J Int Neuropsychol Soc 2004;10:962–75.

36. Miano S, Paolino MC, Urbano A, et al. Neurocognitive assessment and sleep analysis in children with sleep-disordered breathing. Clin Neurophysiol 2011; 122:311–9.
37. Gislason T, Benediktsdottir B. Snoring, apneic episodes, and nocturnal hypoxemia among children 6 months to 6 years old. An epidemiologic study of lower limit of prevalence. Chest 1995;107:963–6.
38. Castronovo V, Zucconi M, Nosetti L, et al. Prevalence of habitual snoring and sleep-disordered breathing in preschool-aged children in an Italian community. J Pediatr 2003;142(4):377–82.
39. Spruyt K, O'Brien LM, Macmillan Coxon AP, et al. Multidimensional scaling of pediatric sleep breathing problem and bio-behavioral correlates. Sleep Med 2006;7(3):269–80.
40. Montgomery-Downs HE, Gozal D. Sleep habits and risk factors for sleep-disordered breathing in infants and young toddlers in Louisville, Kentucky. Sleep Med 2006;7:211–9.
41. Weissbluth M, Davis AT, Poncher J. Night waking in 4- to 8-month-old infants. J Pediatr 1984;104:477–80.
42. Ng DK, Kwok KL, Cheung JM, et al. Prevalence of sleep problems in Hong Kong primary school children: a community-based telephone survey. Chest 2005;128: 1315–23.
43. Rosen CL, Larkin EK, Kirchner HL, et al. Prevalence and risk factors for sleep-disordered breathing in 8- to 11-year-old children: association with race and prematurity. J Pediatr 2003;142:383–9.
44. Smedje H, Broman JE, Hetta J. Parents' reports of disturbed sleep in 5-7-year-old Swedish children. Acta Paediatr 1999;88:858–65.
45. Kaditis A, Finder J, Alexopoulos E, et al. Sleep-disordered breathing in 3,680 Greek children. Pediatr Pulmonol 2004;37:499–509.
46. Liu X, Ma Y, Wang Y, et al. Brief report: an epidemiologic survey of the prevalence of sleep disorders among children 2 to 12 years old in Beijing, China. Pediatrics 2005;115:266–8.
47. Schlaud M, Urschitz MS, Urschitz-Duprat PM, et al. The German study on sleep-disordered breathing in primary school children: epidemiological approach, representativeness of study sample, and preliminary screening results. Paediatr Perinat Epidemiol 2004;18:431–40.
48. Shine NP, Coates HL, Lannigan FJ. Obstructive sleep apnea, morbid obesity, and adenotonsillar surgery: a review of the literature. Int J Pediatr Otorhinolaryngol 2005;69:1475–82.
49. Ali NJ, Pitson DJ, Stradling JR. Snoring, sleep disturbance, and behavior in 4-5 year olds. Arch Dis Child 1993;68(3):360–6.
50. Redline S, Tishler PV, Schluchter M, et al. Risk factors for sleep-disordered breathing in children: associations with obesity, race, and respiratory problems. Am J Respir Crit Care Med 1999;159(5 Pt 1):1527–32.
51. Anuntaseree W, Rookkapan K, Kuasirikul S, et al. Snoring and obstructive sleep apnea in Thai school-age children: prevalence and predisposing factors. Pediatr Pulmonol 2001;32(3):222–7.
52. Brunetti L, Rana S, Lospalluti ML, et al. Prevalence of obstructive sleep apnea syndrome in a cohort of 1,207 children of southern Italy. Chest 2001;120(6): 1930–5.
53. Young T, Peppard PE, Taheri S. Excess weight and sleep-disordered breathing. J Appl Physiol (1985) 2005;99(4):1592–9.

54. Palmer LJ, Buxbaum SG, Larkin E, et al. A whole-genome scan for obstructive sleep apnea and obesity. Am J Hum Genet 2003;72:340–50.
55. Ruiter ME, DeCoster J, Jacobs L, et al. Sleep disorders in African Americans and Caucasian Americans: a meta-analysis. Behav Sleep Med 2010;8:246–59.
56. Ong KC, Clerk AA. Comparison of the severity of sleep-disordered breathing in Asian and Caucasian patients seen at a sleep disorders center. Respir Med 1998;92(6):843–8.
57. Lee RW, Vasudavan S, Hui DS, et al. Differences in craniofacial structures and obesity in Caucasian and Chinese patients with obstructive sleep apnea. Sleep 2010;33:1075–80.
58. Sutherland K, Lee RW, Cistulli PA. Obesity and craniofacial structure as risk factors for obstructive sleep apnoea: impact of ethnicity. Respirology 2012;17: 213–22.
59. Schwab RJ, Pasirstein M, Pierson R, et al. Identification of upper airway anatomic risk factors for obstructive sleep apnea with volumetric magnetic resonance imaging. Am J Respir Crit Care Med 2003;168:522–30.
60. Leach J, Olson J, Hermann J. Polysomnographic and clinical findings in children with obstructive sleep apnea. Arch Otolaryngol Head Neck Surg 1992; 118:741–4.
61. Keefe R, Rachi NP, Live R. The shifting relationship between weight and pediatric obstructive sleep apnea: a historical review. Laryngoscope 2018;00:1–6.
62. Whitaker R, Pepe M, Wright J, et al. Early adiposity rebound and the risk of adult obesity. Pediatrics 1998;101(3):E5.
63. Gozal D, Simakajornboon N, Holbrook CR, et al. Secular trends in obesity and parentally reported daytime sleepiness among children referred to a pediatric sleep center for snoring and suspected sleep-disordered breathing (SDB). Sleep 2006;29:A74.
64. Dayyat E, Kheirandish-Gozal L, Gozal D. Childhood obstructive sleep apnea: one or two distinct disease entities? Sleep Med Clin 2007;2:433–44.
65. Schrader H, Bovim G, Sand T. The prevalence of delayed and advanced sleep phase syndromes. J Sleep Res 1993;2:51–5.
66. Yazaki M, Shirakawa S, Okawa M, et al. Demography of sleep disturbances associated with circadian rhythm disorders in Japan. Psychiatry Clin Neurosci 1999;53:267–8.
67. Nesbitt A. Delayed sleep-wake phase disorder. J Thorac Dis 2018;10(Suppl 1): S103–11.
68. Murray JM, Sletten TL, Magee M, et al. Prevalence of circadian misalignment and its association with depressive symptoms in delayed sleep phase disorder. Sleep 2017;40(1):10.
69. Wyatt JK. Circadian rhythms sleep disorders in children and adolescents. Sleep Med Clin 2007;2:387–96.
70. Ohayon MM. Epidemiology of restless legs syndrome: a synthesis of the literature. Sleep Med Rev 2012;16(4):283–95.
71. Saxvig IW, Pallesen S, Wilhelmsen-Langeland A, et al. Prevalence and correlates of delayed sleep phase in high school students. Sleep Med 2012;13(2): 193–9.
72. Sivertsen B, Pallesen S, Stormark KM, et al. Delayed sleep phase syndrome in adolescents: prevalence and correlates in a large population based study. BMC Public Health 2013;13:1163.
73. Thorpy MJ, Korman E, Spielman AJ, et al. Delayed sleep phase syndrome in adolescents. J Adolesc Health Care 1988;9:22–7.

74. Reid KJ, Jaksa AA, Eisengart JB, et al. Systematic evaluation of Axis-I DSM diagnoses in delayed sleep phase disorder and evening-type circadian preference. Sleep Med 2012;13:1171.

75. Glozier N, O'Dea B, McGorry PD, et al. Delayed sleep onset in depressed young people. BMC Psychiatry 2014;14:33.

76. Schubert JR, Coles ME. Obsessive-compulsive symptoms and characteristics in individuals with delayed sleep phase disorder. J Nerv Ment Dis 2013;201: 877–84.

77. Nota JA, Sharkey KM, Coles ME. Sleep, arousal, and circadian rhythms in adults with obsessive-compulsive disorder: a meta-analysis. Neurosci Biobehav Rev 2015;51:100–7.

78. Kooij JJ, Bijlenga D. The circadian rhythm in adult attention-deficit/hyperactivity disorder: current state of affairs. Expert Rev Neurother 2013;13:1107–16.

79. Kotagal S, Broomall E. Sleep in children with autism spectrum disorder. Pediatr Neurol 2012;47:242–51.

80. Curtis BJ, Ashbrook LH, Young T, et al. Extreme morning chronotypes are often familial and not exceedingly rare: the estimated prevalence of advanced sleep phase, familial advanced sleep phase, and advanced sleep-wake phase disorder in a sleep clinic population. Sleep 2019;42(10):zsz148.

81. Flynn-Evans EE, Tabandeh H, Skene DJ, et al. Circadian rhythm disorders and melatonin production in 127 blind women with and without light perception. J Biol Rhythms 2014;29:215–24.

82. Hayakawa T, Uchiyama M, Kamei Y, et al. Clinical analyses of sighted patients with non-24-hour sleep-wake syndrome: a study of 57 consecutively diagnosed cases. Sleep 2005;28:945–52.

83. Endara-Bravo AS, Thammasitboon S, Thomas A. Free-running disorder in a sighted adolescent. J Pediatr 2012;160(5):877.

84. Allen RP, Picchietti D, Hening WA, et al. Restless legs syndrome: diagnostic criteria, special considerations, and epidemiology. A report from the restless legs syndrome diagnosis and epidemiology workshop at the National Institutes of Health. Sleep Med 2003;4:101–19.

85. Montplaisir J, Boucher S, Poirier G, et al. Clinical, polysomnographic, and genetic characteristics of restless legs syndrome: a study of 133 patients diagnosed with new standard criteria. Mov Disord 1997;12:61–5.

86. Picchietti D, Bruni O, de Weerd A, et al. Pediatric restless legs syndrome diagnostic criteria: an update by the International Restless Legs Syndrome Study Group. Sleep Med 2013;14:1253–9.

87. Kotagal S, Silber MH. Childhood-onset restless legs syndrome. Ann Neurol 2004;56:803–7.

88. Chervin RD, Archbold KH, Dillon JE, et al. Associations between symptoms of inattention, hyperactivity, restless legs, and periodic leg movements. Sleep 2002;25:213–8.

89. Picchietti D, Allen RP, Arthur S, et al. Restless legs syndrome: prevalence and impact in children and adolescents—the peds REST study. Pediatrics 2007; 120(2):253–66.

90. Yilmaz K, Kilincaslan A, Aydin N, et al. Prevalence and correlates of restless legs syndrome in adolescents. Dev Med Child Neurol 2011;53:40–7.

91. Turkdogan D, Bekiroglu N, Zaimoglu S. A prevalence study of restless legs syndrome in Turkish children and adolescents. Sleep Med 2011;12:315–21.

92. Simakajornboon N. Periodic limb movement disorder in children. Paediatr Respir Rev 2006;7:S55–7.

93. Picchietti D, Stevens HE. Early manifestations of restless legs syndrome in child-hood and adolescence. Sleep Med 2008;9:770–81.
94. Rajaram SS, Walters AS, England SJ, et al. Some children with growing pains may actually have restless legs. Sleep 2004;27(4):767–73.
95. Davis ID, Baron J, O'Riordan MA, et al. Sleep disturbances in pediatric dialysis patients. Pediatr Nephrol 2005;20:69–75.
96. Pullen SJ, Wall CA, Angstman ER, et al. Psychiatric comorbidity in children and adolescents with restless legs syndrome: a retrospective study. J Clin Sleep Med 2011;7(6):587–96.
97. Walter AS. Simple sleep-related movement disorders of childhood including benign sleep myoclonus of infancy, rhythmic movement disorder, and childhood restless legs syndrome and periodic limb movements in sleep. Sleep Med Clin 2007;2(3):419–32.
98. Picchietti MA, Picchietti DL. Restless legs syndrome and periodic limb move-ment disorder in children and adolescents. Semin Pediatr Neurol 2008; 15(2):91–9.
99. Guilleminault C, Palombini L, Pelayo R, et al. Sleepwalking and sleep terrors in prepubertal children: what triggers them? Pediatrics 2003;111:e17–25.
100. Winkelmann J, Polo O, Provini F, et al. Genetics of restless legs syndrome (RLS): state-of-the-art and future directions. Mov Disord 2007;22(Suppl 18):S449–58.
101. Schormair B, Zhao C, Bell S, et al. Identification of novel risk loci for restless legs syndrome in genome-wide association studies in individuals of European ancestry: a meta-analysis. Lancet Neurol 2017;16:898–907.
102. Winkelmann J, Muller-Myhsok B, Wittchen HU, et al. Complex segregation anal-ysis of restless legs syndrome provides evidence for an autosomal dominant mode of inheritance in early age at onset families. Ann Neurol 2002;52(3): 297–302.
103. Gingras J, Gaultney J, Picchietti D. Pediatric periodic limb movement disorder: sleep symptom and polysomnographic correlates compared to obstructive sleep apnea. J Clin Sleep Med 2011;7(6):603–9.
104. Chervin RD, Archbold KH. Hyperactivity and polysomnographic findings in chil-dren evaluated for sleep-disordered breathing. Sleep 2001;24:313–20.
105. Crabtree VM, Ivanenko A, O'Brien LM, et al. Periodic limb movement disorder of sleep in children. J Sleep Res 2003;12:73–81.
106. Martinez S, Guilleminault C. Periodic leg movements in prepubertal children with sleep disturbance. Dev Med Child Neurol 2004;46:765–70.
107. Dollinger SJ. On the varieties of childhood sleep disturbance. J Clin Child Psy-chol 1982;1:107–15.
108. Petit D, Touchette E, Tremblay RE, et al. Dyssomnias and parasomnias in early childhood. Pediatrics 2007;119(5):e1016–25.
109. Furet O, Goodwin JL, Quan SF. Incidence and remission of parasomnias among adolescent children in the Tucson Children's Assessment of Sleep Apnea (Tu-CASA) study. Southwest J Pulm Crit Care 2011;2:93.
110. Kales JD, Kales A, Soldatos CR, et al. Night terrors. Arch Gen Psychiatry 1980; 37:1413–7.
111. Reimão RN, Lefévre AB. Prevalence of sleep-talking in childhood. Brain Dev 1980;2:353–7.
112. Klackenberg G. Somnambulism in childhood-prevalence, course and behav-ioral correlations. Acta Paediatr 1982;71:495–9.
113. Essen J, Peckham C. Nocturnal enuresis in childhood. Dev Med Child Neurol 1976;18:577–89.

114. Klackenberg G. Nocturnal enuresis in a longitudinal perspective. Acta Paediatr 1981;70:453–7.

115. Feehan M, McGee R, Stanton W, et al. A 6-year follow-up of childhood enuresis: prevalence in adolescence and consequences for mental health. J Paediatr Child Health 1990;26:75–9.

116. Byrd RS, Weitzman M, Lanphear NE, et al. Bed-wetting in U.S. children: epidemiology and related behavior problems. Pediatrics 1996;98:414–9.

117. Shreeram S, He JP, Kalaydjian A, et al. Prevalence of enuresis and its association with attention-deficit/hyperactivity disorder among U.S. children: results from nationally representative study. J Am Acad Child Adolesc Psychiatry 2009;48(1):35–41.

118. Reding GR, Zepelin H, Monroe LJ. Incidence of bruxism. J Dent Res 1966;45: 1198–204.

119. Fisher BE, Wilson AE. Selected sleep disturbances in school children reported by parents: prevalence, interrelationships, behavioral correlates and parental attributions. Percept Mot Skills 1987;64:1147–57.

120. Hawkins C, Williams TI. Nightmares, life events and behavior problems in preschool children. Child Care Health Dev 1992;18:117–28.

121. Vela-Bueno A, Bixler EO, Dobladez-Blanco B, et al. Prevalence of night terrors and nightmares in elementary school children: a pilot study. Res Commun Psychol Psychiatr Behav 1985;10:177–88.

122. Simonds JF, Parraga H. Prevalence of sleep disorders and sleep behaviors in children and adolescents. J Am Acad Child Psychiatry 1982;21:383–8.

123. Schredl M, Fricke-Oerkermann A, Mitschke A, et al. Longitudinal study of nightmares in children: stability and effect of emotional symptoms. Child Psychiatry Hum Dev 2009;40:439–49.

124. Carlson CR, Cordova MJ. Sleep disorders in childhood and adolescence. Child and adolescent psychological disorders: a comprehensive textbook. New York: Oxford University Press; 1999. p. 415–38.

125. Nielsen T, Carr M, Picard-Deland C, et al. Early childhood adversity associations with nightmare severity and sleep spindles. Sleep Med 2019;56:57–65.

126. Terr LC. Chowchilla revisited: the effect of psychic trauma four years after a school bus kidnapping. Am J Psychiatry 1983;140(12):1543–50.

127. Dollinger SL, Molina BS, Monteiro JM. Sleep anxieties in Brazilian children: the role of cultural and environmental factors in child sleep disturbance. Am J Orthop 1996;66(2):252–61.

128. Finkelhor D, Araji S, Baron L, et al. A sourcebook on child sexual abuse. Beverly Hills (CA): Sage; 1986.

129. Dunn KK, Barrett D. Characteristics of nightmare sufferers. Psychiatr J Univ Ott 1988;13(2):91–3.

130. Levin R. Relations among nightmare frequency and ego strength, death anxiety, and sex in college students. Percept Mot Skills 1989;69:1107–13.

131. Wood JM, Bootzin RR. The prevalence of nightmares and their independence from anxiety. J Abnorm Psychol 1990;99(1):64–8.

132. Nader K. Children's traumatic dreams. In: Barrett D, editor. Trauma and dreams. Cambridge (MA): Harvard University Press; 1996. p. 9–24.

133. Chayon MM, Shapiro CM. Sleep disturbances and psychiatric disorders associated with posttraumatic stress disorder in the general population. Compr Psychiatry 2000;41:469–78.

134. Thabet AA, Ibraheem AN, Shivram R, et al. Parenting support and PTSD in children of a war zone. Int J Soc Psychiatry 2009;55:226–37.

135. Carrion VG, Weems CF, Ray R, et al. Toward an empirical definition of pediatric PTSD: the phenomenology of PTSD symptoms in youth. J Am Acad Child Adolesc Psychiatry 2002;41:166–73.

136. Kotagal S. Rapid eye movement sleep behavior disorder during childhood. Sleep Med Clin 2015;10(2):163–7.

137. De Barros-Ferreira M, Chodkiewicz JP, Lairy GC, et al. Disorganized relations of tonic and phasic events of REM sleep in a case of brain-stem tumour. Electroencephalogr Clin Neurophysiol 1975;38:203–7.

138. Thirumalai SS, Shubin RA, Robinson R. Rapid eye movement sleep behavior disorder in children with autism. J Child Neurol 2002;17:173–8.

139. Lloyd R, Tippmann-Peikert M, Slocumb N, et al. Characteristics of REM sleep behavior disorder in childhood. J Clin Sleep Med 2012;8:127–31.

140. Rye B, Johnston LH, Watts RL, et al. Juvenile Parkinson's disease with REM sleep behavior disorder, sleepiness, and daytime REM onset. Neurology 1999;53(8):1868–70.

141. Henriques-Filho PS, Sergio PA, Pratesi R. Sleep apnea and REM sleep behavior disorder in patients with Chiari malformations. Arq Neuropsiquiatr 2008;66: 344–9.

142. Trajanovic NN, Volch I, Shapiro CM, et al. REM sleep behavior disorder in a child with Tourette syndrome. Can J Neurol Sci 2004;31:572–5.

143. Teman PT, Tippmann-Piekert M, Silber MH, et al. Idiopathic rapid eye movement disorder: associations with antidepressants psychiatric diagnoses, and other factors in relation to age of onset. Sleep Med 2009;10:60–5.

144. Gropman AL, Duncan WC, Smith AC. Neurological and developmental features of the Smith Magenis syndrome (del 17 p11.2). Pediatr Neurol 2006;34:337–50.

145. Nevsimalova S, Prihodova I, Kemlink D, et al. REM sleep behavior disorder (RBD) can be one of the first symptoms of childhood narcolepsy. Sleep Med 2007;8:784–6.

146. Sheldon SH, Jacobsen J. REM-sleep motor disorder in children. J Child Neurol 1998;13:257–60.

147. Maski KP, Jeste SS, Spence SJ. Common neurological co-morbidities in autism spectrum disorders. Curr Opin Pediatr 2011;23:609–15.

148. Simonds JF, Parraga H. Prevalence of sleep disorders and sleep behaviors in children and adolescents. J Am Acad Child Adolesc Psychiatry 1982;21:383–8.

149. Van Dyk TR, Becker SP, Byars KC. Rates of mental health symptoms and associations with self-reported sleep quality and sleep hygiene in adolescents presenting for insomnia treatment. J Clin Sleep Med 2019;15(10):1433–42.

150. Van Dyk TR, Becker SP, Byars KC. Mental health diagnoses and symptoms in preschool and school age youth presenting to insomnia evaluation: prevalence and associations with sleep disruption. Behav Sleep Med 2019;17(6):790–803.

151. Corkum P, Tannock R, Moldofsky H. Sleep disturbances in children with attention-deficit/hyperactivity disorder. J Am Acad Child Adolesc Psychiatry 1998;37:637–46.

152. Cortese S, Faraone SV, Konofal E, et al. Sleep in children with attention-deficit/hyperactivity disorder: meta-analysis of subjective and objective studies. J Am Acad Child Adolesc Psychiatry 2009;48:894–908.

153. Cortese S, Konofal E, Yateman N, et al. Sleep and alertness in children with attention-deficit/hyperactivity disorder: a systematic review of the literature. Sleep 2006;29(4):504–11.

154. Sedky K, Bennett DS, Carvalho KS. Attention deficit hyperactivity disorder and sleep disordered breathing in pediatric populations: a meta-analysis. Sleep Med Rev 2014;18(4):349–56.

155. Alfano CA, Ginsburg GS, Kingery JN. Sleep-related problems among children and adolescents with anxiety disorders. J Am Acad Child Adolesc Psychiatry 2007;46:224–32.

156. Alfano CA, Pina AA, Zerr AA, et al. Pre-sleep arousal and sleep problems of anxiety-disordered youth. Child Psychiatry Hum Dev 2010;41(2):156–67.

157. Mullin BC, Pyle L, Haraden D, et al. A preliminary multimethod comparison of sleep among adolescents with and without generalized anxiety disorder. J Clin Child Adolesc Psychol 2017;46(2):198–210.

158. Rosen G, Mahowald MW, Ferber R. Sleepwalking, confusional arousals, and sleep terrors in the child. In: Ferber R, Kryger M, editors. Principles and practice of sleep disorders in the child. Philadelphia: WB Saunders Co; 1995. p. 45–53.

159. Rona RJ, Li L, Chinn S. Determinants of nocturnal enuresis in England and Scotland in the '90s. Dev Med Child Neurol 1997;39:677–81.

160. Díaz-Román A, Zhang J, Delorme R, et al. Sleep in youth with autism spectrum disorders: systematic review and meta-analysis of subjective and objective studies. Evid Based Ment Health 2018;21(4):146–54.

161. Souders MC, Zavodny S, Eriksen W, et al. Sleep in children with autism spectrum disorder. Curr Psychiatry Rep 2017;19(6):34.

162. Liu X, Buysse DJ, Gentzler AL, et al. Insomnia and hypersomnia associated with depressive phenomenology and comorbidity in childhood depression. Sleep 2007;30:83–90.

163. Wong MM, Brower KJ, Zucker RA. Sleep problems, suicidal ideation, and self-harm behaviors in adolescence. J Psychiatr Res 2011;45(4):505–11.

164. Mars B, Heron J, Klonsky ED, et al. Predictors of future suicide attempt among adolescents with suicidal thoughts on non-suicidal self-harm: a population-based birth cohort study. Lancet Psychiatry 2019;6(4):327–37.

# Screening and Evaluation of Sleep Disturbances and Sleep Disorders in Children and Adolescents

Suman K.R. Baddam[a,*], Craig A. Canapari[b],
Jenna Van de Grift[c], Christopher McGirr[a], Alexandra Y. Nasser[d],
Michael J. Crowley[a]

## KEYWORDS

- Sleep • Screening • Sleep disturbances • Sleep disorders • Consumer wearables
- Evaluation • Polysomnography • Tele-sleep

## KEY POINTS

- Sleep disturbances and disorders are prevalent in children and adolescents and are affected by sleep hygiene, circadian abnormalities, medical disorders, and psychiatric disorders.
- There is inadequate screening of sleep disturbances in pediatric clinics because of limited training and scarcity of pediatric sleep specialists.
- Daytime sleepiness questionnaires, BEARS screening, and comprehensive sleep instruments may be used to increase screening for sleep disturbances.
- Children and adolescents who screen positive for sleep disturbances and sleep disorders not corrected by sleep hygiene should be referred to a sleep specialist for comprehensive clinical sleep evaluation and polysomnography.
- Consumer wearables may play an adjunct role in screening and evaluating sleep disturbances, but they are not substitutes for the evaluation and diagnosis of sleep problems in children and adolescents.

This article originally appeared in *Child and Adolescent Psychiatric Clinics*, Volume 30 Issue 1, January 2021.
Funding: No funding was provided for this article.
[a] Yale Child Study Center, Yale School of Medicine, 230 South Frontage Road, New Haven, CT 06519, USA; [b] Pediatric Pulmonology, Allergy, Immunology & Sleep Medicine, PO Box 208064, New Haven, CT, 06520-8064, USA; [c] Yale University School of Medicine, 230 South Frontage Road, New Haven, CT 06519, USA; [d] Midstate Medical Center, 435 Lewis Avenue, Meriden, CT 06451, USA
* Corresponding author.
*E-mail address:* Suman.Baddam@yale.edu

## INTRODUCTION

Optimal sleep duration and sleep quality are necessary for medical and emotional health in children and adolescents.[1] Sleep problems are common in pediatric medical[2,3] and mental health disorders,[4] and the two are known to have a bidirectional relationship. Child mental health disorders are prevalent,[5,6] with the most common being anxiety disorders followed by mood and disruptive disorders.[5,7] Self-reports of difficulty falling asleep and staying asleep are commonly reported in mental health disorders, but specific objective markers of sleep in these disorders have not been identified.[4] Lower nighttime sleep duration, higher daytime sleepiness, and higher weekend sleep duration is being observed as compared with several decades ago,[8] raising concerns of disrupted academic, medical, and emotional function.

Sleep disorders are common and underdiagnosed in children and adolescents. About 25% of children have a sleep problem in childhood.[9] In various studies, symptoms of insomnia are reported in 19% of children[10] and 10% of adolescents,[11] whereas snoring is reported in 3.4% to 34.0% of elementary school children and severe sleep-disordered breathing in 1.0% of children.[12] However, only 3.7% of children are diagnosed with sleep disorders in pediatric primary care centers, which is significantly lower than the prevalence of these disorders.[13] The screening of sleep problems also varies with age. Only 61.7% of infants, 48.8% of preschoolers, 36.5% of children, and 35.3% of adolescents are screened for sleep disorders by pediatric nurse practitioners.[14] The identification of a "sleep problem" by parents at screening is related to their cultural background.[15] Even when screening for sleep problems is performed, it is often abbreviated, with the screening being highest for sleep patterns, moderate for snoring, and low for sleep movement disorders.[16] Limited screening is compounded by the scarce training opportunities in pediatric sleep medicine[16–18] and the consequent scarcity of pediatric sleep specialists.[16] To put this in perspective, only 313 of 125,332 pediatricians[19] and only around 20 psychiatrists are board certified in sleep medicine in North America.[20] Specialized pediatric sleep medicine training is just beginning to increase in other countries.[21] Considering the low rates of identification of sleep problems in pediatric clinics, we present this review to guide pediatric primary and mental health clinicians in the screening and evaluation of sleep disturbances and sleep disorders.

## SLEEP DISTURBANCES IN THE PEDIATRIC POPULATION

"Sleep patterns," "sleep problems," and "sleep disturbances" are commonly used to describe sleep in the pediatric sleep literature and in the clinical setting. "Sleep patterns" refer to bedtimes, waketimes, sleep duration, and wake after sleep onset duration. "Sleep problems" or "sleep disturbances" are used interchangeably for various sleep abnormalities[22–27] and refer to disruption of bedtimes, waketimes, wake after sleep onset, abnormal behaviors during sleep, and poor sleep quality. Children and adolescents present to primary care and mental health clinics commonly with difficulty falling asleep and daytime sleepiness.[1,28]

The usual presenting pediatric sleep problems—difficulty falling asleep and daytime sleepiness—may be secondary to inadequate sleep quality and quantity, poor sleep hygiene, circadian abnormalities or sleep disorders of insomnia, obstructive sleep apnea, restless legs syndrome, periodic limb movement disorder, and narcolepsy (**Fig. 1**). The specific diagnostic criteria for sleep disorders are coded in the *International Classification of Sleep Disorders*, 3rd edition, and in the *Diagnostic and Statistical Manual of Mental Disorders*, 5th edition. The sleep disorder diagnoses across these 2 diagnostic systems are broadly consistent. The specific differences between

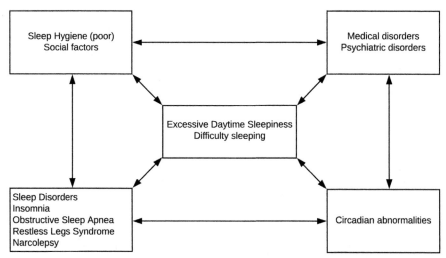

**Fig. 1.** Multiple factors affect common sleep problems.

sleep disorders across various diagnostic systems are beyond the goals of this review (for details, refer to Thorpy 2017).[29] The diagnostic features of common pediatric sleep disorders are presented in abbreviated form in **Box 1**. The full diagnostic criteria for sleep disorders are available in the *Diagnostic and Statistical Manual of Mental*

---

**Box 1**
**Diagnostic criteria of common sleep disorders (criteria in bullet points)**

Insomnias
  Short-term insomnia disorder
    Difficulty initiating or maintaining sleep; waking up early
    Daytime symptoms (fatigue, attention problems)
    Three times per week in less than 3 months
    Not explained by inadequate sleep, poor sleep hygiene, substance, or medical condition
  Chronic insomnia (symptoms ≥3 mo)
  Other insomnia disorder

Central disorders of hypersomnolence
  Insufficient sleep syndrome
    Daily periods of irrepressible need to sleep, daytime lapses, or behaviors attributed to sleepiness
    Patient's sleep time shorter than expected for age
    Symptoms not explained by drugs, medical, neurological, mental disorders
  Narcolepsy (types 1 and 2)
    Daily periods of irrepressible need to sleep or daytime lapses
    Mean sleep latency ≤8 min and 2 REM periods on polysomnography with multiple sleep latency test and cataplexy (cataplexy present in type 1 narcolepsy)
  Idiopathic hypersomnia
    Diagnosis of exclusion (exclude insufficient sleep and narcolepsy)
    Criteria same as narcolepsy without cataplexy and without REM periods (on polysomnography and multiple sleep latency test)
  Hypersomnia related to medical disorder
  Hypersomnia related to medication or substance
  Hypersomnia related to psychiatric disorder

Sleep-disordered breathing
Obstructive sleep apnea, pediatric
Snoring, labored breathing, or sleepiness and behaviors related to sleepiness
One or more obstructive, mixed or hypopneas on polysomnography
Snoring

Parasomnias
Sleepwalking
Arousals involving ambulation and complex behaviors out of bed
Sleep terrors
Episodes of terror associated with autonomic arousal
Confusional arousals
Episodes of mental confusion in bed without terror or ambulation
Nightmares
Repeated dreams at night that are well remembered and dysphoric
Usually oriented and alert after awakening from dreams
Parasomnia related to medical disorder
Parasomnia related to medication or substance
Parasomnia, unspecified

Circadian rhythm sleep–wake disorders
Delayed sleep–wake phase disorder
Delay in major sleep period in relation to desired bedtime and wake time
Presents with symptoms of insomnia or daytime sleepiness and longer than 3 mo
Not explained by poor sleep hygiene, substance, or medical condition
Advanced sleep–wake phase disorder
Circadian sleep–wake disorder not otherwise specified
Sleep-related movement disorders
Restless legs syndrome
Urge to move the legs, partially resolved by moving and symptoms worse in the evening or night
Twice weekly for the past year
Associated with difficulty falling asleep and staying asleep at night, and excessive daytime sleepiness
Periodic limb movement disorder
Increased leg movements during sleep
Number of leg movements >5/h
Associated symptoms of daytime sleepiness or sleep disruption not attributable to another sleep disorder.
Sleep-related rhythmic movement disorder
Repetitive stereotyped rhythmic movements at sleep onset and during sleep
Usually benign
Sleep-related bruxism
Presence of frequent tooth grinding sounds during sleep
Abnormal tooth wear, jaw muscle pain, or jaw locking
Sleep-related movement disorder due to a medical disorder
Sleep-related movement disorder due to a medication or substance
Sleep-related movement disorder, unspecified

*Data from* American Psychiatric Association. Diagnostic and statistical manual of mental disorders. 5th ed. Washington D.C.: 2013; and American Academy of Sleep Medicine. International classification of sleep disorders. 3rd edition. Darien (IL); 2014.

*Disorders*, 5th edition,[30] and the *International Classification of Sleep Disorders*, 3rd edition.[31]

## SCREENING OF SLEEP DISTURBANCES

Difficulty falling asleep, daytime sleepiness, and other sleep disturbances are associated with decreased sleep duration, unhealthy sleep habits, and the presence of sleep disorders,[28,32,33] which are, in turn, exacerbated by the use of electronic media in children and adolescents.[34,35] Sleep hygiene, sleep habits, and sleep disorders interact with each other and worsen sleep problems (see **Fig. 1**). A key goal of screening is to identify sleep disorders that might otherwise go undetected. For example, in a pediatric primary care clinic, the use of a simple screening tool, BEARS, increases the detection of sleep problems by 4-fold compared with usual care.[36] Clinicians working with children and adolescents should universally screen their patients for sleep disturbances and sleep disorders. We recommend that clinicians become especially familiar with the use of BEARS as a screening tool.

## BEARS Screening

BEARS is an acronym that stands for bedtime problems, excessive daytime sleepiness, awakenings and abnormal behaviors at night, regularity and duration of sleep, and snoring. Each item is expanded and used as a screening question in a developmentally appropriate manner. Initial questions may then be followed by specific follow-up questions (for example questions refer to **Box 2**). Parents answer the questions for infants and children; adolescents usually answer themselves.

---

**Box 2**
**BEARS sample questions**

In the examples for each category, the top questions are directed to the parent and the bottom questions are directed to the child/teenager.

*Bedtime*

- Does your child have any trouble falling asleep?
- Does your child resist going to sleep at bedtime?
- Do you have any trouble falling asleep?
- Do you resist going to bed?

*Excessive daytime sleepiness*

- Does your child feel sleepy during the day?
- Does your child fall asleep in class or while watching TV?
- Does your child need to take naps during the day (children >5 years of age)?
- Do you feel very sleepy during the day?
- Do you fall asleep in class?
- Do you nap during the day?

*Awakenings and abnormal behaviors at night*

- Does your child wake up many times in the middle of the night?
- Does your child display any abnormal or problematic behaviors during sleep, for example, sleepwalking or frequent nightmares?
- Do you wake up a lot during your sleep?
- Do you have nightmares during sleep or any other unusual behaviors?

*Regularity of sleep*

- Does your child have regular bedtimes and waketimes on schooldays and weekends?
- Do you have regular bedtimes and waketimes on schooldays and weekends?

*Sleep-disordered breathing*

- Does your child snore loudly or stop breathing at night?
- Have you been told that you snore loudly or stop breathing at night?

### Sleep Screening Questionnaires

Several sleep questionnaires are available to screen daytime sleepiness, sleep hygiene, sleep disturbances, and sleep disorders, although not all have been validated.[37,38] In **Tables 1–3**, we present sleep screening questionnaires (daytime sleepiness, sleep hygiene, comprehensive sleep questionnaires) validated in healthy and pediatric clinical populations (for details, refer to Lewandowski and colleagues,[39] 2017). Daytime sleepiness questionnaires are a simple and effective way to identify if sleepiness is pathologic, and they may be administered and scored with little expertise or training. Comprehensive sleep questionnaires identify sleep disturbances and sleep disorders in children and adolescents, but they require training on how to properly administer and score them. Sleep hygiene scales are primarily used in research and are helpful tools for identifying sleep hygiene difficulties. Refer to **Box 3** for a summary of sleep screening questionnaires.

## COMPREHENSIVE CLINICAL SLEEP EVALUATION

Children who screen positive for sleep disturbances and disorders on BEARS and sleep screening questionnaires should undergo a thorough clinical sleep evaluation. The clinical sleep interview is similar to other clinical interviews and involves obtaining a detailed sleep history and a physical examination to generate a differential diagnosis from the history and understanding of normal sleep physiology.[1] Understanding normal sleep patterns (**Box 4, Table 4**) helps to identify deviations from normal during the clinical interview. Usually both parents and children are interviewed to obtain a full picture of the sleep symptoms. Clinicians should initially identify the specific sleep problem, which could broadly fall in one of the following 4 categories—difficulty initiating or maintaining sleep, bedtime resistance, excessive daytime sleepiness, or symptoms suggestive of specific sleep disorders (snoring, leg movements, and abnormal behaviors during sleep).[1]

The sleep history for all children and adolescents should include detailed information about sleep–wake habits—bedtimes and waketimes on school and nonschool days, time to fall asleep, number and duration of awakenings at night, naps, 24-hour sleep duration and sleepiness during the day. Detailed information about sleep hygiene—regularity of sleep–wake patterns, sleeping environment, use of caffeine, naps, use of technology—is important to assess because they may adversely affect daily and weekday-to-weekend sleep patterns (refer to **Box 4** for sleep hygiene). A history of daytime activities and their specific role in causing sleep problems is important to identify as sleep–wake patterns in children and adolescents should be evaluated in the context of the 24-hour day.[1,40]

Sleep complaints and disruption of sleep patterns may be secondary to an underlying sleep disorder. The clinical history should evaluate for symptoms of sleep disorders that includes symptoms of insomnia, sleep apnea, restless legs syndrome, periodic limb movement syndrome, and narcolepsy. The temporal onset of individual symptoms, frequency of symptoms, and day-to-day variability should be ascertained along with their effects on social and occupational functioning.

Of the different age groups, preschool-aged children are more likely to present with bedtime resistance and night wakings and associate bedtime and sleep with parental presence. In these children, a detailed history of bedtime routines and behavioral associations with sleep can clarify if the conditioned associations are the cause of sleep disturbances and disrupted sleep.[40]

The most common sleep disturbances among preschool- and school-aged children are night terrors, confusional arousals, sleepwalking, sleep talking, and nightmares. A

**Table 1**
Daytime sleepiness questionnaires

| Scale | Age Groups | No. of Questions | Assesses | Psychometrics | Usefulness |
|---|---|---|---|---|---|
| Pediatric Daytime Sleepiness Scale[71] | 11–15 y | 8 | Sleepiness-related behaviors | Total: $\alpha$ = 0.80 Split-half: $\alpha$ = 0.81 Scores = 0–32, Cutoff 15 | Daytime sleepiness for adolescents |
| Cleveland Adolescent Sleepiness Questionnaire[72] | 11–17 y | 16 | Daytime sleepiness, daytime and nighttime alertness | Total: $\alpha$ = 0.89 | Daytime sleepiness for adolescents |
| Epworth Sleepiness Scale for Children[73–75] | 2–18 y | 8 | Propensity to fall asleep | Total: $\alpha$ = 0.75 Scores = 10 | Daytime sleepiness for children and adolescents |
| Teacher's Daytime Sleepiness Questionnaire[73] | 4–10 y | 10 | Daytime sleepiness | Total: $\alpha$ = 0.80 | Daytime sleepiness assessed by the teacher |

**Table 2**
Sleep hygiene scales

| Scale | Age Groups | Number of Questions | Assesses | Psychometrics | Usefulness |
|---|---|---|---|---|---|
| Children's Sleep Hygiene Scale[76] | 2–8 y | 25 items | Bedtime routines, sleep environment, behaviors and emotions surrounding sleep | Total: $\alpha$ = 0.76 | Assesses children's sleep hygiene |
| Bedtime Routines Questionnaire[77] | 2–8 y | 31 items | Weekday and weekend routines, reactivity to changes in routine, frequency of adaptive and maladaptive activities before bedtime | Total: $\alpha$ = 0.88 subscales: $\alpha$ = 0.69–.90 | Assesses children's sleep hygiene |
| Adolescent Sleep Hygiene Scale[78] | 12–18 y | 28 items | Bedtime routines, sleep environment, behaviors and emotions surrounding sleep | Total: $\alpha$ = 0.80 subscales: $\alpha$ = 0.46–0.71 | Measures teenagers' sleep hygiene |

**Table 3**
Comprehensive sleep questionnaires

| Scale | Age Groups | Number of Questions | Assesses | Psychometrics | Usefulness |
|---|---|---|---|---|---|
| Sleep Disturbance Scale for Children[79] | 5–15 y | 26 items | Sleep initiation and maintenance, sleep–wake transition disorders, excessive sleepiness, sleep breathing disorders, disorders of arousal | Total: $\alpha = 0.79$ $\alpha = 0.71$ for sleep disorder test–retest: 0.71 total, 0.21–0.66 (single items) Range = 26–130 Cutoff score = 39 | Screen for sleep disorders in children and adolescents |
| Children's Sleep Habits Questionnaire[80] | 4–10 y | 45 items | Bedtime resistance, sleep onset delay, Sleep duration, sleep anxiety, night wakings, parasomnias, sleep disordered breathing, daytime sleepiness | Total: $\alpha = 0.68$ community; $\alpha = 0.78$ clinical subscales: $\alpha = 0.36$–0.70 community; $\alpha = 0.56$–0.93 clinical test–retest: 0.62–0.79 Cutoff score = 41 | Screen for sleep disturbances and sleep disorders in children and adolescents |
| Pediatric Sleep Questionnaire[81] | 2–18 y | 22 items | Sleep-related breathing disorders, snoring, daytime sleepiness, inattention | Subscale $\alpha = 0.77$–0.89 Test–retest: 0.66–0.92 | Screen for sleep apnea, inattention and sleepiness |

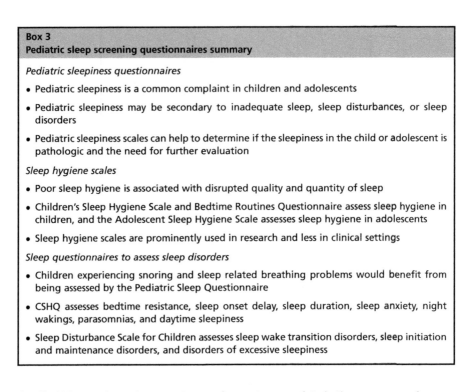

**Box 3**
**Pediatric sleep screening questionnaires summary**

*Pediatric sleepiness questionnaires*

- Pediatric sleepiness is a common complaint in children and adolescents
- Pediatric sleepiness may be secondary to inadequate sleep, sleep disturbances, or sleep disorders
- Pediatric sleepiness scales can help to determine if the sleepiness in the child or adolescent is pathologic and the need for further evaluation

*Sleep hygiene scales*

- Poor sleep hygiene is associated with disrupted quality and quantity of sleep
- Children's Sleep Hygiene Scale and Bedtime Routines Questionnaire assess sleep hygiene in children, and the Adolescent Sleep Hygiene Scale assesses sleep hygiene in adolescents
- Sleep hygiene scales are prominently used in research and less in clinical settings

*Sleep questionnaires to assess sleep disorders*

- Children experiencing snoring and sleep related breathing problems would benefit from being assessed by the Pediatric Sleep Questionnaire
- CSHQ assesses bedtime resistance, sleep onset delay, sleep duration, sleep anxiety, night wakings, parasomnias, and daytime sleepiness
- Sleep Disturbance Scale for Children assesses sleep wake transition disorders, sleep initiation and maintenance disorders, and disorders of excessive sleepiness

detailed history about the prevalence of symptoms, safety in the presence of symptoms, and any disruptions in social and occupational functioning should be assessed. Head banging and teeth grinding are also reported in this age group. The presence of other sleep disorders, the inability to sleep, and/or excessive daytime sleepiness in these children should lead to further evaluation by a sleep specialist and polysomnography.[40]

The prevalence of insomnia disorder increases after puberty and presents with difficulty falling asleep, staying asleep, and social and occupational deficits during the day. Insomnia may start in teenagers after a stressful precipitating event, and it may be perpetuated by irregular sleep habits and poor sleep hygiene. In particular, after puberty adolescents may present with extremely delayed bedtimes, waketimes that do not fit with the typical school day, difficulty falling asleep, and daytime sleepiness. Such adolescents should be evaluated for delayed sleep phase disorder.[40]

Sleep apnea is common in children and adolescents who present with snoring, breathing pauses, mouth breathing, and nasal obstruction. Sleep apnea is also comorbid in several medical and psychiatric disorders, and obesity.

Unpleasant sensations in the legs, the urge to move the legs before and during sleep period, and the urge to move the legs during inactivity, all of which resolve with movement, is characteristic of restless legs syndrome.[33] Children and adolescents with leg symptoms are encouraged to describe the symptoms in their own words, prompted by open-ended questions, because of the heterogeneous presentations of restless legs symptoms. Clinicians should be vigilant, as restless legs symptoms are commonly missed and may present as insomnia or excessive daytime sleepiness.[40]

Teenagers presenting with excessive daytime sleepiness, fragmented sleep, sleep paralysis, hallucinations before sleep and while coming out of sleep, and/or sudden loss of muscle tone should raise suspicion for narcolepsy. It is critical to rule out

---

**Box 4**
**Sleep hygiene**

*Bedtimes, waketimes, and consistency*

- •. Age appropriate need for sleep duration (12–16 hours for infants, 11–14 hours for toddlers, 10–13 hours for preschool, 9–13 hours for school aged children, and 8–10 hours for teenagers)

- • Regular bedtimes and waketimes (typically no later than 9 PM for younger children and 10 PM for teenagers), and consistent naptimes for younger children

*Bedtime routines*

- • Relaxing and consistent bedtime routines

- • For younger children: Bedtime routines include brushing teeth, taking a bath, reading stories, limiting access to electronics.

- • For teenagers: limiting access to electronics in bedrooms during and after bedtime, and relaxing bedtime routines

- • Dark and quiet rooms

*Exercise and diet*

- • No large meals before bedtime, limiting caffeine consumption, healthy and balanced diet, and daily physical activity

- • Create a positive atmosphere in the child's living environment

*Emotional needs*

- • Help children learn to settle down to sleep in their own beds without parents before bedtime and after night wakings

- • Make sure emotional needs are met during the day

*Data from* Paruthi S, Brooks LJ, D'Ambrosio C, et al. recommended amount of sleep for pediatric populations: a consensus statement of the American Academy of Sleep Medicine. J Clin Sleep Med. 2016;12(6):785–6; and Allen SL, Howlett MD, Coulombe JA, Corkum PV. ABCs of SLEEPING: A review of the evidence behind pediatric sleep practice recommendations. Sleep Medicine Rev. 2016;29:1-14.

---

sleepiness related to insufficient sleep before suspecting narcolepsy. The criteria to diagnose these sleep disorders are presented in **Box 1**.

Ascertaining a complete medical history is essential as allergies, lung diseases, and obesity are comorbidly present and worsen sleep apnea. Children with cancer, diabetes, gastroesophageal reflux disease, headaches, sickle cell disease, seizure disorder, headaches, and kidney problems have varied sleep disturbances. Children with Down syndrome should be screened for sleep apnea, which is commonly comorbid secondary to hypotonia. Craniofacial, neurogenetic, hematologic, and metabolic syndromes have a high likelihood of associated sleep disturbances and sleep disorders. The presence of sleep disorders, in turn, can worsen medical disorders. For example, sleep disruption is associated with increased seizures and headaches. Seizures may occur during sleep and can be identified on polysomnography.[40]

A detailed history of pediatric psychiatric disorders and neurodevelopmental disorders is essential to obtain as sleep disturbances and mental health disorders are comorbid and adversely affect each other. Children with attention deficit/hyperactivity disorder have bedtime resistance as well as a higher likelihood of sleep apnea and restless legs syndrome. Mood and anxiety disorders similarly are associated with insomnia and disrupted sleep patterns. Children with autism commonly have sleep

**Table 4**
Normal sleep patterns in children and adolescents

| Age | Toddlers (1–2 y) | Preschool Aged Children (3–5 y) | School Aged Children (6–12 y) | Adolescents (13–18 y) |
|---|---|---|---|---|
| Normal sleep duration/24 h | 12–16 h | 10–13 h | 9–13 h Decrease from | 8–10 h |
| Bedtimes | No later than 8 PM, no weekday–weekend differences | No later than 9 PM on school nights, school night to nonschool night bedtime variability of <2 h | No later than 9 PM on school nights, school night to nonschool night bedtime variability of <2 h | No later than 10 PM on school nights, school night to nonschool night bedtime variability of <2 h |
| Naps | 1–2 naps decreasing with age | Decrease from 1 nap to 0 with age | No naps | No naps |
| Sleep latency | <20 min | <20 min | <30 min | <30 min |
| **Normal polysomnography values** | | | | |
| Sleep efficiency (total sleep time/time in bed) | >85% | >85% | >85% | >85% |
| Rapid eye movement latency | >80 min | >80 min | >80 min | >80 min |
| Obstructive apnea hypopnea index | <1/h | <1/h | <1/h | <1/h |
| Oxygen saturation | >90% | >90% | >90% | >90% |
| Mean end-tidal $CO_2$ | <50 mm Hg | <50 mm Hg | <50 mm Hg | <50 mm Hg |
| Periodic limb movement index | <5/h | <5/h | <5/h | <5/h |
| Common sleep problems | Bedtime resistance, awakenings at night, sleep related rhythmic movements (head banging, body rocking, body rolling) | Bedtime resistance, awakenings at night, sleep apnea, disorders of arousal (sleepwalking, night terrors), sleep related rhythmic movements (head banging, body rocking, body rolling) | Insufficient sleep, unhealthy sleep habits, sleep enuresis, disorders of arousal (sleepwalking, night terrors)sleep apnea, restless legs syndrome | Insufficient sleep, unhealthy sleep patterns, daytime sleepiness, insomnia, delayed sleep wake phase disorder, sleep apnea, restless legs syndrome, narcolepsy |

*Data from* Mindell JA, Owens JA. A clinical guide to pediatric sleep: diagnosis and management of sleep problems. Philadelphia: Lippincott Williams & Wilkins; 2015; and Paruthi S, Brooks LJ, D'Ambrosio C, et al. Recommended amount of sleep for pediatric populations: a consensus statement of the American Academy of Sleep Medicine. J Clin Sleep Med. 2016;12(6):785–6.

disturbances and sleep disorders. For a detailed review, please refer to Baddam and colleagues 2018.[4]

A current and past medication history should be obtained in children and adolescents, because many medications may affect sleep symptoms and sleep architecture. Medications used for asthma and allergies are associated with insomnia and disruption of sleep. Selective serotonin reuptake inhibitors, monoamine oxidase inhibitors, and selective noradrenergic reuptake inhibitors are all associated with disruption of REM sleep. Antipsychotics, especially atypical antipsychotics, and anticonvulsants are associated with daytime somnolence and weight gain and increase the likelihood of developing sleep apnea. Stimulants used to treat attention deficit/hyperactivity disorder may interfere with sleep initiation.[40]

Familial clustering of sleep disorders is common, so it is important to inquire about any family history of sleep disorders. A detailed social history includes family environment, school history including school start times, and academic functioning, because sleep disorders may compromise cognitive functioning and adversely affect academic performance. The social history should also document the number of people living at home, room sharing, and socioeconomic status because sleep disturbances are more common in lower socioeconomic status populations. A concomitant developmental history will highlight if there are any developmental delays secondary to chronic sleep complaints that in turn contribute to sleep disturbances and sleep disorders. Last, it is important to inquire about recreational drug use in teenagers (alcohol, nicotine, stimulants, etc) because these substances can adversely affect sleep.[40]

### Physical Evaluation

A comprehensive clinical history is followed by a physical examination to identify specific physical abnormalities that can help to narrow the differential diagnosis of sleep problems and the etiology of the disorder. Children with daytime sleepiness may present with physical signs of yawning, droopy eyelids, and irritability. Children with undiagnosed sleep problems may have failure to thrive with lower height, weight, and body mass index; hence, it is important to monitor the growth chart. Physical examination may reveal abnormal facial features (craniofacial abnormalities such as micrognathia or midfacial hypoplasia), enlarged tongue base, adenoid facies, high arched palate, adenotonsillar hypertrophy, and mouth breathing. The examination of ear, nose and throat, respiratory (lung disease), endocrine (thyroid problems), gastrointestinal (reflux symptoms affecting sleep), cardiovascular, infectious (Lyme disease), neurologic (seizures, headache), neuromuscular (muscular dystrophy), and psychiatric systems (anxiety, depression, or autism) for abnormal signs is essential because sleep disturbances are commonly associated with pediatric medical and mental health disorders.[1]

### Laboratory Tests

Typical laboratory tests may be required for sleep disturbances if there is suspicion for medical disorders (thyroid-stimulating hormone, growth hormone, albumin) and associated sleep difficulties. Inflammatory markers (C-reactive protein and IL-6) may be elevated in the presence of sleep disorders, but do not add any clinical value. Low ferritin is common in restless legs syndrome and important to assess as correction of low ferritin (to >50 ng/mL) may improve restless legs syndrome.[41] Human leukocyte antigen and cerebrospinal fluid hypocretin levels are assessed in narcolepsy but are used primarily for research purposes and do not add clinical value.[40]

### Sleep Diary

The sleep–wake schedules reported by children and adolescents should be verified by asking parents to maintain a sleep log or sleep diary for a period of 2 weeks. Sleep logs capture the day-to-day variation in sleep patterns and provide a self-report of sleep patterns. Standardized sleep diaries are unavailable for children and adolescents, but they are nevertheless commonly used in clinical practice. The expert developed Expanded Consensus Sleep Diary in adults identifies the following: time of getting into bed, time to fall asleep, number and duration of awakenings at night, time of final awakening, time of getting out of bed, early morning awakenings, estimated total sleep time, perceived sleep quality (on a Likert scale), naps, and alcohol, caffeine, and medication use.[42] Sleep logs are filled out by parents for children, whereas adolescents fill out the sleep logs themselves. Parent filled sleep diaries have been shown to agree well with those of children.[43–45] Assessment of sleep using sleep diaries or sleep logs (nonstandardized versions) is the gold standard for subjective sleep assessment and essential for the evaluation of insomnia, hypersomnia, and circadian disorders[42] despite the inaccuracies observed in sleep duration and awakenings. Alternatives to paper sleep diaries include electronic or web-based sleep diaries and mobile applications that have the advantages of taking less time to complete, time stamps of reports, and automatic scoring.[46] In summary, a sleep diary is a simple, cost-effective, and reliable way to assess multiple sleep features and should be used routinely in sleep assessments. Please refer to a summary of sleep diaries in **Box 5**.

### WHEN TO REFER TO A SLEEP SPECIALIST: COMPLEX CASES AND POLYSOMNOGRAPHY

Sleep disturbances may be transient and resolve or can become chronic and develop into severe sleep disorders. It is essential to use an initial open-ended question about sleep in the patient's intake paperwork to assess the need for further screening. We propose an initial open-ended question such as, "Does your child have a problem with sleep? If yes, please explain." Clinicians (nonsleep specialists) should be able to evaluate further using the BEARS screening questions in **Box 2**. Alternately, clinicians who are trained to use comprehensive sleep questionnaires may use them to screen for sleep disturbances. Clinicians should use the sleep log to identify if the presenting sleep symptoms are secondary to irregular sleep patterns and poor sleep hygiene based on the knowledge of typical sleep patterns (**see Table 4**). Clinicians should be able to recommend simple sleep hygiene interventions to improve sleep difficulties (see **Box 4**).

Of the pediatric sleep disorders, sleep association insomnia in preschool children can be easily diagnosed by obtaining a detailed history surrounding bedtime associations. Further management may be conducted by clinicians skilled in sleep

---

**Box 5**
**Sleep diaries/logs summary**

- Sleep logs are a cost effective, gold standard method for assessing subjective sleep duration and sleep patterns
- Paper and electronic sleep logs should include bedtimes, time to initiate sleep, awakenings at night, waketimes, naps and sleep quality
- Future research should focus on developing standardized sleep logs and sleep diaries

behavioral techniques. The evaluation and treatment of adolescent insomnia may be conducted by a clinician skilled in cognitive behavioral therapy for insomnia. Disorders of arousal (sleep walking, sleep talking, night terrors, nightmares, and confusional arousals) do not need further evaluation if they are infrequent and not associated with daytime deficits. Clinicians should be able to diagnose restless legs syndrome as it is a clinical diagnosis based on clinical history and ferritin level.

Children and adolescents with snoring and suspicion for sleep apnea, excessive daytime sleepiness with suspicion for narcolepsy, insomnia not improved by sleep hygiene measures, the presence of 2 or more sleep disorders, or comorbid sleep and medical or psychiatric disorders should be further evaluated by a sleep specialist.

### Polysomnography

Polysomnography is the gold standard method for the diagnosis of sleep disorders in children and adolescents.[47] Polysomnography is an all-night procedure conducted in an outpatient setting with sleep technologists; it is indicated for suspected sleep apnea, periodic limb movement syndrome, narcolepsy, and atypical parasomnias. It is not indicated for insomnia, circadian rhythm disorders, or sleep disturbances secondary to behavioral complaints.[1] Polysomnography involves video monitoring during sleep and measuring electroencephalography (brain waves), electromyogram (muscle tone), electrooculogram (eye movements), electrocardiogram (heart rate and rhythm), leg movements, snoring, airflow, and exhaled oxygen and carbon dioxide.[48] The overnight sleep recordings are scored by a technician or sleep specialist using the standardized criteria for scoring sleep provided by the American Academy of Sleep Medicine. The objective measurement of excessive daytime sleepiness is conducted by polysomnography followed by a multiple sleep latency test. Polysomnography with a multiple sleep latency test is commonly used as a diagnostic tool for narcolepsy or idiopathic hypersomnia. The lower end of normal polysomnography values is presented in **Table 4**. Home sleep testing is not validated in the pediatric population.[49] **Box 6** provides a summary of the evaluation and diagnosis of sleep disorders.

## ACTIGRAPHY, CONSUMER WEARABLES, AND MOBILE SLEEP APPLICATIONS

Actigraphy, a movement sensor-based estimation of sleep patterns, may be used to record sleep duration, bedtimes, and waketimes, in children suspected of having excessive daytime sleepiness, narcolepsy and delayed sleep phase syndrome. Actiwatches used in actigraphy are wrist-worn, watch-like devices using piezoelectric accelerometers to measure movement and light levels.[50] Movement is interpreted as wakefulness and lack of movement as sleep. Actiwatches have high sensitivity (high ability to identify sleep) and poor specificity (poor ability to identify wake by overestimating sleep during inactivity)[51,52] and are validated against polysomnography and

---

**Box 6**
**Sleep evaluation and diagnosis summary**

- Detailed information about sleep history includes sleep–wake history, symptoms of sleep disorders, and associated medical disorders

- Physical examination is essential to identify the signs in sleep disorders such as sleep apnea, narcolepsy

- Sleep log, laboratory tests, and polysomnography are used for the confirmation and diagnosis of sleep disorders

sleep diaries across pediatric age groups.[53] A recent meta-analysis showed actigraphy is a reliable tool for measuring sleep parameters, has good correlation with sleep logs and polysomnography, and provides unique information about sleep.[54]

Other consumer wearables include smartwatches (including Apple and Fitbit), embedded devices (mattress and bed), and smartphone applications.[55] These consumer wearables (Smartwatches, Fitbit, Jawbone UP, Apple Watch, etc) and sleep applications are widely available and advertised directly to consumers.[56] Consumer wearables calculate sleep duration and sleep stages from manufacturer developed algorithms using movement and heart rate sensors. Sleep trackers worn on the finger use pulse rate (variation in interbeat intervals and pulse amplitude), motion, and body temperature to estimate sleep and sleep stages using machine learning algorithms.[57] Comparative studies of consumer wearables against actigraphy and polysomnography are inconsistently available and the effects of periodic software updates on manufacturer developed algorithms are unknown.[58] Smart phone applications are available to record and measure snoring and video record apneic episodes. Similar to the consumer wearables; however, these applications have not been validated for clinical use.[59]

Consumer wearables are easily accessible, have the potential for long-term data collection, provide real-time feedback to patients, increase awareness about sleep, and may help patient–provider engagement. However, the majority of consumer wearables and technology are not validated for clinical use, and sleep estimation algorithms are not public. Consumer wearables may also be expensive and inaccessible to lower socioeconomic groups, thus limiting their usefulness. The American Academy of Sleep Medicine recommends that consumer wearables and sleep applications may be used as an adjunct within the context of comprehensive sleep evaluation, but they should not replace or substitute existing instruments that are validated for clinical use.[60] Please refer to **Box 7** for a summary.

## PEDIATRIC TELE-SLEEP EVALUATION

Telemedicine, the delivery of health care services using communication technologies where distance is a critical factor,[61] has taken a new significance during the novel

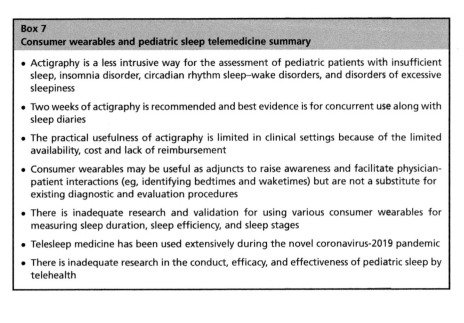

**Box 7**
**Consumer wearables and pediatric sleep telemedicine summary**

- Actigraphy is a less intrusive way for the assessment of pediatric patients with insufficient sleep, insomnia disorder, circadian rhythm sleep–wake disorders, and disorders of excessive sleepiness

- Two weeks of actigraphy is recommended and best evidence is for concurrent use along with sleep diaries

- The practical usefulness of actigraphy is limited in clinical settings because of the limited availability, cost and lack of reimbursement

- Consumer wearables may be useful as adjuncts to raise awareness and facilitate physician-patient interactions (eg, identifying bedtimes and waketimes) but are not a substitute for existing diagnostic and evaluation procedures

- There is inadequate research and validation for using various consumer wearables for measuring sleep duration, sleep efficiency, and sleep stages

- Telesleep medicine has been used extensively during the novel coronavirus-2019 pandemic

- There is inadequate research in the conduct, efficacy, and effectiveness of pediatric sleep by telehealth

coronavirus-2019 pandemic. The American Academy of Sleep Medicine, Committee on Pediatric Workforce at the American Academy of Pediatrics, and American Academy of Child and Adolescent Psychiatry all recommend tele-sleep medicine to provide greater access to sleep medicine experts[62] and specialist shortages.[63,64]

Before the novel coronavirus-2019 pandemic, few tele-sleep programs existed for children and adolescents. A pilot program developed to provide tele-sleep in Alberta, Canada, used a 2-week sleep diary, the Children's Sleep Habits Questionnaire, and pediatric quality of life (a questionnaire of pediatric general well-being) for screening followed by a tele-sleep interview (lasting 1 hour) to diagnose and develop an individualized medical and psychological treatment plan. The telehealth team included a board-certified pediatric sleep specialist, a pediatrician, a child psychologist, and a pediatric nurse.[65]

Even though telemedicine is promising and cost effective, the evidence related to its therapeutic effectiveness is limited.[66] In adults, sleep telemedicine used for the evaluation and management of insomnia and sleep apnea[67] save time for patients and clinicians and increase accessibility.[68] Pilot programs with an intraoral camera have been used for the assessment of oral cavities in remote sleep interviews in adults.[69] Technology for the remote recording of sleep—polygraphy, actigraphy, and continuous positive airway pressure compliance[70]—is available but has not been validated in children and adolescents. The ability to integrate screening tools and sleep logs, conduct a comprehensive evaluation, and provide treatments via telemedicine are essential for effective pediatric telesleep screening programs. Please refer to **Box 7** for a summary.

## SUMMARY

Sleep problems are prevalent, highly comorbid with medical and psychiatric disorders, underdiagnosed, and associated with adverse medical and social problems. Sleep disturbances are underdiagnosed owing to a lack of adequate training and the scarcity of specialists in pediatric sleep medicine. Screening in pediatric clinics is essential as child and adolescent sleep problems are widely underrecognized. We propose starting with an open-ended sleep question in the initial clinical paperwork that, if positive, can lead to BEARS screening. Screening questionnaires exist for the assessment of daytime sleepiness, sleep hygiene/environment, and sleep disorders, but these modalities require some training in scoring and interpretation. Sleep logs should be used in primary mental health and pediatric clinics and can identify underlying sleep hygiene and sleep duration difficulties which are correctable with sleep hygiene education. An in-depth clinical evaluation by a sleep specialist is recommended for snoring, excessive daytime sleepiness, abnormal movements during sleep, and sleep disturbances not improved by sleep hygiene recommendations. Consumer wearables are useful as adjuncts for sleep screening and evaluation, but are not effective as the only tools for sleep evaluation. Further research is needed for the effective use of screening tools in pediatric sleep medicine and tele-screening of sleep to improve pediatric sleep services.

## CLINICS CARE POINTS

- Evaluation of sleep disturbances and sleep disorders is pivotal in mental health and pediatric clinics

- Clinicians in pediatric mental health clinics should learn to screen for sleep disturbances and sleep disorders because of the scarcity of sleep specialists, and refer complex co-morbid sleep and mental health disturbances to sleep specialists
- Clinicians should learn to use the paper based sleep logs or sleep diaries and improve poor sleep hygiene in children and adolescents
- Tele-sleep programs should only be used after rigorous evaluation of efficacy and effectiveness in pediatric clinics
- Consumer wearables should not be used as the primary tools to identify sleep disturbances

## DISCLOSURE

The authors have nothing to disclose.

## REFERENCES

1. Gruber R, Carrey N, Weiss SK, et al. Position statement on pediatric sleep for psychiatrists. J Can Acad Child Adolesc Psychiatry 2014;23(3):174–95.
2. Lewandowski AS, Ward TM, Palermo TM. Sleep problems in children and adolescents with common medical conditions. Pediatr Clin North Am 2011;58(3):699–713.
3. Matricciani L, Paquet C, Galland B, et al. Children's sleep and health: a meta-review. Sleep Med Rev 2019;46:136–50.
4. Baddam SKR, Canapari CA, van Noordt SJR, et al. Sleep disturbances in child and adolescent mental health disorders: a review of the variability of objective sleep markers. Med Sci (Basel) 2018;6(2). https://doi.org/10.3390/medsci6020046.
5. Merikangas KR, He J, Burstein M, et al. Lifetime prevalence of mental disorders in U.S. adolescents: results from the national comorbidity survey replication–adolescent supplement (NCS-A). J Am Acad Child Adolesc Psychiatry 2010;49(10):980–9.
6. Polanczyk GV, Salum GA, Sugaya LS, et al. Annual research review: a meta-analysis of the worldwide prevalence of mental disorders in children and adolescents. J Child Psychol Psychiatry 2015;56(3):345–65.
7. Merikangas KR, He J-P, Brody D, et al. Prevalence and treatment of mental disorders among US children in the 2001-2004 NHANES. Pediatrics 2010;125(1):75–81.
8. Gradisar M, Gardner G, Dohnt H. Recent worldwide sleep patterns and problems during adolescence: a review and meta-analysis of age, region, and sleep. Sleep Med 2011;12(2):110–8.
9. Owens J. Classification and epidemiology of childhood sleep disorders. Sleep Med Clin 2007;2(3):353–61.
10. Calhoun SL, Fernandez-Mendoza J, Vgontzas AN, et al. Prevalence of insomnia symptoms in a general population sample of young children and preadolescents: gender effects. Sleep Med 2014;15(1):91–5.
11. Johnson EO, Roth T, Schultz L, et al. Epidemiology of DSM-IV insomnia in adolescence: lifetime prevalence, chronicity, and an emergent gender difference. Pediatrics 2006;117(2):E247–56.
12. Bixler EO, Vgontzas AN, Lin H-M, et al. Sleep disordered breathing in children in a general population sample: prevalence and risk factors. Sleep 2009;32(6):731–6.

13. Meltzer LJ, Johnson C, Crosette J, et al. Prevalence of diagnosed sleep disorders in pediatric primary care practices. Pediatrics 2010;125(6):e1410–8.

14. Mindell JA, Owens JA. Sleep problems in pediatric practice: clinical issues for the pediatric nurse practitioner. J Pediatr Health Care 2003;17(6):324–31.

15. Sadeh A, Mindell J, Rivera L. "My child has a sleep problem": a cross-cultural comparison of parental definitions. Sleep Med 2011;12(5):478–82.

16. Honaker SM, Meltzer LJ. Sleep in pediatric primary care: a review of the literature. Sleep Med Rev 2016;25:31–9.

17. Faruqui F, Khubchandani J, Price JH, et al. Sleep disorders in children: a national assessment of primary care pediatrician practices and perceptions. Pediatrics 2011;128(3):539–46.

18. Rosen R, Mahowald M, Chesson A, et al. The taskforce 2000 survey on medical education in sleep and sleep disorders. Sleep 1998;21(3):235–8.

19. Current pediatric physicians workforce data book. the American board of pediatrics. Available at: https://www.abp.org/content/recent-publications-annual-workforce-data-book-and-archived-data. Accessed March 12, 2020.

20. American board of psychiatry and neurology. Available at: https://application.abpn.com/verifycert/verifycert.asp. Accessed March 12, 2020.

21. Katz SL, Weiss SK, Fleetham JA. Pediatric sleep disorder medicine training in Canada: past, present and future. Sleep Med 2019;56:38–40.

22. Sadeh A, Raviv A, Gruber R. Sleep patterns and sleep disruptions in school-age children. Dev Psychol 2000;36(3):291–301.

23. Alfano CA, Pina AA, Zerr AA, et al. Pre-sleep arousal and sleep problems of anxiety-disordered youth. Child Psychiatry Hum Dev 2010;41(2):156–67.

24. Camhi SL, Morgan WJ, Pernisco N, et al. Factors affecting sleep disturbances in children and adolescents. Sleep Med 2000;1(2):117–23.

25. Liu X, Liu L, Owens JA, et al. Sleep patterns and sleep problems among school-children in the United States and China. Pediatrics 2005;115(1 Suppl):241–9.

26. Lund HG, Reider BD, Whiting AB, et al. Sleep patterns and predictors of disturbed sleep in a large population of college students. J Adolesc Health 2010;46(2):124–32.

27. Wolfson AR, Carskadon MA. Understanding adolescents' sleep patterns and school performance: a critical appraisal. Sleep Med Rev 2003;7(6):491–506.

28. Owens J. Insufficient Sleep in adolescents and young adults: an update on causes and consequences. Pediatrics 2014;134(3):e921–32.

29. Thorpy MJ. International Classification of Sleep Disorders. In: Chokroverty S, editor. Sleep Disorders Medicine: Basic Science, Technical Considerations and Clinical Aspects. New York: Springer; 2017. p. 475–84.

30. Association AP. Diagnostic and statistical manual of mental disorders (DSM-5®). Washington, DC: American Psychiatric Pub; 2013.

31. International classification of sleep disorders. 3rd edition. American Academy of Sleep Medicine; 2014. Available at: https://europepmc.org/article/med/25367475. Accessed April 9, 2020.

32. Millman RP. Excessive sleepiness in adolescents and young adults: causes, consequences, and treatment strategies. Pediatrics 2005;115(6):1774–86.

33. Hoban TF, Chervin RD. Assessment of sleepiness in children. Semin Pediatr Neurol 2001;8(4):216–28.

34. Arora T, Broglia E, Thomas GN, et al. Associations between specific technologies and adolescent sleep quantity, sleep quality, and parasomnias. Sleep Med 2014;15(2):240–7.

35. Poulain T, Vogel M, Buzek T, et al. Reciprocal longitudinal associations between adolescents' media consumption and sleep. Behav Sleep Med 2019;17(6): 763–77.
36. Owens J, Dalzell V. Use of the 'BEARS' sleep screening tool in a pediatric residents' continuity clinic: a pilot study. Sleep Med 2005;6(1):63–9.
37. Spruyt K, Gozal D. Pediatric sleep questionnaires as diagnostic or epidemiological tools: a review of currently available instruments. Sleep Med Rev 2011;15(1): 19–32.
38. Spruyt K, Gozal D. Development of pediatric sleep questionnaires as diagnostic or epidemiological tools: a brief review of Dos and Don'ts. Sleep Med Rev 2011; 15(1):7–17.
39. Lewandowski AS, Toliver-Sokol M, Palermo TM. Evidence-based review of subjective pediatric sleep measures. J Pediatr Psychol 2011;36(7):780–93.
40. Mindell JA, Owens JA. A clinical guide to pediatric sleep: diagnosis and management of sleep problems. Philadelphia: Lippincott Williams & Wilkins; 2015.
41. Meltzer LJ, Mindell JA. Sleep and sleep disorders in children and adolescents. Psychiatr Clin 2006;29(4):1059–76.
42. Carney CE, Buysse DJ, Ancoli-Israel S, et al. The consensus sleep diary: standardizing prospective sleep self-monitoring. Sleep 2012;35(2):287–302.
43. Werner H, Molinari L, Guyer C, et al. Agreement rates between actigraphy, diary, and questionnaire for children's sleep patterns. Arch Pediatr Adolesc Med 2008; 162(4):350–8.
44. Tetreault E, Belanger M-E, Bernier A, et al. Actigraphy data in pediatric research: the role of sleep diaries. Sleep Med 2018;47:86–92.
45. Short MA, Gradisar M, Lack LC, et al. The discrepancy between actigraphic and sleep diary measures of sleep in adolescents. Sleep Med 2012;13(4):378–84.
46. Tonetti L, Mingozzi R, Natale V. Comparison between paper and electronic sleep diary. Biol Rhythm Res 2016;47(5):743–53.
47. Marcus CL, Brooks LJ, Draper KA, et al. Diagnosis and management of childhood obstructive sleep apnea syndrome. Pediatrics 2012;130(3):576–84.
48. Beck SE, Marcus CL. Pediatric polysomnography. Sleep Med Clin 2009;4(3): 393–406.
49. Massicotte C, Al-Saleh S, Witmans M, et al. The utility of a portable sleep monitor to diagnose sleep-disordered breathing in a pediatric population. Can Respir J 2014;21(1):31–5.
50. Rothney MP, Apker GA, Song Y, et al. Comparing the performance of three generations of ActiGraph accelerometers. J Appl Phys 2008;105(4):1091–7.
51. Meltzer LJ, Montgomery-Downs HE, Insana SP, et al. Use of actigraphy for assessment in pediatric sleep research. Sleep Med Rev 2012;16(5):463–75.
52. Sadeh A. The role and validity of actigraphy in sleep medicine: an update. Sleep Med Rev 2011;15(4):259–67.
53. Shelgikar AV, Anderson PF, Stephens MR. Sleep tracking, wearable technology, and opportunities for research and clinical care. Chest 2016;150(3):732–43.
54. Smith MT, McCrae CS, Cheung J, et al. Use of actigraphy for the evaluation of sleep disorders and circadian rhythm sleep-wake disorders: an American Academy of Sleep Medicine clinical practice guideline. J Clin Sleep Med 2018;14(7): 1231–7.
55. Ko P-RT, Kientz JA, Choe EK, et al. Consumer sleep technologies: a review of the landscape. J Clin Sleep Med 2015;11(12):1455–61.
56. Lee J, Finkelstein J. Consumer sleep tracking devices: a critical review. Stud Health Technol Inform 2015;210:458–60.

57. de Zambotti M, Rosas L, Colrain IM, et al. The sleep of the ring: comparison of the ŌURA sleep tracker against polysomnography. Behav Sleep Med 2017;21:1–15. Published online March.

58. Walch O, Huang Y, Forger D, et al. Sleep stage prediction with raw acceleration and photoplethysmography heart rate data derived from a consumer wearable device. Sleep 2019;42(12):zsz180.

59. Behar J, Roebuck A, Domingos JS, et al. A review of current sleep screening applications for smartphones. Physiol Meas 2013;34(7):R29–46.

60. Seema K, Deak Maryann C, Dominic Gault, et al. Consumer sleep technology: an American Academy of Sleep Medicine position statement. J Clin Sleep Med 2018;14(05):877–80.

61. Kruse CS, Karem P, Shifflett K, et al. Evaluating barriers to adopting telemedicine worldwide: a systematic review. J Telemed Telecare 2016. https://doi.org/10.1177/1357633X16674087. Published online October 16.

62. Singh Jaspal, Safwan Badr M, Wendy Diebert, et al. American academy of sleep medicine (AASM) position paper for the use of telemedicine for the diagnosis and treatment of sleep disorders. J Clin Sleep Med 2015;11(10):1187–98.

63. Committee on Pediatric Workforce, Marcin JP, Rimsza ME, Moskowitz WB. The use of telemedicine to address access and physician workforce shortages. Pediatrics 2015;136(1):202–9.

64. Myers K, Cain S. Practice parameter for telepsychiatry with children and adolescents. J Am Acad Child Adolesc Psychiatry 2008;47(12):1468–83.

65. Witmans MB, Dick B, Good J, et al. Delivery of pediatric sleep services via telehealth: the Alberta experience and lessons learned. Behav Sleep Med 2008;6(4):207–19.

66. Ekeland AG, Bowes A, Flottorp S. Effectiveness of telemedicine: a systematic review of reviews. Int J Med Inf 2010;79(11):736–71.

67. Zia S, Fields BG. Sleep telemedicine: an emerging field's latest frontier. Chest 2016;149(6):1556–65.

68. Murphie P, Paton R, Scholefield C, et al. Telesleep medicine review - patient and clinician experience. Eur Respir J 2014;44(Suppl 58). Available at: https://erj.ersjournals.com/content/44/Suppl_58/P3283. Accessed June 4, 2020.

69. Spaulding R, Stevens D, Velasquez SE. Experience with telehealth for sleep monitoring and sleep laboratory management. J Telemed Telecare 2011;17(7):346–9.

70. Penzel T, Glos M, Schöbel C, et al. Telemedizin und telemetrische Aufzeichnungsmethoden zur Diagnostik in der Schlafmedizin. Somnologie 2018;22(3):199–208.

71. Drake C, Nickel C, Burduvali E, et al. The pediatric daytime sleepiness scale (PDSS): sleep habits and school outcomes in middle-school children. Sleep 2003;26(4):455–8.

72. Spilsbury JC, Drotar D, Rosen CL, et al. The Cleveland adolescent sleepiness questionnaire. J Clin Sleep Med 2007;3(6):603–12.

73. Janssen KC, Phillipson S, O'Connor J, et al. Validation of the Epworth Sleepiness Scale for children and adolescents using Rasch analysis. Sleep Med 2017;33:30–5.

74. Amschler DH, McKenzie JF. Elementary students' sleep habits and teacher observations of sleep-related problems. J Sch Health 2005;75(2):50–6.

75. Owens J, Spirito A, McGuinn M, et al. Sleep habits and sleep disturbance in elementary school-aged children. J Dev Behav Pediatr 2000;21(1):27–36.

76. Harsh J, Easley A, Lebourgeois M. A measure of sleep hygiene. Sleep 2002;25: A316.
77. Henderson JA, Jordan SS. Development and preliminary evaluation of the bedtime routines questionnaire. J Psychopathol Behav Assess 2010;32(2): 271–80.
78. Storfer-Isser A, LeBourgeois M, Harsh J, et al. Psychometric properties of the adolescent sleep hygiene scale (ASHS). J Sleep Res 2013;22(6). https://doi. org/10.1111/jsr.12059.
79. Bruni O, Ottaviano S, Guidetti V, et al. The sleep disturbance scale for children (SDSC). Construction and validation of an instrument to evaluate sleep distur- bances in childhood and adolescence. J Sleep Res 1996;5(4):251–61.
80. Owens J, Spirito A, McGuinn M. The children's sleep habits questionnaire (CSHQ): psychometric properties of a survey instrument for school-aged chil- dren. Sleep 2000;23(8):1043–51.
81. Chervin RD, Hedger K, Dillon JE, et al. Pediatric sleep questionnaire (PSQ): val- idity and reliability of scales for sleep-disordered breathing, snoring, sleepiness, and behavioral problems. Sleep Med 2000;1(1):21–32.

# Medications Used for Pediatric Insomnia

Vijayabharathi Ekambaram, MD, MPH[a],*, Judith Owens, MD, MPH[b]

## KEYWORDS

- Insomnia • Sleep disorders • Pharmacotherapy • Medications • Pediatrics
- Children

## KEY POINTS

- There are no Food and Drug Administration–approved medications for pediatric insomnia.
- Pharmacologic interventions derived mostly from adult data or case reports in pediatric populations.
- Medication selection should be based on the clinician's judgment of the best possible match between the clinical circumstances and the properties of currently available drugs.
- Pharmacologic management should be considered in combination with behavior therapy, which proven to have long-lasting patient outcomes.

## INTRODUCTION

Insomnia in children and adolescents can be related to many different etiologic factors, and often there is more than 1 contributing condition. These include behavioral issues, psychiatric conditions such as anxiety and mood disorders, underlying medical disorders including chronic pain and sleep-disrupting medications, primary sleep disorders such as restless legs syndrome, and neurodevelopmental disorders, including autism.[1]

The prevalence of pediatric insomnia varies across age groups; frequent night awakenings are reported among 40% of infants, disruptive nighttime awakenings are seen in 25% to 50% of preschoolers, bedtime resistance in school-age children ranges from 15% to 27%, and insomnia in adolescents is reported to be as high as 11%.[1–3] In the case of children with special needs, a higher prevalence rate of 50% to 75% has been reported owing to sleep dysregulation caused by several factors

This article originally appeared in *Child and Adolescent Psychiatric Clinics*, Volume 30 Issue 1, January 2021.

[a] Department of Psychiatry, University of Central Florida, HCA Florida Healthcare Program, 8383 N. Davis Hwy, Pensacola, FL 32514, USA; [b] Department of Neurology, Boston Children's Hospital, Harvard Medical School, Boston, MA 02115, USA
* Corresponding author.
*E-mail address:* ekambaram.md@gmail.com

such as increased arousals, delayed sleep onset latencies, sleep deprivation, and concomitant medication use.[2,4]

Pediatric insomnia can significantly affect physical health, mental health, and can result in daytime sleepiness, mood dysregulation, impulsivity, hyperactivity, cognitive deficits, social deficits, and decreased quality of life.[1,2]

Behavioral interventions such as sleep hygiene education (eg, consistent sleep schedule, avoidance of electronic devices before bedtime), sleep restriction (matching time in bed with time asleep), relaxation techniques, and cognitive restructuring are considered the mainstays of treatment for pediatric insomnia.[1] Pharmacotherapy should only be considered when behavioral techniques are ineffective and should be used in combination with behavioral interventions.

Furthermore, there is a lack of evidence-based literature related to efficacy, safety, and tolerability of medications used in treating children with insomnia, and it is noteworthy to point out that currently, there are no medications approved by the US Food and Drug Administration (FDA) for pediatric insomnia. Pharmacologic intervention for pediatric insomnia derived mostly from adult data or case reports or small case series in pediatric populations. Very few published studies have documented the effectiveness of hypnotic/sedative use in children using randomized placebo-controlled clinical trials.[1,2,5]

Despite the dearth of data, off-label medications and over-the-counter (OTC) sleep aids are prescribed frequently by practitioners. In a national survey, about 88% of the child psychiatry practitioners recommended OTC medicines for the treatment of insomnia in a typical month.[3,6] Because many prescribing pediatric health care providers, including those in primary care and mental health settings, lack sufficient education in the use of sedative/hypnotics, incorrect medication selection, overdosing, or underdosing can occur. Therefore, providers must learn general principles, practice guidelines, and pharmacologic considerations for treatment selection in insomnia.[5]

This review article provides general principles of medication use for insomnia in children, followed by a discussion of specific features of those sleep medications that have been identified as commonly used in pediatric settings. Thus, although whenever possible empirical data will be included, this review primarily focuses on general principles, rather than empirically based guidelines for the rational use of these medications in clinical practice.

## GENERAL PRINCIPLES FOR MEDICATION USE IN PEDIATRIC INSOMNIA
### Clinical Considerations

1. Treatment strategies should always be diagnostically driven and based on the systematic evaluation of possible etiologic factors.
2. Medication is rarely a first choice or sole treatment. In almost all cases, the medication should be used in combination with nonpharmacologic behavioral management strategies. Although pharmacologic interventions may have a more rapid effect, nonpharmacologic treatments have been shown to result in more sustained improvement.[7,8] Combining therapies also helps to minimize side effects.
3. Existing unhealthy sleep practices should be addressed, and treatment recommendations must include the institution of more appropriate sleep behaviors. Healthy sleep practices, commonly referred to as "good sleep hygiene," include modifiable daytime, bedtime, and within-sleep practices that positively impact sleep to wake transitions, psychophysiological arousal, and the sleep environment.
4. Psychoeducation regarding the basics of sleep and sleep regulation is a critical component of responsible medication management. For example, a late-day nap

may decrease the sleep drive such that even large doses of medication are ineffective in facilitating sleep initiation at the desired bedtime. Clinicians can help parents to understand the appropriate role of pharmacotherapy by explaining that sleep is a biological function that is influenced by multiple internal and external facilitating and inhibiting factors and that medication acts to facilitate but does not cause sleep.

5. Clear, well-defined treatment goals must be established with the patient and family. Treatment outcomes should be realistic, clearly defined, and measurable. Caregiver expectations regarding the potential impact of pharmacotherapy must be explicitly stated and appropriate. For example, the immediate goal of treatment should be to alleviate or improve rather than eliminate sleep problems.

6. Potential modifications in dosage and timing should be reviewed ahead of time with the family. For example, is the medication to be given on a nightly or an intermittent as-needed basis? If the latter, what are the criteria for administering the medication on any given night (eg, sleep onset latency >45 minutes)? If middle-of-the-night dosing for night wakings is to be used, what parameters govern this dosing (eg, there must be at least a 4-hour remaining sleep opportunity)?

7. Any hypnotics, particularly those with high toxicity levels in overdose, should be used with extreme caution in patients with a history of depression owing to the risk of nonaccidental overdose.

8. Adolescents should be screened for alcohol and drug use before initiation of sleep medication, as many recreational substances may have additive effects when combined with sedatives/hypnotics.

### Pharmacologic Considerations

1. Treatment selection should be based on the clinician's judgment of the best possible match between the clinical circumstances (the type of sleep problem, patient characteristics, etc) and the properties of currently available drugs (onset of action, safety, tolerability, etc). Medication selection, particularly onset and duration of action, should be appropriate for the presenting complaint. For example, for children with sleep-onset problems, a shorter acting medication is generally desirable, whereas longer acting medications should be considered for sleep maintenance problems.

2. Consideration should be given to the timing of drug administration relative to the targeted time of sleep onset (eg, within 30 minutes of lights out) and to the second-wind phenomenon. Circadian-mediated alertness in adults and children typically increases in the evening hours just before sleep onset, making it more difficult to fall asleep during this 1- or 2-hour window. Most hypnotic medications have their onset of action within 30 minutes of administration and peak within 1 to 2 hours. Thus, giving the medication too early (eg, 2 hours before sleep onset) is not only less likely to be effective than dosing closer to bedtime, but may induce a dissociative phenomenon (ie, disinhibition, hallucinations) when administered during this window of increased circadian alertness.[5]

3. Dosing should be initiated at the lowest level likely to be effective and increased as necessary. There should be clearly defined criteria for dose escalation with simultaneous monitoring for side effects. Close communication with the family with frequent follow-up visits is key to successful and safe management.

4. Medication should be used with caution when there is a potential for pharmacodynamic drug–drug interaction with concurrent medications (eg, opiates) or pharmacokinetic drug–drug interaction (eg, fluoxetine, a CYP2D6 and -2C19 inhibitor and diphenhydramine).

5. Caregivers and patients should be questioned regarding concurrent use of parent or self-initiated nonprescription sleep medications (acetaminophen with diphenhydramine [Tylenol PM], melatonin, herbals), as well as other OTC medications. In some cases, OTC sleep medications may interact with other prescription or OTC drugs or may exacerbate an underlying medical condition. Although generally viewed by parents as safe, the potential drug–drug interactions between most OTC and complementary and alternative therapies (ie, herbal preparations) and sedative/hypnotics, as well as with other medications is largely unknown and thus should be approached with caution.
6. In general, abrupt discontinuation of medications, especially those that are being used on a nightly basis over a period of time, should be avoided. Drugs should be tapered gradually to decrease the possibility of rebound insomnia. This phenomenon is especially prevalent at higher doses and with short or intermediate half-life drugs
7. It is essential at the outset of treatment to have a defined exit strategy in terms of expectations regarding the duration of treatment; the clinician should begin planning for discontinuation of medication at the time of initiation. The length of therapy should be discussed and clarified with the family at the outset.

### Tolerability

1. All medications prescribed for sleep problems should be closely monitored for the emergence of adverse effects. Some medications may also precipitate or exacerbate coexisting sleep problems such as sleepwalking and daytime sleepiness. Furthermore, discontinuation of these agents may also result in increased sleep problems. For example, an increase in nightmares may be seen when REM-suppressing medication is abruptly withdrawn as a result of a subsequent rebound REM sleep.
2. Insomnia in children commonly occurs with other primary sleep disorders (eg, obstructive sleep apnea, restless legs syndrome). Thus, the presence of both medically based and behaviorally based sleep disorders warrants attention. Also, the pharmacologic treatment of insomnia could exacerbate the coexisting sleep problems. For example, sedative/hypnotics with respiratory depressant properties (eg, benzodiazepines [BZDs]) and medications that may cause significant weight gain (eg, mirtazapine) should be avoided if the insomnia occurs in the presence of obstructive sleep apnea, and sedating selective serotonin reuptake inhibitors should be used with caution in the presence of insomnia, as they may increase symptoms of restless legs syndrome.

## SPECIFIC FEATURES OF MEDICATIONS USED FOR PEDIATRIC INSOMNIA

The discussion is focused mainly on 3 major categories of medications: (I) FDA-approved prescription drugs (in adults), (II) OTC drugs, and (III) off-label pediatric insomnia drugs. The clinical properties of selected medications are summarized in **Table 1**.

### Prescription Drugs Approved by the US Food and Drug Administration (in Adults)

#### Benzodiazepine receptor agonists and benzodiazepines

BZDs act primarily through gamma-aminobutyric acid (GABA).[9] The inhibitory neurotransmitter GABA's action on the central nervous system contributes to anxiolytic, anticonvulsant, sedative, and muscle-relaxing effects of BZDs.[4,9] The shorter acting BZDs are used in treating sleep-onset insomnia, and longer acting BZDs are used

**Table 1**
Clinical properties of selected medications used for pediatric insomnia

| Medications | Mechanism of Action | Suggested Pediatric Dosing Range (mg/d)[a] | Formulations | Common Side Effects | Comments |
|---|---|---|---|---|---|
| Benzodiazepine receptor agonists Clonazepam (Klonopin)[b] | Bind to central GABA receptors | 0.5–2.0 | Tablet, orally disintegrating tablet | Residual daytime sedation, rebound insomnia on discontinuation, psychomotor impairment, anterograde amnesia (dose dependent); respiratory impairment function | Also used to control partial arousal parasomnias (night terrors, sleepwalking) |
| Nonbenzodiazepine receptor agonists Zolpidem (Ambien)[b] Zaleplon (Sonata)[b] | Bind to $\alpha_1$-subunits GABA receptors | 5–10 | Tablet, oral spray, sublingual tablet | Headache, retrograde amnesia; few residual next-day effects | Little clinical experience in children |
| Synthetic melatonin receptor agonist Ramelteon (Rozerem)[b] | Selective affinity $MT_1$, $MT_2$ receptors | 4–8 | Tablet | Fatigue, headache, and dizziness | Avoid coadministration with fluvoxamine |
| Selective histamine receptor antagonist Doxepin (Silenor)[b] | Selective antagonism of the histamine receptor | 3–6 | Tablet, capsule, oral liquid concentrate | Daytime somnolence and residual next-day effect | Used for sleep maintenance insomnia |
| Dual orexin receptor antagonists Suvorexant (Belsomra)[b] Lemborexant (Dayvigo)[b] | Bind to OX1 R and OX2 R receptors and inhibit the activation of the arousal system | 5–20 5–10 | Tablet | Daytime somnolence and abnormal dreams | Schedule IV drugs |

(continued on next page)

**Table 1**
*(continued)*

| Medications | Mechanism of Action | Suggested Pediatric Dosing Range (mg/d)[a] | Formulations | Common Side Effects | Comments |
|---|---|---|---|---|---|
| Antihistamines Diphenhydramine (Benadryl) Cyproheptadine (Periactin) Hydroxyzine (Atarax) | Competitive histamine receptor blocker in the central nervous system | 25–50 4–8 25–100 | Tablet, capsule, syrup, injectable | Daytime drowsiness, gastrointestinal (appetite loss, vomiting, constipation, dry mouth), paradoxic excitation | Weak soporifics; high-level parental/ practitioner acceptance |
| Hormone analog Melatonin | Main effect suprachiasmatic nucleus; nonselective action at $MT_1$ and $MT_2$ receptors | 2.5–5.0 (0.3–25.0) | Tablet; various strengths | Headache, nightmares, morning grogginess; Possible exacerbation of comorbid autoimmune diseases | Used in children with developmental disabilities, autism, neurologic impairment, blindness; jet lag |
| α-Agonists Clonidine (Catapres) Guanfacine (Tenex) | α-Adrenergic receptor agonists; (guanfacine more selective) decrease NE release | 0.050–0.225 0.5–2.0 | Tablet, transdermal patch | Dry mouth, bradycardia, hypotension, rebound hypertension on discontinuation | Also used in daytime treatment of attention-deficit/ hyperactivity disorder |
| Atypical antidepressants Trazodone | $5\text{-}HT_{2A/C}$ antagonist | 25–50 | Tablet | Dizziness, central nervous system overstimulation, cardiac arrhythmias, hypotension, priapism | May be used with comorbid depression |

*Abbreviations:* GABA, gamma-aminobutyric acid; SOL, sleep-onset latency; SWS, slow-wave sleep (stage 3–4).
[a] When available.
[b] FDA-approved medications in adults.

for sleep maintenance. Despite the widespread use of BZDs in adults, their use in the pediatric population is limited owing to their risk of addiction and concerning side effects profile, include morning hangover, daytime sleepiness, dizziness, headaches, anterograde amnesia, rebound insomnia, and withdrawal phenomena. In patients with suspected sleep-disordered breathing, BZDs should be used in caution owing to their muscle relaxant properties.[2] Additionally, BZDs are known to cause alteration of normal sleep state architecture, causing slow-wave sleep suppression in polysomnographic studies.[4]

In children, BZDs are used only for short-term insomnia or in comorbid conditions such as anxiety disorder, seizure disorder, and some parasomnias (eg, refractory sleep terrors) in which their other properties (eg, anxiolytic, anticonvulsant, muscle relaxant) are known to be beneficial in the treatment.[2]

Few pediatric studies have documented BZDs use in children with the exception of the intermediate-acting BZD, clonazepam. Clonazepam is known to be effective in the treatment of periodic limb movement disorder and parasomnias such as sleepwalking.[2,4] The half-life of clonazepam ranges from 18 to 39 hours and reaches its maximum plasma concentration within 1 to 4 hours after oral administration. Clonazepam is also available as disintegrating tablets that are easily dissolvable when placed under the tongue.[5]

### Nonbenzodiazepine receptor agonists

Nonbenzodiazepines referred to as "Z-drugs" include zaleplon, zolpidem, and eszopiclone. Z-drugs have similar pharmacology to BZDs but with different chemical structures.[4] They selectively bind and activate the $\alpha_1$ subunits of the GABA-A receptor complex.[10]

Zaleplon (ultra short acting, 1- to 2-hour half-life) and zolpidem (short acting, 2- to 3-hour half-life) are primarily used in sleep initiation. Sublingual forms of zolpidem and zaleplon are also used in middle of the night insomnia (if $\geq 5$ hours remain before the desired wake time).[11] The intermediate-to-long acting forms (5- to 7-hour half-life), eszopiclone, and zolpidem-CR are used in sleep maintenance.[2,12]

Zaleplon can trigger sleepwalking in adolescents and is reported to cause drowsiness, ataxia, dizziness, confusion, and blurred speech in nonaccidental overdose.[13] Zolpidem-induced complex sleep-related behaviors such as sleep eating, sleepwalking, and sleep driving have been documented extensively in adult studies, which raise concerns about its use in the pediatric population.[2,14,15] Eszopiclone can cause an unpleasant metallic taste and headaches.[2,12]

Unlike BZDs, z-drugs in their recommended doses do not typically cause rebound insomnia (a worsening of insomnia on abrupt cessation of a hypnotic) with abrupt discontinuation.[5] Longer duration trials of z-drugs in adults suggest continued hypnotic benefit at 6 months, without the development of tolerance.[12] The potential side effects of z-drugs include headaches, dizziness, anterograde amnesia, confusion, and hallucinations.[13] Z-drugs are contraindicated in patients with sleep apnea because they blunt the arousal response to hypoxemia and can deteriorate apnea.[2]

**Melatonin receptor agonists.** Ramelteon is the only FDA-approved synthetic melatonin receptor agonist used in the treatment of insomnia in adults.[16] It has a high affinity for melatonin-1 and melatonin-2 receptors located in the suprachiasmatic nucleus; melatonin-1 promotes sleep initiation whereas melatonin-2 regulates the circadian sleep–wake cycle.[16–18] Ramelteon seems to act primarily through action on melatonin-1.[16–18] Clinical studies of ramelteon have shown a reduction in sleep latency compared with placebo, but subjective improvements are less consistently reported than objective (ie, polysomnography) improvements in sleep onset latency.[19] Ramelteon has rapid oral absorption, short elimination half-life (1.0 to 2.6 hours), and its pharmacokinetics are altered by high-fat meals.[16]

Pediatric case series have documented ramelteon to be quite effective in the treatment of insomnia in children; it is well-tolerated without any daytime sedation.[17,20,21] Frequently reported adverse events include fatigue, headache, and dizziness.[20] Adult data suggest there was no evidence of next-day impairment associated with the use of ramelteon.[16,20] In contrast with GABA modulators, ramelteon has not shown potential for abuse, dependence, withdrawal, and rebound insomnia, and it is not a scheduled drug.[16,17,21]

**Selective histamine receptor antagonists.** The old tricyclic antidepressant, doxepin (Silenor) at a low dose (3–6 mg), is FDA approved for sleep maintenance insomnia but not for sleep-onset insomnia. At this low dose, doxepin exerts its sedative effect through selective antagonism of the histamine H1 receptor.[22] It has a longer time to maximum plasma concentration of 2 to 8 hours and its elimination half-life is close to 24 hours.[22–24] The drug has not been studied in the pediatric population. Adult clinical studies have documented improvement in total sleep time, quality of sleep, and a decrease in wake after sleep onset compared with placebo.[19] The common adverse effects reported were daytime somnolence and residual next-day effect with the 6 mg dose.[22]

Doxepin is not a scheduled drug, and it does not have any abuse potential. It is available in a generic formulation as 10 mg capsules or 10 mg/mL oral liquid concentrate, but these formulations have not been approved by the FDA for insomnia treatment.[19,22,23]

**Dual orexin receptor antagonists.** Suvorexant, a dual orexin receptor antagonist, blocks orexin receptors (OX1R and OX2R) and promotes sleep by reducing wakefulness and arousal.[24–26] It is classified under schedule IV drugs owing to its potential for addiction. Owing to its higher cost and addictive potential, it is not recommended as a first-line treatment for insomnia.[25] Clinical studies of suvorexant have documented improvement in total sleep time and a decrease in wake after sleep onset compared with placebo.[19] A small trial of suvorexant in adolescents found it to be relatively safe. The most noticeable side effects reported in the trial were daytime somnolence and abnormal dreams; otherwise, it was well-tolerated.[25]

A newer dual orexin receptor antagonist, lemborexant, was approved by the FDA on December 20, 2019 under scheduled IV category.[26,27] Lemborexant has more OX2R inhibition, and it dissociates rapidly from orexin receptors compared with suvorexant, so it is expected to have less risk of daytime sedation.[26,27]

### Over-the-Counter Drugs

#### Antihistamines

Antihistamines are often considered acceptable choices for families and health care providers owing to their familiarity, low cost, and availability.[3] First-generation antihistamines (eg, diphenhydramine, cyproheptadine, hydroxyzine) act as competitive histamine receptor blockers in the central nervous system and peripheral nervous system. They are lipid soluble, rapidly absorbed, can easily pass through the blood–brain barrier, causing significant sedative and hypnotic effects compared with second- and third-generation antihistamines.[2,4]

Antihistamines are generally well-tolerated in children, and their effects on sleep architecture seem to be minimal. A randomized controlled trial in school-aged children documented subjective improvement in sleep latency and night waking.[28] However, another more recent pediatric study found that antihistamines were not more effective than placebo in decreasing nighttime awakening in young children.[29]

Both diphenhydramine and cyproheptadine are available OTC medications; hydroxyzine requires a prescription.[2,4,30] The potential side effects include daytime drowsiness, fever, blurred vision, dry mouth, constipation, urinary retention, tachycardia, and confusion. Diphenhydramine can also exacerbate restless legs syndrome symptoms. Tolerance can develop quickly with these medications and often require higher dosing, which in turn leads to worsening adverse effects.[2,4,30] These properties make them poorly suited for long-term use.

### Melatonin

Melatonin, a pineal hormone, plays a significant role in the regulation of circadian sleep–wake cycles and core body temperature rhythms. The sedative property of melatonin is through nonselective action at $MT_1$, and $MT_2$ receptors located within the suprachiasmatic nucleus in the hypothalamus and its production is inhibited by exposure of the retina to light.[2,4]

Melatonin promotes sleep through both chronobiotic (ie, shifts the circadian sleep–wake cycle) and hypnotic (ie, sedating) effects, depending on the dose and timing of administration. For example, a relatively larger hypnotic dose of melatonin (ie, 3–5 mg) can be administered close to bedtime (30 minutes prior) for the decrease of sleep-onset latency in insomnia.[2] Alternatively, in children with circadian phase delay, a smaller chronobiotic dose of melatonin (eg, 0.3–0.5 mg) can be administered earlier in the evening.

Melatonin is generally well-tolerated, and there is considerable empirical evidence for the use of melatonin in the pediatric population, especially in children with special needs.[31,32] Studies have documented that significant reduction in sleep-onset latency both in healthy children[33] and in children with attention-deficit/hyperactivity disorder, based on the premise that some of these children have a circadian-mediated phase delay (ie, delayed sleep onset and offset compared with developmental norms).[34,35] Melatonin is also clinically used in the correction of chronic or acute circadian rhythm disturbances in healthy children (eg, delayed sleep phase syndrome, jet lag) and in children with neurodevelopmental disorders (eg, blindness, Rett syndrome, autism).[36]

Melatonin is commercially available over the counter in different formulations, and it is not regulated by the FDA. Melatonin is also available in liquid preparations. These formulations often vary in strength, purity, and efficacy of melatonin. A concern is often raised regarding the actual content of melatonin in these commercial brands.

A recent study that analyzed a total of 31 commercial supplements by chromatography, documented that actual melatonin content ranged from −83% to +478% of the labeled content; in addition, serotonin (5-hydroxytryptamine) was identified in more than one-quarter of the commercially available brands.[37] Because of these variations, the use of pharmaceutical-grade melatonin (available on the Internet) should be considered. Melatonin has low and variable bioavailability owing to extensive first-pass metabolism, and younger children seem to metabolize it more rapidly than older children.

The immediate release form of melatonin has a half-life of close to 45 minutes, and it reaches its peak plasma concentration within 1 hour of administration.[24] There are no clear-cut dosing guidelines for melatonin, and its effective dosing varies across studies. Based on the 2012 recommendations of a Canadian Pediatric Society study, a 2014 European expert consensus treatment guidelines, and an open-label study of melatonin for children with insomnia, the commonly recommended doses of melatonin are 1 mg in infants, 2.5 to 3.0 mg in older children, and 5.0 mg in adolescents.[38–40] In children with special needs, the reported dosing ranges from 0.5 to 10.0 mg, irrespective of age[5,38]; however, it should be noted that the 2014 treatment guidelines recommend a maximum dose: less than 40 kg, 3 mg, and greater than 40 kg, 5 mg.[40] As noted elsewhere in this article, a delay in sleep-onset initiation owing to a circadian-based phase delay may respond better to a small dose (0.5 mg) in the evening; although studies (largely in adults) vary somewhat with regard to timing of melatonin administration as a chronobiotic, recommendations are typically12 hours before desired bedtime or 4 to 5 hours before actual bedtime.[1,2,41,42]

Melatonin is also available in controlled release formulations with prolonged half-life of 3.5 to 4.0 hours, which may be used for sleep maintenance.[24] Although clinical trials of the controlled release melatonin minitablet (Circadin-CR) have yielded promising results, in the EU, use of extended-release preparations in the United States is limited by the lack of formulations that do not require swallowing a pill or capsule.

Melatonin generally has a low side effect profile and generally considered safe even under conditions of long-term use.[43] However, prospective longitudinal studies are lacking, and a theoretic side effect of suppression of the hypothalamic–gonadal axis by melatonin has been proposed based on increased endogenous melatonin in males with delayed puberty.[44] Owing to its immunomodulating properties, melatonin should be used with caution in children with some immune disorders or who are on immuno-suppressants (ie, corticosteroids).[2,45]

### Herbal preparations

The commonly used herbal supplements for sleep disorders include valerian, chamomile, kava-kava, tryptophan, and lavender.[46] Valerian root and chamomile bind to BZD receptors and produce mild sedating effects.[46] Valerian has been documented in several adult studies to have sleep promotion without the hangover effects seen with the BZDs.[47]

Kava-kava and lavender have a depressive effect on the central nervous system. Aromatherapy with volatilized lavender has been reported in several small studies to improve sleep quality.[46] L-Tryptophan, an essential amino acid, has been documented in the treatment of insomnia in adults. Pediatric studies of L-tryptophan have shown sleep promotion and improvement in childhood parasomnias by decreasing the sleep fragmentation.[48] Herbal supplements are generally considered safe in adults; however, owing to the lack of data in the pediatric population, their safety and efficacy are unknown. Kava-kava and tryptophan have been associated with hepatotoxicity and eosinophilic myalgia syndrome, respectively, which raise significant safety concerns.[47]

### Off-Label Pediatric Insomnia Drugs

### Alpha agonists

Clonidine is a central and peripheral $\alpha2$-adrenergic receptor agonist that decreases adrenergic tone, generally used in the treatment of attention-deficit/hyperactivity disorder, and pediatric insomnia.[49] Despite its widespread use[3,6] in pediatric and psychiatry practice, the clinical data regarding safety and efficacy in children are limited.

The 2 open-label retrospective studies of clonidine in children with neurodevelopmental disorders have documented improvement in both sleep initiation and maintenance insomnia with good tolerability and few adverse events.[50,51] Owing to its rapid absorption, it has an onset of action within 1 hour, and it reaches peak effects within 2 to 4 hours. Clonidine causes minimal disruption in sleep architecture, but sometimes it may decrease both REM and slow-wave sleep. Thus, its discontinuation can cause vivid dreams, increased sleepwalking and sleep terrors (owing to a rebound increase in REM, and slow-wave sleep, respectively).[2,4]

Despite its relatively low adverse effect profile,[50] clonidine has a narrow therapeutic index, and there have been reports of overdose with this medication.[52] The potential side effects of clonidine include dry mouth, bradycardia, irritability, and hypotension; abrupt discontinuation can cause rebound hypertension. Clonidine should be avoided in patients with diabetes and Raynaud syndrome.[2,4]

Guanfacine, a selective $\alpha$2A-adrenergic receptor agonist, has less sedation and fewer cardiovascular side effects compared with clonidine owing to its $\alpha$2A-receptor selectivity.[2] Despite of lack of clinical studies in children, immediate-release guanfacine (Tenex) is frequently used for treating insomnia in pediatric and psychiatric practices. In a recent randomized, placebo-controlled trial of children with attention-deficit/hyperactivity disorder, extended-release guanfacine (Intuniv) was reported to cause an increase in wake after sleep onset, a decrease in total sleep time, and overall sleep reduction in participants.[4,53] More clinical studies are needed to evaluate the efficacy of extended-release guanfacine use in pediatric insomnia.

### Antidepressants

Tricyclic antidepressants (amitriptyline and doxepin) and atypical antidepressants (trazodone and mirtazapine) are commonly used for treating insomnia in both pediatric and adult populations.[24] Despite their widespread use, there is a lack of methodologically studies in support of their use in insomnia. Therefore, their use should generally be limited to clinical situations in which there are concurrent mood disorders with insomnia. The dosage of antidepressants for insomnia is typically less than the dosage used to treat mood disorders. Owing to their anticholinergic effects, the majority of these antidepressants suppress REM sleep, and their abrupt withdrawal may lead to REM rebound and increased nightmares.[2]

Amitriptyline (dosing, 10–25 mg) is one of the most sedating tricyclic antidepressants frequently used for insomnia. The most commonly reported side effects include blurred vision, dry mouth, urinary retention, orthostatic hypotension. Tricyclic antidepressants may also exacerbate restless legs syndrome symptoms.[2,24]

Mirtazapine, an $\alpha_2$-adrenergic, 5-HT antagonist, has a high degree of sedation at low doses (eg, 7.5 mg), and potential side effects include residual daytime sleepiness and weight gain.[2,24,54]

Trazodone, a $5-HT_{2A/C}$ antagonist, is one of the most sedating antidepressants and seems to inhibit postsynaptic binding of serotonin and block histamine receptors.[54] It can cause a morning hangover and has been associated with hypotension, arrhythmias, and serotonin syndrome; in the 50- to 150-mg dose range, it has been associated with reports of priapism in adults.[2,24]

### Antipsychotics

Atypical antipsychotics (risperidone, olanzapine, and quetiapine) are used for sleep disturbances in children with underlying psychiatric disorders (eg, bipolar disorder, mood dysregulation, and aggression). Their effect on multiple neurotransmitters (muscarinic, histaminergic, and serotoninergic) promotes sleep.[24,55] Most of these antipsychotics decrease sleep-onset latency, increase sleep continuity, and suppress REM sleep (in higher doses). Their sedating effects may also interfere with daytime functioning and learning. They can cause weight gain and thus worsen obstructive sleep apnea.[2]

### Anticonvulsants

Carbamazepine, phenobarbital, and valproic acid are all associated with increased daytime somnolence. Newer anticonvulsants have varying degrees of daytime sedation. For example, sedation rates with topiramate are 15% to 25% and 5% to 15% with gabapentin.

Gabapentin, which has effects on dopamine, serotonin, and norepinephrine, also seems to increase slow-wave sleep and improve sleep maintenance, and has been shown to decrease restless legs syndrome symptoms. In children with neurodevelopmental disorders, gabapentin (dosing range, 5–15 mg/kg) has shown promising results in improving refractory insomnia.[56] Anticonvulsants typically cause dose-dependent sedation, although tolerance to this effect may develop.

## SUMMARY

Clinicians working in pediatric settings need to evaluate all factors potentially contributing to the development and persistence of insomnia, including comorbid medical, psychiatric and neurodevelopmental disorders, coexisting sleep disorders, caregiver behaviors, and patient practices interfering with sleep before considering sedative/hypnotic medication use. Behavior therapy should always be considered as the first modality of treatment; when behavior treatment is ineffective, pharmacologic management should be considered in combination with behavior therapy, which is proven to have long-lasting patient outcomes. Overall, there are limited data in regard to medication use for pediatric insomnia. Selection of medication, when determined to be appropriate, should be based on pharmacokinetic and pharmacodynamic profiles of the individual drugs and the specific clinical circumstances (age, presence of comorbid medical or psychiatric conditions, concomitant medications, abuse potential, etc).

## CLINICS CARE POINTS

- There are currently no FDA-approved medications for pediatric insomnia.
- Recommendations for pharmacologic interventions are derived mostly from adult data, and case reports and limited randomized clinical trials in pediatric populations, as well as clinical experience.
- Medication selection should be based on the clinician's judgment of the best possible match between the clinical circumstances and the properties of currently available drugs.
- Pharmacologic management should be considered in combination with behavior therapy, which is proven to have long-lasting patient outcomes.
- Medications such as SSRIs have been shown to improve both youth anxiety as well as associated SRPs.
- OTC medications (eg, melatonin and antihistamines), and prescription medications (eg, α-agonists and antidepressants) are commonly used for treating insomnia in children.
- BZDs should be used with caution owing to their risk of addiction and concerning side effect profiles.
- Given the variability in actual content of melatonin compared with labels, the use of pharmaceutical grade melatonin is recommended.
- Adult data on insomnia medications with novel mechanisms such as suvorexant and lumborexant in the treatment of insomnia are promising. Further research is needed in the pediatric population to evaluate the efficacy and safety of these medications in children.

## DISCLOSURE

The authors have nothing to disclose.

## REFERENCES

1. Owens JA, Mindell JA. Pediatric insomnia. Pediatr Clin North Am 2011;58(3): 555–69.
2. Owens JA, Moturi S. Pharmacologic treatment of pediatric insomnia. Child Adolesc Psychiatr Clin N Am 2009;18(4):1001–16.
3. Owens JA, Rosen CL, Mindell JA. Medication use in the treatment of pediatric insomnia: results of a survey of community-based pediatricians. Pediatrics 2003;111(5 Pt 1):e628–35.
4. Relia S, Ekambaram V. Pharmacological approach to sleep disturbances in autism spectrum disorders with psychiatric comorbidities: a literature review. Med Sci (Basel) 2018;6(4).
5. Pelayo R, Dubik M. Pediatric sleep pharmacology. Semin Pediatr Neurol 2008; 15(2):79–90.
6. Owens JA, Rosen CL, Mindell JA, et al. Use of pharmacotherapy for insomnia in child psychiatry practice: a national survey. Sleep Med 2010;11(7):692–700.
7. Mindell JA, Kuhn B, Lewin DS, et al. Behavioral treatment of bedtime problems and night wakings in infants and young children. Sleep 2006;29(10):1263–76.
8. Mindell JA, Emslie G, Blumer J, et al. Pharmacologic management of insomnia in children and adolescents: consensus statement. Pediatrics 2006;117(6): e1223–32.
9. Griffin CE 3rd, Kaye AM, Bueno FR, et al. Benzodiazepine pharmacology and central nervous system-mediated effects. Ochsner J 2013;13(2):214–23.
10. Möhler H, Fritschy JM, Rudolph U. A new benzodiazepine pharmacology. J Pharmacol Exp Ther 2002;300(1):2–8.
11. Zammit GK, Corser B, Doghramji K, et al. Sleep and residual sedation after administration of zaleplon, zolpidem, and placebo during experimental middle-of-the-night awakening. J Clin Sleep Med 2006;2(4):417–23.
12. Walsh JK, Krystal AD, Amato DA, et al. Nightly treatment of primary insomnia with eszopiclone for six months: effect on sleep, quality of life, and work limitations. Sleep 2007;30(8):959–68.
13. Liskow B, Pikalov A. Zaleplon overdose associated with sleepwalking and complex behavior. J Am Acad Child Adolesc Psychiatry 2004;43(8):927–8.
14. Blumer JL, Reed MD, Steinberg F, et al. Potential pharmacokinetic basis for zolpidem dosing in children with sleep difficulties. Clin Pharmacol Ther 2008;83(4): 551–8.
15. Blumer JL, Findling RL, Shih WJ, et al. Controlled clinical trial of zolpidem for the treatment of insomnia associated with attention-deficit/hyperactivity disorder in children 6 to 17 years of age. Pediatrics 2009;123(5):e770–6.
16. FDA. Highlights of prescribing information rozerem (ramelteon) tablets. 2005. Available at: https://www.accessdata.fda.gov/drugsatfda_docs/label/2010/021782s011lbl.pdf. Accessed July 21, 2020.
17. Stigler KA, Posey DJ, McDougle CJ. Ramelteon for insomnia in two youths with autistic disorder. J Child Adolesc Psychopharmacol 2006;16(5):631–6.
18. Hatta K, Kishi Y, Wada K, et al. Preventive effects of ramelteon on delirium: a randomized placebo-controlled trial. JAMA Psychiatry 2014;71(4):397–403.

19. Sateia MJ, Buysse DJ, Krystal AD, et al. Clinical practice guideline for the pharmacologic treatment of chronic insomnia in adults: an American Academy of Sleep Medicine Clinical Practice Guideline. J Clin Sleep Med 2017;13(2):307–49.

20. Kawabe K, Horiuchi F, Oka Y, et al. The melatonin receptor agonist ramelteon effectively treats insomnia and behavioral symptoms in autistic disorder. Case Rep Psychiatry 2014;2014:561071.

21. Miyamoto A, Fukuda I, Tanaka H, et al. Treatment with ramelteon for sleep disturbance in severely disabled children and young adults. No To Hattatsu 2013; 45(6):440–4 [in Japanese].

22. Weber J, Siddiqui MA, Wagstaff AJ, et al. Low-dose doxepin: in the treatment of insomnia. CNS Drugs 2010;24(8):713–20.

23. Low-dose doxepin (Silenor) for insomnia. Med Lett Drugs Ther 2010;52(1348): 79–80.

24. Dujardin S, Pijpers A, Pevernagie D. Prescription drugs used in insomnia. Sleep Med Clin 2018;13(2):169–82.

25. Kawabe K, Horiuchi F, Ochi M, et al. Suvorexant for the treatment of insomnia in adolescents. J Child Adolesc Psychopharmacol 2017;27(9):792–5.

26. Kishi T, Nomura I, Matsuda Y, et al. Lemborexant vs suvorexant for insomnia: a systematic review and network meta-analysis. J Psychiatr Res 2020;128:68–74.

27. Landry I, Nakai K, Ferry J, et al. Pharmacokinetics, pharmacodynamics, and safety of the dual orexin receptor antagonist lemborexant: findings from single-dose and multiple-ascending-dose phase 1 studies in healthy adults. Clin Pharmacol Drug Dev 2020 (0)1-13.

28. Russo RM, Gururaj VJ, Allen JE. The effectiveness of diphenhydramine HCl in pediatric sleep disorders. J Clin Pharmacol 1976;16(5–6):284–8.

29. Merenstein D, Diener-West M, Halbower AC, et al. The trial of infant response to diphenhydramine: the TIRED study–a randomized, controlled, patient-oriented trial. Arch Pediatr Adolesc Med 2006;160(7):707–71212.

30. Daviss WB, Scott J. A chart review of cyproheptadine for stimulant-induced weight loss. J Child Adolesc Psychopharmacol 2004;14(1):65–73.

31. Jan JE, Wasdell MB, Reiter RJ, et al. Melatonin therapy of pediatric sleep disorders: recent advances, why it works, who are the candidates and how to treat. Curr Pediatr Rev 2007;3:214–24.

32. Bendz LM, Scates AC. Melatonin treatment for insomnia in pediatric patients with attention-deficit/hyperactivity disorder. Ann Pharmacother 2010;44(1):185–91.

33. van Geijlswijk IM, Korzilius HP, Smits MG. The use of exogenous melatonin in delayed sleep phase disorder: a meta-analysis. Sleep 2010;33(12):1605–14.

34. van der Heijden KB, Smits MG, van Someren EJ, et al. Prediction of melatonin efficacy by pretreatment dim light melatonin onset in children with idiopathic chronic sleep onset insomnia. J Sleep Res 2005;14(2):187–94.

35. Van der Heijden KB, Smits MG, Van Someren EJ, et al. Effect of melatonin on sleep, behavior, and cognition in ADHD and chronic sleep-onset insomnia. J Am Acad Child Adolesc Psychiatry 2007;46(2):233–41.

36. Johnson KP, Malow BA. Sleep in children with autism spectrum disorders. Curr Treat Options Neurol 2008;10(5):350–9.

37. Erland LA, Saxena PK. Melatonin natural health products and supplements: presence of serotonin and significant variability of melatonin content. J Clin Sleep Med 2017;13(2):275–81.

38. Andersen IM, Kaczmarska J, McGrew SG, et al. Melatonin for insomnia in children with autism spectrum disorders. J Child Neurol 2008;23(5):482–5.

39. Cummings C, Canadian Paediatric Society CPC. Melatonin for the management of sleep disorders in children and adolescents. Paediatr Child Health 2012;17(6): 331–6.
40. Bruni O, Alonso-Alconada D, Besag F, et al. Current role of melatonin in pediatric neurology: clinical recommendations. Eur J Paediatr Neurol 2015;19(2):122–33.
41. Szeinberg A, Borodkin K, Dagan Y. Melatonin treatment in adolescents with delayed sleep phase syndrome. Clin Pediatr (Phila) 2006;45(9):809–18.
42. Sletten TL, Magee M, Murray JM, et al. Efficacy of melatonin with behavioural sleep-wake scheduling for delayed sleep-wake phase disorder: a double-blind, randomised clinical trial. PLoS Med 2018;15(6):e1002587.
43. Carr R, Wasdell MB, Hamilton D, et al. Long-term effectiveness outcome of melatonin therapy in children with treatment-resistant circadian rhythm sleep disorders. J Pineal Res 2007;43(4):351–9.
44. Luboshitzky R, Lavi S, Thuma I, et al. Increased nocturnal melatonin secretion in male patients with hypogonadotropic hypogonadism and delayed puberty. J Clin Endocrinol Metab 1995;80(7):2144–8.
45. Lin GJ, Huang SH, Chen SJ, et al. Modulation by melatonin of the pathogenesis of inflammatory autoimmune diseases. Int J Mol Sci 2013;14(6):11742–66.
46. Owens JA, Babcock D, Blumer J, et al. The use of pharmacotherapy in the treatment of pediatric insomnia in primary care: rational approaches. A consensus meeting summary. J Clin Sleep Med 2005;1(1):49–59.
47. Meolie AL, Rosen C, Kristo D, et al. Oral nonprescription treatment for insomnia: an evaluation of products with limited evidence. J Clin Sleep Med 2005;1(2): 173–87.
48. van Zyl LT, Chung SA, Shahid A, et al. L-Tryptophan as treatment for pediatric non-rapid eye movement parasomnia. J Child Adolesc Psychopharmacol 2018; 28(6):395–401.
49. Prince JB, Wilens TE, Biederman J, et al. Clonidine for sleep disturbances associated with attention-deficit hyperactivity disorder: a systematic chart review of 62 cases. J Am Acad Child Adolesc Psychiatry 1996;35(5):599–605.
50. Ingrassia A, Turk J. The use of clonidine for severe and intractable sleep problems in children with neurodevelopmental disorders–a case series. Eur Child Adolesc Psychiatry 2005;14(1):34–40.
51. Xue M, Brimacombe M, Chaaban J, et al. Autism spectrum disorders: concurrent clinical disorders. J Child Neurol 2008;23(1):6–13.
52. Kappagoda C, Schell DN, Hanson RM, et al. Clonidine overdose in childhood: implications of increased prescribing. J Paediatr Child Health 1998;34(6):508–12.
53. Rugino TA. Effect on primary sleep disorders when children with ADHD are administered guanfacine extended release. J Atten Disord 2018;22(1):14–24.
54. Younus M, Labellarte MJ. Insomnia in children: when are hypnotics indicated? Paediatr Drugs 2002;4(6):391–403.
55. Keshavan MS, Prasad KM, Montrose DM, et al. Sleep quality and architecture in quetiapine, risperidone, or never-treated schizophrenia patients. J Clin Psychopharmacol 2007;27(6):703–5.
56. Robinson AA, Malow BA. Gabapentin shows promise in treating refractory insomnia in children. J Child Neurol 2013;28(12):1618–21.

# Behavioral Treatment of Insomnia and Sleep Disturbances in School-Aged Children and Adolescents

Jessica R. Lunsford-Avery, PhD[a],*, Tatyana Bidopia, BS[b,1],
Leah Jackson, MS[c,2], Jessica Solis Sloan, PhD[d,3]

## KEYWORDS

- Sleep • Insomnia • Behavioral therapy • Cognitive behavior therapy–insomnia
- Behavioral intervention • Behavioral treatment • Children • Adolescents

## KEY POINTS

- Pediatric sleep disturbances are common but rarely adequately treated.
- Behavioral sleep interventions affect many facets of children's sleep, including duration, efficiency, latency, and regularity.
- Behavioral sleep interventions may have downstream impacts on psychiatric health among youth, including inattention/hyperactivity, depression, and anxiety.
- Future research is needed to clarify the long-term efficacy of behavioral sleep interventions as well as their efficacy across demographic groups of youth.

## INTRODUCTION

Insomnia and related sleep disturbances commonly affect youth, with prevalence rates estimated at ~30% in school-aged children (6–12 years) and ~24% in adolescents (13–18 years).[1,2] Estimates are higher in pediatric populations with psychiatric diagnoses, including attention-deficit/hyperactivity disorder (ADHD), autism spectrum

This article originally appeared in *Child and Adolescent Psychiatric Clinics*, Volume 30 Issue 1, January 2021.
[a] Department of Psychiatry, Duke University School of Medicine, 2400 Pratt Street, Office 7036, 7th Floor, North Pavilion, Durham, NC 27705, USA; [b] Department of Psychology, Fordham University, Bronx, NY, USA; [c] HRC Behavioral Health & Psychiatry, PA, Chapel Hill, NC, USA; [d] Department of OB/GYN, Duke University, Durham, NC, USA
[1] Present address: 21 W 86th St Apt 6B New York, NY 10024.
[2] Present address: 217 Grenoch Valley Lane, Apex, NC 27539.
[3] Present address: 6649 Perry Creek Road, Raleigh, NC 27616.
* Corresponding author.
*E-mail address:* Jessica.r.avery@duke.edu
Twitter: @DukeADHDProgram (J.R.L.-A.)

Psychiatr Clin N Am 47 (2024) 103–120
https://doi.org/10.1016/j.psc.2023.06.007
0193-953X/24/© 2023 Elsevier Inc. All rights reserved.

disorder (ASD), and anxiety and depression.[3–6] Youth with insomnia face many dele-terious consequences, including reduced quality of life, impaired cognition, behav-ioral/emotional problems, greater obesity, poorer performance in school, and greater risk-taking behaviors.[2,7,8] Insomnia also affects family functioning and is asso-ciated with increased stress and disrupted sleep for parents.[9] These negative out-comes, coupled with potential for chronicity and high prevalence in youth, warrant attention on the development and implementation of efficacious treatments for pedi-atric sleep disturbances.[10]

Clinicians frequently rely on pharmacologic interventions when treating pediatric sleep disturbances; however, limited evidence exists for the safety and tolerability of medications for insomnia in youth, and medications also provide short-lived effects not maintained following discontinuation.[11] In adults, behavioral interventions, such as cognitive behavior therapy for insomnia (CBT-I), are considered first line in treating sleep disturbances.[12] In the last decade, a growing literature has suggested that behavioral interventions may be similarly effective for youth[13–16]; however, pediatric sleep assessments and treatments are rarely implemented in medical settings.[17] This article provides essential information regarding the efficacy of behavioral inter-ventions for sleep disturbances in school-aged children and adolescents and further informs psychiatric practice in the treatment of pediatric insomnia.

## BEHAVIORAL TREATMENT OPTIONS
### Patient Evaluation Overview

Diagnostic criteria for insomnia in youth include the presence of 1 or more of the following symptoms for at least 3 nights per week and for at least 3 months: (1) difficulty with sleep onset, commonly manifesting as difficulty in initiating sleep without a caregiver's pres-ence; (2) night awakenings and an inability to return to sleep; and (3) early-morning awak-enings.[18] These symptoms must be accompanied by significant daytime impairment. For this article, it is notable that interventions commonly target a range of sleep disturbances related to insomnia, including sleep duration, sleep-onset latency (ie, length of time to sleep onset), frequency/duration of night awakenings, regularity of bedtimes and wake times, and sleep efficiency (ie, ratio of time asleep to time in bed). An additional childhood sleep complaint is bedtime resistance (ie, bedtime refusal, stalling, and requests for care-giver attention to delay bedtime).[19] Diagnostic tools for assessing sleep disturbances in youth include parent and child questionnaires[20]; clinical interviews querying sleep schedule, habits, and the nature of sleep problems[16]; daily sleep diaries[21]; and objective assessments (eg, actigraphy, polysomnography).[16]

### Behavioral Sleep Intervention Guidelines

#### Developmental considerations
Sleep problems occur throughout early development but manifest differently depending on age. Sleep among school-aged children is characterized by a long duration need (9–12 h/night)[22] and manifestation of circadian preference (morning lark vs night owl).[23] Insufficient sleep duration, as well as desire for parental support for initiating sleep, are common in this period. Adolescence is associated with signif-icant changes in sleep health and behavior, including shifts toward reduced duration and later bedtimes. Given greater academic and social demands in adolescence, as well as the frequent mismatch between early school start times and the preference for delayed bedtimes and wake times, most adolescents do not receive the recom-mended hours of sleep per night.[24] Sleep disturbances are common in both age groups and are connected to poorer psychiatric health and daytime functioning.[2]

Coupled with the lack of approved medications for childhood insomnia, parents' inclination toward behavioral interventions,[25] and potential functional impairment, the need for effective behavioral interventions is paramount for the health and well-being of youth. Behavioral sleep interventions have been developed to target the range of sleep problems occurring during this developmental period, with implications for improved psychiatric health.

### Modes of delivery

Behavioral sleep interventions have been delivered in a range of formats depending on the severity and type of sleep complaints targeted, but all tend to be short term (ie, most ≤6 sessions). At their simplest, interventions are educational and provide information about the importance of sleep, sleep hygiene, and/or basic behavioral strategies to support sleep health.[26–38] Among school-aged children, families have received educational interventions via printed materials (eg, pamphlets, information sheets),[26–29] video[27–38] or phone calls,[30–33] or in person during individual[29–36] or group sessions[30,36–38] led by clinically trained health professionals (eg, nurses, occupational therapists, psychologists, pediatricians)[31–38] or trained research staff.[29,30] Settings for in-person visits included children's homes,[29,31] schools,[33] clinics,[31,32,34,35] and research locations.[30,36] Given parents' important role in establishing and implementing rules at this age, they are most frequently the targeted agents of change. However, an educational intervention delivered by older peers to elementary school students yielded sustained improvement in sleep complaints,[26] suggesting that, as children mature, they should also be educated on healthy sleep habits.[39]

Adolescent interventions invariably engage the teens directly, but may include parent participation.[40–50] In this age group, school-based interventions are often used to improve knowledge of the importance of sleep, sleep habits, and sleep duration in the general adolescent population. These interventions use classroom, lecture, and/or workbook formats and are led by trained school personnel (eg, teachers, athletic trainers, counselors), sometimes in conjunction with clinical psychologists or physicians.[40–44,49,51–57] In addition to didactic formats, strategies such as modeling, role-playing, games or contests, and rewards[43,52,54,57]; peer-to-peer teaching[44]; and digital components (eg, online videos[41]) have been used to bolster adolescent engagement.

Behavioral interventions become more structured and clinically oriented when sleep complaints are severe (ie, insomnia). Among school-aged children, interventions such as CBT-I[58–61] or other formal sleep training programs, such as faded bedtime with response cost and positive reinforcement (FBRC-PR), are frequently used.[36,62] FBRC-PR involves delaying bedtime until the child is likely to fall asleep and subsequently making bedtime earlier by increments of 15 to 30 minutes once the child is able to rapidly initiate sleep at each time point. If unable to fall asleep within 20 minutes, the response cost component has the child (1) removed from bed; (2) engaged in a quiet, unrewarding activity for 20 minutes; and then (3) returned to bed to initiate sleep again. The child is rewarded for meeting FBRC-PR goals, and this strategy is implemented until the child is able to quickly fall asleep at a predetermined bedtime goal.[62,63] Parents, and sometimes their children, participate in these therapeutic interventions via phone or in person (individually or in groups) with psychologists/psychology trainees or paraprofessionals.[58–62,64] In psychiatric populations, sleep interventions for school-aged children are often coupled with CBT strategies for anxiety or depression,[59–61] parenting strategies,[60,61] and/or application of behavior management training to children's sleep problems.[65]

Similarly, for adolescents with insomnia, behavioral therapies including CBT-I are the most commonly used modalities. Behavioral therapy is delivered directly to the teen in individual or group formats, is typically implemented by clinical psychologists or other health care providers,[46–48,50,66–74] and may include supplementary treatments such as bright light therapy for adolescents with delayed sleep phase,[48,66] or, for psychiatric populations, be combined with other CBT treatments, such as treatments of depression.[75] Briefer behavioral therapies focused on sleep hygiene and/or gradual sleep extension have also been implemented with adolescents with problematic sleep.[45,76,77] Notably, several behavioral therapies for adolescents have used Internet, text-messaging, or telephone formats.[45,47,69,76,78,79]

### Common components of treatment

Sleep education and sleep hygiene techniques are the most prevalent components of behavioral sleep interventions, irrespective of modality. Sleep education emphasizes the importance of obtaining sufficient sleep to support health, cognition, and achievement and provides recommended sleep guidelines. Sleep hygiene is a set of practices intended to support optimal sleep health, such as ensuring a dark, quiet sleeping environment.[13–16] Among school-aged children, behavioral principles addressing common sleep complaints for this age group may be included (eg, strategies for reducing bedtime resistance, cosleeping, night waking, and early rising). Notably, when parent-targeted interventions include specific behavioral strategies, rather than just a presentation of general behavioral principles, these programs are typically tailored to the specific child/family, including use of comprehensive sleep assessments,[29,31,35,36,38] individualized sleep management plans,[31,33,35,36] and monitoring tools, such as sleep diaries[29–31,35,36,38] or actigraphy.[30,38] For adolescents, who have frequent smartphone/electronics use and tend to sleep later/longer on weekends compared with weekdays, stabilizing bedtimes and wake times and limiting presleep electronics and substance use (eg, caffeine, nicotine) are particularly critical aspects of sleep hygiene.[40]

Therapies for clinical insomnia, such as CBT-I, incorporate these techniques in addition to specific behavioral interventions (eg, goal setting, stimulus control, bedtime fading, graduated extinction, sleep restriction) and cognitive restructuring.[46–48,50,58–62,66–75] Among school-aged children, behavioral therapy may also address parent and child anxiety about sleep/bedtime (eg, relaxation, positive self-instructions, nightmare rescripting) and parenting (eg, effective instructions, differential attention, token economy).[58–62] Given that adolescents often express ambivalence regarding alterations to sleep behavior,[53] such as reducing presleep electronics use,[78] motivational interviewing techniques may be useful for supporting adoption of new sleep behaviors in this age group.[41,52] Additional techniques, including mindfulness,[66–68,71–73] hypnotherapy,[46,60] and adjunct bright light therapy[36,48,66] or melatonin,[58] may also be useful for youth with insomnia (**Table 1**).

For examples of behavioral techniques targeting sleep, see **Table 1**. For more details about implementation of these strategies, see the behavioral sleep manuals and resource texts targeting insomnia and sleep disturbances (**Table 2**).

### Clinical Outcomes for Sleep Health

Behavioral interventions have a positive impact on sleep health in childhood and adolescence, although the magnitude of the effect has differed across mode of delivery, treatment content, and target population (general vs clinical). Among school-aged children, educational interventions have shown improvements in daytime sleepiness,[34] earlier bedtimes,[26,34] sleep duration,[26,28,34] nighttime awakenings,[26] sleep-onset latency,[34] and bedtime resistance[26]; however, they are more likely to be effective if they are delivered by an individual rather than solely through printed materials.[27,28] When

**Table 1**
Examples of behavioral techniques to address insomnia and sleep disturbances in youth

| Target | Technique | Examples for Practice |
|---|---|---|
| General sleep health | Sleep education | • Information about sleep (eg, need, architecture, homeostasis), circadian rhythms, and their interaction<br>• Importance of sleep for health, cognition, achievement<br>• American Academy of Pediatrics Guidelines: 9–12 h/night (school age), 8–10 h/night (adolescents)[22] |
|  | Sleep hygiene | • Set/maintain regular bedtimes and wake times<br>• Set/maintain regular bedtime routine<br>• Avoid stimulating play, electronics 1 h before bed<br>• Eliminate napping<br>• Ensure dark/quiet sleep environment<br>• Exercise daily, but avoid exercise close to bedtime<br>• For children, ensure child falls asleep in own bed<br>• For adolescents, eliminate caffeine, nicotine, and alcohol, particularly in evenings |
|  | Goal setting/tracking | • Set specific goal (eg, 10 PM bedtime each day)<br>• Tailor to personal sleep need and circadian preference, as appropriate<br>• Monitor adherence to goal using sleep logs |
|  | Motivational interviewing | • Assess ambivalence about changing sleep behaviors<br>• Explore pros/cons<br>• Experiment with changing a sleep behavior<br>• Explore consequences |
|  | Sleep extension (adolescents) | • Assess current sleep schedule using sleep logs<br>• Advance bedtime 5 min/night until desired sleep length is achieved |
| Clinical sleep complaints (eg, insomnia) | Stimulus control | • Increase association between the bed and sleep; reduce association between bed and other activities<br>• Use bed only for sleeping<br>• If cannot sleep, leave bed for 15 min and engage in calming activity in a different space<br>• Return to bed when sleepy |
|  | Sleep restriction (adolescents) | • Assess amount of sleep occurring each night using sleep logs (eg, 6 h of sleeping during 9 h of time in bed)<br>• Restrict time in bed to equal current sleep amount (eg, 6 h), typically by going to bed later |

(continued on next page)

**Table 1**
*(continued)*

| Target | Technique | Examples for Practice |
|---|---|---|
| | Bedtime fading (children) | • Monitor using sleep logs until 85% of time in bed is spent asleep (sleep efficiency = 85%)<br>• Gradually advance sleep time until desired sleep length is met while maintaining sleep efficiency<br>• Assess current sleep schedule using sleep diaries<br>• Determine bedtime based on when child is likely to fall asleep within 15 min<br>• Set bedtime earlier after several successful nights until reaching the desired bedtime<br>• Avoid sleeping outside prescribed times |
| | Graduated extension (children) | • For children sleeping with parents, gradually separate parent from child (eg, move parent from bed to sitting next to bed, next to door, outside door, and so forth) |
| | Parenting/behavioral management training (children) | • Positive attention<br>• Differential attention<br>• Effective instructions<br>• Token economy system |
| | Relaxation | • Progressive relaxation techniques (eg, body scan)<br>• Deep breathing techniques<br>• Recognize emotions associated with sleep (eg, anxiety) |
| | Cognitive restructuring | • Identify sleep-interfering thoughts (eg, "If I don't fall asleep soon, I won't do well at school tomorrow!")<br>• Assess evidence for/against thought<br>• Replace with coping thought (eg, "Sleep will happen when it needs to happen.")<br>• Nightmare rescripting (eg, change anxiety-provoking elements of nightmare, rehearse altered dream script while awake) |
| | Mindfulness | • Short meditation practices (eg, 3-min breathing space) |

Note: strategies included in the table are consolidated from studies included in this article.

**Table 2**
Examples of behavioral sleep intervention manuals and resources

| Audience | Reference | Title |
|---|---|---|
| Pediatrics | Mindell & Owens,[80] 2015 | *A Clinical Guide to Pediatric Sleep: Diagnosis and Management of Sleep Problems* (third edition) |
| | Meltzer & Crabtree,[81] 2015 | *Pediatric Sleep Problems: A Clinician's Guide to Behavioral Interventions* (first edition) |
| Adolescents[a] | Edinger & Carney,[82] 2014 | *Overcoming Insomnia: A Cognitive-Behavioral Therapy Approach, Therapist Guide* (second edition) |
| | Perlis et al,[83] 2005 | *Cognitive Behavioral Treatment of Insomnia: A Session-by-Session Guide* (first edition) |
| | Manber & Carney,[84] 2015 | *Treatment Plans and Interventions for Insomnia: A Case Formulation Approach* (first edition) |
| | Morin & Espie,[85] 2003 | *Insomnia: A Clinical Guide to Assessment and Treatment* (2004 edition) |
| | Harvey & Buysse,[86] 2017 | *Treating Sleep Problems: A Transdiagnostic Approach* (first edition) |
| All ages | Attarian,[87] 2016 | *Clinical Handbook of Insomnia* (third edition) |
| | Chopra et al,[88] 2020 | *Management of Sleep Disorders in Psychiatry* |

[a] With the exception of Harvey & Buysse,[86] 2017, CBT-I manuals have been developed for use with adults. However, strategies may be implemented with adolescents.

interventions expand on education to include specific behavioral strategies, sleep outcomes also improve in this age group. Interventions that use individualized approaches tailored to the child/family (eg, sleep assessments, sleep plans, sleep diaries) show both immediate and long-term (eg, 3–6 months after treatment) improvements in sleep duration,[29,35,38] nighttime awakenings,[29] sleep-onset latency,[29,35,38] earlier bedtimes,[38] bedtime resistance,[38] sleep anxiety,[38] sleeping in own bed,[38] and overall sleep problems.[31–33,36,37] Interestingly, sleep problems sometimes worsened before improving in the long term.[37]

Among adolescents, school-based interventions using education and hygiene techniques improve sleep knowledge,[49,52,53,55,57] self-efficacy[43] and motivation[52] to modify sleep behaviors, sleep practices (eg, reducing presleep electronics/caffeine use, earlier bedtimes),[40,43,57,78] and sleep health (eg, duration, time in bed, sleep-onset latency, and regularity of bedtimes/wake times).[43,44,54,57,78,79] One study showed that typical trends occurring in adolescence, including shifts toward shorter duration and later bedtimes/wake times, were lessened among adolescents participating in a sleep education program.[49] It is notable that improvements in sleep knowledge[55] and self-efficacy in supporting sleep health[43] seem to be sustained over several months' follow-up. However, the impact of behavioral interventions on sleep habits and duration is not consistently shown in the general adolescent population.[42,52,53,56] Specifically, effects seem to be stronger with longer-term interventions, such as those with booster sessions across the school year,[43] than for briefer (eg, 1 session) treatments,[40] and for adolescents with greater sleep difficulties (eg, delays in sleep timing[53]) than those who already have good sleep habits.[51]

Behavioral therapies, such as CBT-I, frequently produce improvements in school-aged children's sleep health, including sleep duration,[58,60–62,64] sleep efficiency,[59–61] nighttime awakenings,[58–62,64,65] sleep-onset latency,[58–60,62] sleep anxiety,[60,64,65] sleeping in own bed,[61,65] and consistent bedtimes[61] and waketimes.[61,64] These positive outcomes may be sustained up to 12 months after treatment[60] and may improve when combined with melatonin (eg, greater improvements in sleep efficiency and sleep-onset latency).[58]

Among adolescents with problematic sleep, brief behavioral interventions focused on sleep hygiene and/or gradual sleep extension have been shown to increase sleep duration and time in bed; improve sleep hygiene (eg, earlier bedtimes, reduced time in bed before/after sleeping) and subjective sleep quality; stabilize sleep-wake rhythms; and reduce insomnia symptoms, sleep disturbances, and daytime sleepiness,[45,76,77] with 1 study showing sustained improvements at 20-week follow-up.[45] Behavioral therapies, such as CBT-I, have been shown to shorten sleep latency; reduce nocturnal awakenings and insomnia symptoms; and increase sleep efficiency, duration, regularity, and perceptions of sleep quality/feeling rested among adolescents with insomnia,[46,50,66,68–71,73–75] and there is evidence for efficacy using digital/telephone formats.[47,69] In addition, CBT-I may be superior to sleep hygiene techniques alone for improving sleep health in clinical samples,[75] and 1 study has shown sustained improvements in sleep 6 to 12 months after treatment completion.[47] In addition, another study showed that combining CBT-I with bright light therapy resulted in earlier bedtimes and wake times, reduced latency and awakenings, longer sleep time, and reduced sleepiness and fatigue for adolescents with delayed sleep phase, with gains maintained 6 months later.[48]

### Application to Psychiatric Populations

Sleep problems are associated with a variety of emotional and behavioral issues. Among school-aged children, programs that introduced specific behavioral strategies, including behavioral therapy (eg, CBT-I), have sought to characterize the impact of these interventions on parent and child well-being. Specifically, studies have found a positive impact on parent[32,33] and child[30,59,62] internalizing symptoms (eg, anxiety, depression), child externalizing problems,[62] parent[32,61] and child[30,32,35,64] quality of life, child emotional functioning,[35] and child social functioning.[35,64] In addition, several studies found a reduction in specific psychiatric symptoms of ADHD (eg, inattention, hyperactivity)[30,31,35,37,61,62] and ASD.[30,38,61] Often, this was due to the study sample testing these behavioral sleep interventions for these specific or other psychiatric populations (eg, neurodevelopmental disorders,[29,36,37,65] disruptive behavior disorders[32,62]). Overall, of the studies evaluating the effect of behavioral interventions on emotional and behavioral well-being, many did not investigate[30,37,38,62,64] or reported null findings[32,61] with regard to sustained psychiatric improvement in the long term.

Among adolescents, studies have similarly sought to understand the potential downstream impact of behavioral sleep interventions on psychiatric and psychosocial functioning. In the general adolescent population, school-based sleep interventions have been associated with decreased externalizing (eg, conduct, hyperactivity)[49] and internalizing (eg, depressive) symptoms and improved academic performance[43]; however, improvements in mental health are not consistently found,[53] particularly for very short-term interventions (eg, 1 session of sleep education) or among adolescents who already report good overall sleep habits.[51] Behavioral therapies have a more consistent positive impact on psychiatric health. Brief behavioral therapies and/or CBT-I have been associated with reduced stress, anxiety, rumination, and depression; improved coping; and improved overall emotional well-being among adolescents,[46,50,66,68,70,71,73–77] and 1 study showed that improvements in social, attentional, and aggressive behaviors resulting from CBT-I combined with mindfulness training were mediated by improvements in self-reported sleep quality.[67] Regarding substance use, behavioral therapy including mindfulness reduced substance abuse and improved self-efficacy about substance use, with gains maintained 12 months later.[66,71] In addition, initial evidence suggests CBT-I may be effective in reducing paranoia and hallucinations among adolescents at ultrahigh risk for psychosis.[74]

Given the prevalence and complexity of sleep problems in youth experiencing psychiatric symptoms, there has been recent interest in the development of a transdiagnostic intervention designed to flexibly treat the range of sleep problems experienced by this population. The Transdiagnostic Sleep and Circadian Intervention (TranS-C) involves a combination of CBT-I, delayed sleep phase treatment strategies, and interpersonal and social rhythms therapy (IPSRT) to treat sleep disturbances in youth with psychiatric diagnoses.[89] The TranS-C program consists of a total of 12 modules, 4 that define treatment goals and rationale (eg, functional analysis, sleep/circadian education, motivational interviewing, goal setting), 4 core modules that correct unhealthy sleep habits (eg, irregular sleep-wake times, difficulty winding down, difficulty waking up) and prevent relapse, and 4 optional modules targeting specific sleep disturbances (eg, poor sleep efficiency, too much time in bed, delayed phase, sleep-related worry).

Results from an initial randomized controlled trial (RCT) indicated that TranS-C improved self-reported sleep and reduced daytime sleepiness and weekend-weeknight sleep variability in youth at risk for emotional, behavioral, social, cognitive, and/or physical health problems.[90] In addition, youth participating in TranS-C showed significant improvements in parent-reported cognitive health, thought problems, and rule breaking compared with an educational control condition. Youth receiving TranS-C also showed significantly reduced depression following treatment; however, this improvement was not significantly different from gains observed from the control

**Table 3**
Examples of behavioral sleep interventions targeting psychiatric symptoms in youth

| Intervention Title | Intervention Elements | Impact on Psychiatric Symptoms |
|---|---|---|
| **ASD** | | |
| Parent-based sleep education[30] | Sleep education | Reduced inattention, withdrawal, repetitive behaviors |
| Parent-based sleep education workshops[38] | Sleep education | Reduced hyperactivity, self-stimulatory behavior |
| CBT-I[61] | Parent/child CBT-I | Reduced irritability, lethargy, stereotypy, hyperactivity, inappropriate speech |
| Sleepwise[36,a] | Sleep education, goal setting/tracking | No significant changes |
| **ADHD** | | |
| Sleeping Sound with ADHD[31,32,35,b] | Sleep education, hygiene | Reduced ADHD severity, inattention, emotional and behavioral difficulties |
| Better Nights/Better Days[62] | Sleep education, sleep hygiene, faded bedtime with response cost and positive reinforcement | Reduced internalizing and externalizing behaviors |
| Sleep training[64] | Sleep hygiene, positive reinforcement | Improved prosocial behavior, social acceptance, emotions |
| **Anxiety/Depression** | | |
| Sleep SENSE[67,72,73] | CBT-I, motivational interviewing, mindfulness | Reduced social problems, attention problems, aggressive behaviors, anxiety |
| CBT-I + CBT for depression[75] | CBT (insomnia and depression) | No significant differences in depression diagnosis recovery between conditions, although more participants in the treatment condition recovered at follow-up |
| Sleep extension and sleep hygiene combined intervention[76] | Sleep extension, sleep hygiene | Reduced depression |
| **Substance Abuse** | | |
| Multicomponent small group treatment[66,71] | Stimulus control, bright light therapy, sleep hygiene, sleep education, cognitive therapy, and mindfulness-based stress reduction | Improved mental health, reduced emotional distress, decreased substance use at 12-mo follow-up |

| Psychosis | | |
|---|---|---|
| SleepWell[74] | CBT-I | Reduced depression, anxiety, stress, paranoia, hallucinations, improved well-being, social functioning |
| Transdiagnostic | | |
| TranS-C[90] | CBT-I, delayed sleep phase treatment, IPSRT | Improved cognitive health and reduced thought problems and rule breaking compared with educational control condition, reduced depression but reduction comparable with the control intervention |

*Abbreviation:* SENSE, Sleep and Education: Learning New Skills Early.
[a] Study focused on developmental disabilities, but most participants had ASD.
[b] Study focused on comorbid ADHD and ASD.

intervention. Given the novelty of the TranS-C intervention, more studies are needed to determine the efficacy of this approach in treating sleep disturbances in youth with psychiatric symptoms (**Table 3**).

## Discussion

### Summary

Sleep disturbances are common among children and adolescents and have a detrimental impact on their psychiatric health, suggesting a strong need for effective treatments in this population. Behavioral sleep interventions span several modes of delivery (educational vs behavioral, in person vs digital), include a range of components depending on the severity of the sleep complaint, and are associated with improved sleep knowledge, behavior, and health in youth. In addition, these treatments may benefit children with neurodevelopmental and psychiatric disorders, a group at particular risk for sleep complaints.

### Limitations and future directions

Although behavioral interventions are associated with improved sleep and psychiatric health in youth, there are several important caveats to consider. First, many interventions have been implemented with generally white samples, and their efficacy among children and adolescents from diverse racial/ethnic and socioeconomic backgrounds is largely unknown. In 1 study using a text-messaging format to set individualized bedtime goals, sleep duration increased, but only for non-Hispanic white adolescents and not for racial/ethnic minorities.[79] Given documented sleep disparities across demographic groups of youth,[91] tailored interventions with proven efficacy in minority groups are sorely needed.

Second, it is notable that the body of literature supporting behavioral sleep interventions in youth is young, and there is a need for more studies using high-quality study designs[14] and RCT formats.[16] In addition, insomnia and related sleep problems are multifaceted clinical constructs, and a recent meta-analysis suggested that behavioral therapies, such as CBT-I, may be more effective for treating some symptoms of insomnia, including sleep-onset latency and sleep efficiency, than others, such as sleep duration and night awakenings.[15] Future replication studies using high-quality RCT designs are necessary to further affirm the efficacy of behavioral sleep interventions in youth and to determine which aspects of insomnia may be best targeted by such treatments.

Third, few studies of behavioral sleep interventions have evaluated the long-term impact on sustaining improvement in sleep health and related psychiatric symptoms, and, as noted earlier, some have found null findings. Thus, additional research is needed to determine the effectiveness of sleep treatments in the long term, and which intervention components may be most important for sustaining treatment gains over time. For example, interventions that tailor the treatment to the individual child/adolescent, combine education with behavioral strategies, and include booster sessions may be more effective in the long term, and future studies should clarify the relative efficacy of these and other mechanisms in supporting sustained sleep and psychiatric health.

## CLINICS CARE POINTS

- Comprehensive sleep evaluations, including parent and child report, identify specific sleep problems and can be used to individualize treatment targets.

- Sleep education may improve sleep health of youth; however, adding behavioral strategies to education is likely to further enhance outcomes.
- Tailoring behavioral techniques to the child/family is important to support development of new sleep behaviors.
- Consideration of developmental stage is essential, such as including a parent in treatment of school-aged children and reducing caffeine/electronics use among adolescents.
- For insomnia, CBT-I is clinically indicated and supplemental strategies, such as motivational interviewing, mindfulness, and bright light therapy, may further improve sleep.
- Behavioral sleep interventions are intended to be short term; evidence suggests even a few sessions targeting sleep behaviors reduces insomnia in youth.

## DISCLOSURE

Preparation of this article was supported by the National Institute of Mental Health grant K23 MH108704 to Dr. Lunsford-Avery.

## REFERENCES

1. Combs D, Goodwin JL, Quan SF, et al. Insomnia, health-related quality of life and health outcomes in children: a seven year longitudinal cohort. Sci Rep 2016;6: 27921.
2. de Zambotti M, Goldstone A, Colrain IM, et al. Insomnia disorder in adolescence: diagnosis, impact, and treatment. Sleep Med Rev 2018;39:12–24.
3. Souders MC, Zavodny S, Eriksen W, et al. Sleep in children with autism spectrum disorder. Curr Psychiatry Rep 2017;19(6):34.
4. Lunsford-Avery JR, Krystal AD, Kollins SH. Sleep disturbances in adolescents with ADHD: a systematic review and framework for future research. Clin Psychol Rev 2016;50:159–74.
5. Hvolby A. Associations of sleep disturbance with ADHD: implications for treatment. Atten Defic Hyperact Disord 2015;7(1):1–18.
6. Ramtekkar U, Ivanenko A. Sleep in children with psychiatric disorders. Semin Pediatr Neurol 2015;22(2):148–55.
7. Owens J. Classification and epidemiology of childhood sleep disorders. Prim Care 2008;35(3):533.
8. Donskoy I, Loghmanee D. Insomnia in adolescence. Med Sci (Basel) 2018; 6(3):72.
9. Meltzer LJ, Mindell JA. Relationship between child sleep disturbances and maternal sleep, mood, and parenting stress: a pilot study. J Fam Psychol 2007; 21(1):67–73.
10. Roberts RE, Roberts CR, Duong HT. Chronic insomnia and its negative consequences for health and functioning of adolescents: a 12-month prospective study. J Adolesc Health 2008;42(3):294–302.
11. Owens JA, Moturi S. Pharmacologic treatment of pediatric insomnia. Child Adolesc Psychiatr Clin N Am 2009;18(4):1001.
12. Qaseem A, Kansagara D, Forciea MA, et al. Management of chronic insomnia disorder in adults: a clinical practice guideline from the American College of Physicians. Ann Intern Med 2016;165(2):I26.
13. Meltzer LJ, Mindell JA. Systematic review and meta-analysis of behavioral interventions for pediatric insomnia (vol 39, pg 932, 2014). J Pediatr Psychol 2015; 40(2):262–5.

14. Busch V, Altenburg TM, Harmsen IA, et al. Interventions that stimulate healthy sleep in school-aged children: a systematic literature review. Eur J Public Health 2017;27(1):53–65.

15. Ma ZR, Shi LJ, Deng MH. Efficacy of cognitive behavioral therapy in children and adolescents with insomnia: a systematic review and meta-analysis. Braz J Med Biol Res 2018;51(6):e7070.

16. Dewald-Kaufmann J, de Bruin E, Michael G. Cognitive behavioral therapy for insomnia (CBT-i) in school-aged children and adolescents. Sleep Med Clin 2019;14(2):155.

17. Meltzer LJ, Plaufcan MR, Thomas JH, et al. Sleep problems and sleep disorders in pediatric primary care: treatment recommendations, persistence, and health care utilization. J Clin Sleep Med 2014;10(4):421–6.

18. American Psychiatric Association. DSM-5 Task Force. Diagnostic and statistical manual of mental disorders: DSM-5. 5th edition. Washington, DC: American Psychiatric Association; 2013.

19. Wilson KE, Lumeng JC, Kaciroti N, et al. Sleep hygiene practices and bedtime resistance in low-income preschoolers: does temperament matter? Behav Sleep Med 2015;13(5):412–23.

20. Spruyt.K, Gozal D. Pediatric sleep questionnaires as diagnostic or epidemiological tools: a review of currently available instruments. Sleep Med Rev 2011;15(1):19–32.

21. Carney CE, Buysse DJ, Ancoli-Israel S, et al. The consensus sleep diary: standardizing prospective sleep self-monitoring. Sleep 2012;35(2):287–302.

22. Paruthi S, Brooks LJ, D'Ambrosio C, et al. Recommended amount of sleep for pediatric populations: a consensus statement of the American Academy of Sleep Medicine. J Clin Sleep Med 2016;12(6):785–6.

23. Jenni OG, Carskadon MA. Sleep behavior and sleep regulation from infancy through adolescence: normative aspects. Sleep Med Clin 2007;2(3):321–9.

24. Crowley SJ, Wolfson AR, Tarokh L, et al. An update on adolescent sleep: new evidence informing the perfect storm model. J Adolesc 2018;67:55–65.

25. Goodday A, Corkum P, Smith IM. Parental acceptance of treatments for insomnia in children with attention-deficit/hyperactivity disorder, autistic spectrum disorder, and their typically developing peers. Child Health Care 2014;43(1):54–71.

26. Surani SR, Surani SS, Sadasiva S, et al. Effect of animated movie in combating child sleep health problems. Springerplus 2015;4:343.

27. Adkins KW, Molloy C, Weiss SK, et al. Effects of a standardized pamphlet on insomnia in children with autism spectrum disorders. Pediatrics 2012;130:S139–44.

28. Mindell JA, Sedmak R, Boyle, et al. Sleep Well!: a pilot study of an education campaign to improve sleep of socioeconomically disadvantaged Children. J Clin Sleep Med 2016;12(12):1593–9.

29. Montgomery P, Stores G, Wiggs L. The relative efficacy of two brief treatments for sleep problems in young learning disabled (mentally retarded) children: a randomised controlled trial. Arch Dis Child 2004;89(2):125–30.

30. Malow BA, Adkins KW, Reynolds A, et al. Parent-based sleep education for children with autism spectrum disorders. J Autism Dev Disord 2014;44(1):216–28.

31. Hiscock H, Sciberras E, Mensah F, et al. Impact of a behavioural sleep intervention on symptoms and sleep in children with attention deficit hyperactivity disorder, and parental mental health: randomised controlled trial. BMJ 2015;350:h68.

32. Sciberras E, Fulton M, Efron D, et al. Managing sleep problems in school aged children with ADHD: a pilot randomised controlled trial. Sleep Med 2011;12(9): 932–5.
33. Quach J, Hiscock H, Ukoumunne OC, et al. A brief sleep intervention improves outcomes in the school entry year: a randomized controlled trial. Pediatrics 2011;128(4):692–701.
34. Bastida-Pozuelo MF, Sanchez-Ortuno MM, Meltzer LJ. Nurse-led brief sleep education intervention aimed at parents of school-aged children with neurodevelopmental and mental health disorders: results from a pilot study. J Spec Pediatr Nurs 2018;23(4):e12228.
35. Papadopoulos N, Sciberras E, Hiscock H, et al. The efficacy of a brief behavioral sleep intervention in school-aged children with ADHD and comorbid autism spectrum disorder. J Atten Disord 2019;23(4):341–50.
36. Moss AHB, Gordon JE, O'Connell A. Impact of sleepwise: an intervention for youth with developmental disabilities and sleep disturbance. J Autism Dev Disord 2014;44(7):1695–707.
37. Stuttard L, Beresford B, Clarke S, et al. A preliminary investigation into the effectiveness of a group-delivered sleep management intervention for parents of children with intellectual disabilities. J Intellect Disabil 2015;19(4):342–55.
38. Reed HE, McGrew SG, Artibee K, et al. Parent-based sleep education workshops in autism. J Child Neurol 2009;24(8):936–45.
39. Vriend J, Corkum P. Clinical management of behavioral insomnia of childhood. Psychol Res Behav Manag 2011;4:69–79.
40. Das-Friebel A, Perkinson-Gloor N, Brand S, et al. A pilot cluster-randomised study to increase sleep duration by decreasing electronic media use at night and caffeine consumption in adolescents. Sleep Med 2019;60:109–15.
41. Bonnar D, Gradisar M, Moseley L, et al. Evaluation of novel school-based interventions for adolescent sleep problems: does parental involvement and bright light improve outcomes? Sleep Health 2015;1(1):66–74.
42. Rigney G, Blunden S, Maher C, et al. Can a school-based sleep education programme improve sleep knowledge, hygiene and behaviours using a randomised controlled trial. Sleep Med 2015;16(6):736–45.
43. Wolfson AR, Harkins E, Johnson M, et al. Effects of the young adolescent sleep smart program on sleep hygiene practices, sleep health efficacy, and behavioral well-being. Sleep Health 2015;1(3):197–204.
44. Kira G, Maddison R, Hull M, et al. Sleep education improves the sleep duration of adolescents: a randomized controlled pilot study. J Clin Sleep Med 2014;10(7): 787–92.
45. Tan E, Healey D, Gray AR, et al. Sleep hygiene intervention for youth aged 10 to 18 years with problematic sleep: a before-after pilot study. BMC Pediatr 2012; 12:189.
46. Schlarb AA, Liddle CC, Hautzinger M. JuSt - a multimodal program for treatment of insomnia in adolescents: a pilot study. Nat Sci Sleep 2011;3:13–20.
47. de Bruin EJ, Bogels SM, Oort FJ, et al. Efficacy of cognitive behavioral therapy for insomnia in adolescents: a randomized controlled trial with internet therapy, group therapy and a waiting list condition. Sleep 2015;38(12):1913–26.
48. Gradisar M, Dohnt H, Gardner G, et al. A randomized controlled trial of cognitive-behavior therapy plus bright light therapy for adolescent delayed sleep phase disorder. Sleep 2011;34(12):1671–80.
49. Wing YK, Chan NY, Yu MWM, et al. A school-based sleep education program for adolescents: a cluster randomized trial. Pediatrics 2015;135(3):E635–43.

50. Hendricks MC, Ward CM, Grodin LK, et al. Multicomponent cognitive-behavioural intervention to improve sleep in adolescents: a multiple baseline design. Behav Cogn Psychother 2014;42(3):368–73.

51. Harris A, Gundersen H, Mork-Andreassen P, et al. Restricted use of electronic media, sleep, performance, and mood in high school athletes-a randomized trial. Sleep Health 2015;1(4):314–21.

52. Cain N, Gradisar M, Moseley L. A motivational school-based intervention for adolescent sleep problems. Sleep Med 2011;12(3):246–51.

53. Moseley L, Gradisar M. Evaluation of a school-based intervention for adolescent sleep problems. Sleep 2009;32(3):334–41.

54. de Sousa IC, Araujo JF, de Azevedo CVM. The effect of a sleep hygiene education program on the sleep-wake cycle of Brazilian adolescent students. Sleep Biol Rhythms 2007;5(4):251–8.

55. Cortesi F, Giannotti F, Sebastiani T, et al. Knowledge of sleep in Italian high school students: pilot-test of a school-based sleep educational program. J Adolesc Health 2004;34(4):344–51.

56. Beijamini F, Louzada FM. Are educational interventions able to prevent excessive daytime sleepiness in adolescents? Biol Rhythm Res 2012;43(6):603–13.

57. Sousa IC, Souza JC, Louzada FM, et al. Changes in sleep habits and knowledge after an educational sleep program in 12th grade students. Sleep Biol Rhythms 2013;11(3):144–53.

58. Cortesi F, Giannotti F, Sebastiani T, et al. Controlled-release melatonin, singly and combined with cognitive behavioural therapy, for persistent insomnia in children with autism spectrum disorders: a randomized placebo-controlled trial. J Sleep Res 2012;21(6):700–9.

59. Paine S, Gradisar M. A randomised controlled trial of cognitive-behaviour therapy for behavioural insomnia of childhood in school-aged children. Behav Res Ther 2011;49(6–7):379–88.

60. Schlarb AA, Bihlmaier I, Velten-Schurian K, et al. Short- and long-term effects of CBT-I in groups for school-age children suffering from chronic insomnia: the KiSS-Program. Behav Sleep Med 2018;16(4):380–97.

61. McCrae CS, Chan WS, Curtis AF, et al. Cognitive behavioral treatment of insomnia in school-aged children with autism spectrum disorder: a pilot feasibility study. Autism Res 2020;13(1):167–76.

62. Corkum P, Lingley-Pottie P, Davidson F, et al. Better nights/better days-distance intervention for insomnia in school-aged children with/without ADHD: a randomized controlled trial. J Pediatr Psychol 2016;41(6):701–13.

63. Mindell JA, Kuhn B, Lewin DS, et al. Behavioral treatment of bedtime problems and night wakings in infants and young children. Sleep 2006;29(10):1263–76.

64. Keshavarzi Z, Bajoghli H, Mohamadi MR, et al. In a randomized case-control trial with 10-years olds suffering from attention deficit/hyperactivity disorder (ADHD) sleep and psychological functioning improved during a 12-week sleep-training program. World J Biol Psychiatry 2014;15(8):609–19.

65. Weiskop S, Richdale A, Matthews J. Behavioural treatment to reduce sleep problems in children with autism or fragile X syndrome. Dev Med Child Neurol 2005; 47(2):94–104.

66. Bootzin RR, Stevens SJ. Adolescents, substance abuse, and the treatment of insomnia and daytime sleepiness. Clin Psychol Rev 2005;25(5):629–44.

67. Blake MJ, Snoep L, Raniti M, et al. A cognitive-behavioral and mindfulness-based group sleep intervention improves behavior problems in at-risk adolescents by improving perceived sleep quality. Behav Res Ther 2017;99:147–56.

68. Bei B, Byrne ML, Ivens C, et al. Pilot study of a mindfulness-based, multi-component, in-school group sleep intervention in adolescent girls. Early Interv Psychiatry 2013;7(2):213–20.

69. de Bruin EJ, Oort FJ, Bogels SM, et al. Efficacy of internet and group-administered cognitive behavioral therapy for insomnia in adolescents: a pilot study. Behav Sleep Med 2014;12(3):235–54.

70. Norell-Clarke A, Nyander E, Jansson-Frojmark M. Sleepless in Sweden: a single subject study of effects of cognitive therapy for insomnia on three adolescents. Behav Cogn Psychother 2011;39(3):367–74.

71. Britton WB, Bootzin RR, Cousins JC, et al. The contribution of mindfulness practice to a multicomponent behavioral sleep intervention following substance abuse treatment in adolescents: a treatment-development study. Subst Abus 2010; 31(2):86–97.

72. Waloszek JM, Schwartz O, Simmons JG, et al. The SENSE Study (Sleep and Education: learning New Skills Early): a community cognitive-behavioural therapy and mindfulness-based sleep intervention to prevent depression and improve cardiac health in adolescence. BMC Psychol 2015;3:39.

73. Blake M, Waloszek JM, Schwartz O, et al. The SENSE study: post intervention effects of a randomized controlled trial of a cognitive-behavioral and mindfulness-based group sleep improvement intervention among at-risk adolescents. J Consult Clin Psychol 2016;84(12):1039–51.

74. Bradley J, Freeman D, Chadwick E, et al. Treating sleep problems in young people at ultra-high risk of psychosis: a feasibility case series. Behav Cogn Psychother 2018;46(3):276–91.

75. Clarke G, McGlinchey EL, Hein K, et al. Cognitive-behavioral treatment of insomnia and depression in adolescents: a pilot randomized trial. Behav Res Ther 2015;69:111–8.

76. Dewald-Kaufmann JF, Oort FJ, Meijer AM. The effects of sleep extension and sleep hygiene advice on sleep and depressive symptoms in adolescents: a randomized controlled trial. J Child Psychol Psychiatry 2014;55(3):273–83.

77. Paavonen EJ, Huurre T, Tilli M, et al. Brief behavioral sleep intervention for adolescents: an effectiveness study. Behav Sleep Med 2016;14(4):351–66.

78. Bartel K, Scheeren R, Gradisar M. Altering adolescents' pre-bedtime phone use to achieve better sleep health. Health Commun 2019;34(4):456–62.

79. Tavernier R, Adam EK. Text message intervention improves objective sleep hours among adolescents: the moderating role of race-ethnicity. Sleep Health 2017; 3(1):62–7.

80. Mindell JA, Owens JA. A clinical guide to pediatric sleep: diagnosis and management of sleep problems. 3rd edition. Philadelphia: Wolters Kluwer; 2015.

81. Meltzer LJ, Crabtree V. Pediatric sleep problems: a clinician's guide to behavioral interventions. Washington, DC: American Psychological Association; 2015.

82. Edinger JD, Carney C. Overcoming insomnia: a cognitive-behavioral therapy approach : therapist guide. New York: Oxford University Press; 2014. Available at: https://login.proxy.lib.duke.edu/login?url=https://ebookcentral.proquest.com/lib/duke/detail.action?docID=415620.

83. Perlis ML, Jungquist C, Smith MT, et al. Cognitive behavioral treatment of insomnia: a session-by-session guide. New York: Springer Science & Business Media; 2005.

84. Manber R, Carney CE. Treatment plans and interventions for insomnia: a case formulation approach. New York: Guilford Publications; 2015.

85. Morin CM, Espie CA. Insomnia: a clinical guide to assessment and treatment. New York: Springer Science & Business Media; 2007.

86. Harvey AG, Buysse DJ. Treating sleep problems: a transdiagnostic approach. New York: Guilford Publications; 2017.

87. Clinical handbook of insomnia. In: Attarian HP (Cham), editor. Switzerland: Springer Nature; 2016.

88. Chopra A, Das P, Doghramji K. Management of sleep disorders in psychiatry. Oxford University Press; 2020.

89. Harvey AG. A transdiagnostic intervention for youth sleep and circadian problems. Cogn Behav Pract 2016;23(3):341–55.

90. Harvey AG, Hein K, Dolsen MR, et al. Modifying the impact of eveningness chronotype ("night-owls") in youth: a randomized controlled trial. J Am Acad Child Adolesc Psychiatry 2018;57(10):742–54.

91. Guglielmo D, Gazmararian JA, Chung J, et al. Racial/ethnic sleep disparities in US school-aged children and adolescents: a review of the literature. Sleep Health 2018;4(1):68–80.

# Pediatric Insomnia

Madeline Himelfarb, BFA, Jess P. Shatkin, MD, MPH*

## KEYWORDS

- Insomnia • Pediatric insomnia • Children • Adolescents
- Cognitive behavior therapy for insomnia • Sleep • Sleep hygiene

## KEY POINTS

- Insomnia is prevalent among children and adolescents worldwide, but there is a discrepancy between high prevalence rates and low numbers of diagnoses by clinicians.
- Pediatric insomnia has a 24-hour impact. Although it is a nighttime sleep disorder, daytime functioning (eg, alertness, decision-making, academic functioning, and interpersonal relations) suffers as a result.
- Many factors contribute to pediatric insomnia, including hyperarousal and stress, screen use, and the presence of comorbid psychiatric disorders.
- Cognitive Behavioral Therapy for Insomnia (CBT-I) is the first-line recommendation for the treatment of pediatric insomnia. Melatonin has the best data for efficacy among medications.

## INTRODUCTION

Insomnia is a global epidemic. Insufficient and disordered sleep results in readily observable physical and psychological impairments and subsequent problems in academic, occupational, and interpersonal functioning.[1] Although most studies to date have focused on adult populations, youth are equally affected and, akin to their adult counterparts, often go undiagnosed.[2] Given the importance of sleep for development, the effects of insomnia on children can be particularly detrimental, impacting their ability to learn, manage mood and anxiety, develop relationships, avoid accidents, and stay physically healthy.[3] To ensure the well-being of all children and teens, accurate and thorough screening, diagnosis, and treatment of insomnia is critical. This article describes how insomnia presents, contributing factors, the impact of twenty-first century technology, and most importantly, how pediatric insomnia should be assessed and treated by clinicians.

This article originally appeared in *Child and Adolescent Psychiatric Clinics*, Volume 30 Issue 1, January 2021.
Department of Child & Adolescent Psychiatry, New York University, One Park Avenue, 7th Floor, New York, NY 10016, USA
* Corresponding author.
*E-mail address:* jess.shatkin@nyulangone.org

Psychiatr Clin N Am 47 (2024) 121–134
https://doi.org/10.1016/j.psc.2023.06.008
**psych.theclinics.com**

### Prevalence of Pediatric Insomnia

From infancy through adolescence, sleep is vital for development. Children's brains are malleable, and sleep is necessary to promote the plastic processes that accompany neurodevelopment.[4] Bedtime, however, can be tricky for children and parents. With fear of nightmares and bedtime resistance, ensuring children receive adequate sleep is often stressful for parents. Nearly all children periodically struggle with sleep; yet when we look beyond routine sleep troubles, such as occasional difficulties falling asleep, diagnosable sleep pathologies are pervasive among youth. Depending on factors such as age, gender, and cultural habits, the percentage of sleep complaints in children can reach as high as 80% in various regions of the world.[5] Parental indicators and definitions of sleep problems vary across cultures, but prevalence rates of sleep disturbances among youth populations remain consistently high. Our best data suggests that at least 25% of children suffer a clinically significant sleep pathology at some point in childhood.[6]

Pediatric sleep problems range from night awakenings to sleep-related breathing disorders, hyper and parasomnias, circadian rhythm disorders, and sleep-related movement disorders, with insomnia being the most common. One in 5 young children and preadolescents, in fact, report symptoms of insomnia,[7] and among adolescents, symptoms of insomnia are nearly ubiquitous. A representative US sample of 13-year-olds to 16-year-olds found a 30-day prevalence of insomnia disorder of 9.4% and a lifetime prevalence of 10.7%. In addition, 88% of the adolescents with a lifetime history of insomnia reported current sleep difficulties, further indicating the chronicity of insomnia among youth.[8]

These and other epidemiologic studies demonstrate that prevalence rates of pediatric insomnia and other sleep disorders are high, yet they remain largely underdiagnosed by care providers and parents alike. One of the first studies to review electronic medical records for ICD-9 diagnoses given by primary care providers found that only 3.7% of a sample of more than 150,000 children were diagnosed with a sleep disorder, far below what would be expected.[2] Given the discrepancy between low diagnosis rates and high prevalence rates, it is resoundingly clear that insomnia and other pediatric sleep disorders remain largely neglected.

### Presentation of Pediatric Insomnia

Insomnia is often described as an overall difficulty with sleep, or an inability to turn off the brain at night.[9] The *Diagnostic and Statistical Manual of Mental Disorders* (5th Edition) (DSM) defines insomnia disorder by the following criteria: (1) dissatisfaction with quantity and quality of sleep accompanied with complaints of one or more of the following: difficulty initiating and/or maintaining sleep (in children, this may manifest as difficulty initiating/maintaining sleep *without caregiver intervention*), and early morning awakenings; (2) significant distress or interference with personal functioning in daily living caused by sleep difficulty; (3) sleep difficulty occurring at least 3 nights a week; (4) sleep difficulty present for at least 3 months; (5) sleep difficulties occurring despite adequate circumstances and opportunity for sleep; (6) coexisting mental and/or sleep disorders do not explain the predominant insomnia complaint; and (7) symptoms cannot be attributed to physiologic effects of a drug or other substance.[10] Although symptoms may begin at bedtime, daytime symptoms often include mood disturbances, fatigue, excessive daytime sleepiness, and decreased daytime alertness.[10] These daytime symptoms prove the extent of this disorder's 24-hour reach; although insomnia may be a sleep disorder, it causes problems around the clock.

The presentation of pediatric insomnia will vary depending on the age of the child. Behaviorally, insomnia among toddlers and preschoolers most often presents with bedtime stalling and resistance; sleep-onset associations such as sucking thumbs, nursing, rocking, or driving in the car to induce sleep; night awakenings; and/or refusal. Night awakenings and sleep-onset associations are believed to occur in 25% to 50% of children between 6 and 12 months, 30% of 1-year-olds, and 15% to 20% of children between 1 and 3 years of age. Bedtime resistance and stalling is found in 10% to 30% of children.[11]

As children grow into adolescents, both their autonomy and expectations increase. Unlike children, teens are expected to juggle hours of nightly homework, earlier school start times, an increase in responsibilities, time-consuming extracurricular activities, and an active social life. These demands, compounded by adolescents' natural tendency toward a delayed circadian rhythm, typically result in later bedtimes and excessive daytime sleepiness, which have been well studied. Compared with children and even adults, adolescents exhibit higher levels of sleep deprivation.[12] Among a sample of more than 10,000 adolescents, roughly two-thirds reported a sleep-onset latency exceeding 30-minutes and a sleep deficiency of 2 hours on weekdays.[13] Adolescents, overall, are struggling to receive adequate amounts of sleep, and as a result, their daytime attentiveness is suffering.[14] Lower grade point averages and standardized test scores, more automobile accidents, increased risky behavior, and higher rates of anxiety and depression are but a few of the many well-established consequences of inadequate sleep during adolescence.[15–18]

These observations further demonstrate the pressing need for health care providers and parents to treat pediatric insomnia appropriately. Although not every sleep-deprived adolescent meets criteria for a diagnosis of insomnia, poor sleep habits can, over time, increase the likelihood of a diagnosis if left untreated. Among the aforementioned sample of more than 10,000 adolescents exhibiting sleep deficiency, there was a high rate of insomnia, ranging from 13.6% to 23.6% depending on diagnostic criteria. Insomnia disorder among adolescents is often characterized by nonrestorative sleep, difficulty maintaining sleep, anxiety around the inability to fall asleep, excessive napping, and the aforementioned sleep phase delay.[19,20] As symptoms of the disorder are ubiquitous among adolescents, it is the responsibility of the clinician to pay close attention to reports of prolonged symptoms, be familiar with DSM criteria, monitor their patients long-term, and address early symptoms. To assist clinicians, many comprehensive screening assessments have been designed to help recognize insomnia and other sleep disorders among children and adolescents, two of which are discussed further in this article.

### Predisposing, Precipitating, and Perpetuating Factors

To treat pediatric insomnia comprehensively, it is imperative to understand the multifactorial nature of the disorder's etiology. Insomnia represents a "constellation of symptoms" that arise from a wide range of medical, behavioral, and biological causes.[21] Hyperarousal, comorbid sleep and/or mental health disorders, stress, trauma, screen-time and other environmental factors have been shown to predispose, precipitate, and perpetuate symptoms of insomnia.[3] Here, we address a few of these factors in depth (**Box 1**).

#### → Hyperarousal and stress-responses
Hyperactive neurobiological and psychological systems contribute to difficulty with sleeping, driven, at least in part, by the hypothalamic-pituitary-adrenal axis. As our research tools have improved in recent years, so too has our understanding of

---

**Box 1**
**Predisposing, precipitating, and perpetuating factors**

Contributing Factors
- Predisposing factors
  - Personality/genetic
  - Sleep-wake cycle
  - Circadian rhythm
  - Coping mechanisms
  - Age
- Precipitating factors
  - Situational
  - Environmental
  - Medical
  - Psychiatric
  - Medications
- Perpetuating factors
  - Conditioning
  - Substance abuse
  - Performance anxiety
  - Poor sleep hygiene

*Data from* Brown KM, MD, Malow BA, MD. Pediatric insomnia. Chest. 2016;149(5):133–9; and Spielman AJ, Caruso LS, Glovinsky PB. A behavioral perspective on insomnia treatment. Psychiatr Clin North Am. 1987;10(4):541–53.

---

hyperarousal.[22] We now know that patients with insomnia commonly experience atypical hormone secretion, increased metabolic activity, an increase in sympathetic nervous system engagement, elevated heart rate, and unexpected electroencephalogram (EEG) activation patterns during sleep.[23,24] One study discovered that pediatric insomnia is associated with increased beta activity (as observed on EEG) during sleep, suggesting that cortical hyperarousal occurs in individuals with insomnia as early as adolescence.[25]

Stressors vary greatly in terms of source, potency, and duration.[22] Generally, those who suffer from insomnia demonstrate exaggerated and dysfunctional neurobiological and cognitive-emotional reactivity to stressors, which contributes to hyperarousal. One study found that 37% of the variance in vulnerability to stress-induced insomnia in siblings was accounted for by familial aggregation.[26] Although it may be assumed that a larger number of stressful events would correspondingly increase the vulnerability to insomnia, studies have contradicted this notion by finding that, rather, vulnerability is heightened based on the "appraisal of stressors and the perceived lack of control over stressful events."[27] This observation mirrors precisely what is known about anxiety: it is not so much the worry itself, it is one's appraisal of the value of the worry that causes problems.[28]

These findings are particularly pertinent for clinicians, as treatment plans for pediatric insomnia must include helping children to accurately appraise stress and enhance their coping skills. Hyperarousal and stress reactivity are key players in the onset and exacerbation of insomnia, and must not be overlooked by parents, educators, and clinicians.

### → *Comorbid mental health disorders*
Prevalence rates of insomnia are highest among youth with comorbid mental health disorders. Among a representative US sample of adolescents, 52.8% of those diagnosed with insomnia had a comorbid psychiatric disorder.[8] Insomnia is highly prevalent among children with autism spectrum disorder, with estimates ranging from 50%

to 80%.[29] In addition, at least 50% of children and adolescents with attention-deficit/hyperactivity disorder are affected by sleep problems, making them 2 to 3 times more likely to suffer than typical youth, and further exacerbating their symptoms of inattention and hyperactivity.[30,31]

Insomnia has traditionally been conceptualized as a symptom of other disorders; however, longitudinal studies now suggest that insomnia is also a risk factor for new onset of psychiatric disorders, including depression, anxiety, and substance use disorders. In a study conducted at a pediatric sleep center, 50% of the youth patients presenting for insomnia had an existing psychiatric diagnosis, and the remaining 50% had elevated psychological impairment scores.[32] As with most psychiatric disorders, we are learning that the onset of insomnia during childhood is more commonly the rule than the exception.[33] With 1 in 4-to-5 youth in the United States meeting criteria for a psychiatric disorder over the course of their lifetime, the "chicken and egg" bidirectional relationship between sleep and mental health is critical for clinicians to understand.[34] A thorough sleep history must be a key component of every psychiatric evaluation.

The relationship between sleep and mental health extends as far as suicide. Plentiful evidence points to a strong relationship between poor sleep and suicidal behavior in individuals with comorbid psychiatric disorders.[35,36] Numerous explanations have been offered to explain the association between suicide and insomnia. Most obviously, individuals with insomnia are at higher risk for experiencing a depressive episode, which is a well-recognized risk factor for suicidal ideation; alternatively, with less sleep, we become more impulsive and have greater difficulty making decisions.[37] Regardless, mounting data support the correlation of suicide and insomnia, which demands that clinicians always screen for insomnia among their youth with mental illness.

### → Screen-time

Technological advancements over the past several decades have propelled screen use among youth to an all-time high. *We Are Social's* 2019 Global Statshot reports that 5.11 billion individuals own a cell phone, representing roughly 66% of the world's population, and the United Nations estimates that more people worldwide have access to smartphones than toilets.[38,39] The statistics on technology use among children and adolescents are staggering. A 2019 Census examined a nationally representative sample of more than 1600 youths and discovered that technology ownership is near universal: 53% have their own smartphone by age 11, and 69% by age 12 (**Fig. 1**). The census paints a vivid picture of a typical day for an American child, finding that on average 62% spend more than 4 hours a day on screen media, and 29% use screens for upward of 8 hours a day.[40]

As technology among youth populations becomes ubiquitous, there has been an increase in research exploring the effect of screen use on sleep habits and sleep efficiency.[41,42] Among a large sample of American youth in 2011, 90% reported using a cell phone in the hour before bed, including a preponderance of adolescents (72%). The amount of technology used in the hour before bed was significantly related to both difficulty falling asleep and the frequency of reports of "unrefreshing" sleep, suggesting that cognitive and physiologic stimulation from these devices almost certainly interferes with sleep. In addition, 57% of these individuals left their cell phones and ringers on overnight, with 1 in 10 reporting an inability to maintain sleep a few nights per week.[43]

In addition to psychological and physiologic arousal, the bright light from screens offers yet another explanation for screens' negative effects on sleep. Light moderates

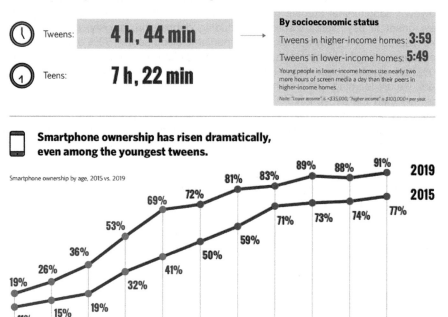

2019
# THE COMMON SENSE CENSUS: MEDIA USE BY TWEENS AND TEENS

**Amount of daily screen use**, not including for school or homework

Tweens: **4 h, 44 min**

Teens: **7 h, 22 min**

**By socioeconomic status**

Tweens in higher-income homes: **3:59**

Tweens in lower-income homes: **5:49**

Young people in lower-income homes use nearly two more hours of screen media a day than their peers in higher-income homes.

Note: "Lower income" is <$35,000, "higher income" is $100,000+ per year.

**Smartphone ownership has risen dramatically, even among the youngest tweens.**

Smartphone ownership by age, 2015 vs. 2019

2019: 19%, 26%, 36%, 53%, 69%, 72%, 81%, 83%, 89%, 88%, 91%

2015: 11%, 15%, 19%, 32%, 41%, 50%, 59%, 71%, 73%, 74%, 77%

AGE, IN YEARS (8, 9, 10, 11, 12, 13, 14, 15, 16, 17, 18)

**Fig. 1.** Statistics on screen use among tweens and teens. (*From* Rideout V, Robb MB. The common sense census: Media use by tweens and teens. 2019. https://sleepeducation.org/resources/sleep-diary/; with permission.)

the circadian rhythms that organize our 24-hour sleep and wake patterns.[44,45] When light is removed and we are in darkness, our bodies secrete melatonin, a naturally occurring hormone that decreases alertness and promotes sleep.[46] In addition to window or lamp light, exposure to luminous devices suppresses melatonin levels, which shifts our circadian clock, elongates sleep onset, and decreases morning alertness levels.[47,48]

The growing literature on the negative relationship between screen use and sleep for adolescents indicates a pressing need for intervention.[49] Poor quality of sleep diminishes every adolescent's potential to excel, and therefore it is every clinician and parent's duty to educate their teens on the detriments of screen use and to monitor electronic device usage.

### Screening and Assessment

Despite the importance of sleep in the healthy development of children and adolescents, only approximately one-third of pediatricians routinely ask about sleep habits.[50] Numerous tools are available, however, to aid practitioners in this endeavor.

The user-friendly "BEARS" pediatric sleep screening tool is the easiest place to start. This validated survey addresses 5 domains of common sleep irregularities: bedtime problems, excessive daytime sleepiness, awakenings, regularity and duration of sleep, and snoring. Each domain includes a set of both parent-oriented and child-oriented questions (**Table 1**). Clinicians can use this survey during clinical sessions to obtain sleep-related information and identify potential sleep problems. Using BEARS has been shown to double the likelihood that primary care physicians will identify sleep problems.[46,51] Further assessment and treatment planning is advised if difficulties within 2 or more domains are identified.

To gather more precise information about a patient's sleep, clinicians will find a sleep diary highly effective.[52] Many varieties of sleep logs are available, but each tracks sleep and habits that affect sleep, such as exercise, caffeine-use, and medications (**Fig. 2**).

Many additional sleep screening tools are available with varying validity and psychometric measurements.[53] After completing a routine screening such as the BEARS, clinicians may consider a survey such as the Insomnia Severity Index (ISI), which maps symptoms onto DSM-IV criteria for insomnia and measures 7 items using a 5-point Likert scale. One particular benefit to the ISI is its demonstrated validity in measuring the efficacy of CBT-I treatment (see later in this article).[54] The ISI is freely available for providers to download online.

For an objective assessment of a patient's sleep, actigraphy is an outstanding choice, although most clinicians do not have access to this technology. Actigraphs are wearable devices that, unlike the aforementioned assessments, gather objective data on an individual's sleep timing and duration based on movement tracking. The main limitation of actigraphy is that waking motionless states cannot be differentiated from sleep, but when used in conjunction with a sleep diary, it can prove to be a thorough assessment measure.[55] As personal fitness trackers such as Fitbits improve, they will undoubtedly also assist in gathering accurate data on sleep; however, to date, fitness trackers have generally shown great variability and inaccuracy.[56]

### Current Approaches to Treatment

Behavioral treatments are preferred as the first-line treatment for children and adolescents because they are effective, lead to rapid improvements, and have long-lasting results.[57] CBT-I is an evidence-based method particularly effective at treating the psychological and behavioral factors that perpetuate insomnia once it has begun. CBT-I includes components of sleep education, stimulus control, sleep restriction therapy, sleep hygiene, cognitive therapy, and relaxation training, and routinely leads to improvements in sleep latency, wake-after sleep onset, and sleep efficiency. Numerous trials have demonstrated that CBT-I can benefit adolescents and that many of its component parts can be applied to the treatment of prepubertal insomnia as well.[58,59] See **Table 2** for further details on the treatment.

Proper sleep hygiene education, a component of CBT-I, is essential to use to effectively treat insomnia and educate patients about various behavioral practices that interfere with sleep. Limiting exposure to blue light via screens, caffeine, and alcohol and drugs, such as marijuana, along with managing the timing of exercise and creating a comfortable sleep environment with limited light and noise are additional strategies that augment the techniques of CBT-I.[46] Although sleep hygiene alone has not been shown to be adequately effective for the treatment of pediatric insomnia, sleep hygiene is often advised by practitioners as part of a treatment plan.[60]

Pharmacologic interventions are a second line of treatment for pediatric insomnia, and despite the lack of medications approved by the Food and Drug Administration,

**Table 1**
**BEARS sleep screening tool**

| | Toddler/Preschooler (Questions to Parents) | School-Aged (Questions to Parents) | Adolescent (Questions to Patient) |
|---|---|---|---|
| Bedtime problems | • Any problems going to bed or falling asleep? | • Any problems at bedtime? | • Any problems falling asleep at bedtime? |
| Excessive daytime sleepiness | • Napping or seeming overtired or sleepy a lot during the day? | • Difficulty waking in the morning, feels sleepy during the day or naps? | • Very sleepy during the day? At school? While driving? |
| Awakenings | • Waking up a lot at night? | • Waking up a lot at night or having trouble getting back to sleep?<br>• Sleepwalking or nightmares? | • Do you wake up a lot at night or have trouble getting back to sleep? |
| Regularity and duration of sleep | • Regular bedtime and wake up time? What are they? | • At what time does your child go to bed and get up on school days? Weekends?<br>• Is this enough sleep? | • What time do you usually go to bed on school nights? Weekends?<br>• How much sleep do you usually get? |
| Snoring | • Snoring a lot or having difficulty breathing at night? | • Snoring loudly or having breathing difficulties at night? | • Snoring loudly? (question to parent) |

*From* Owens JA, Dalzell V. Use of the 'BEARS' sleep screening tool in a pediatric residents' continuity clinic: A pilot study. Sleep Med. 2005;6(1):68–9; with permission.

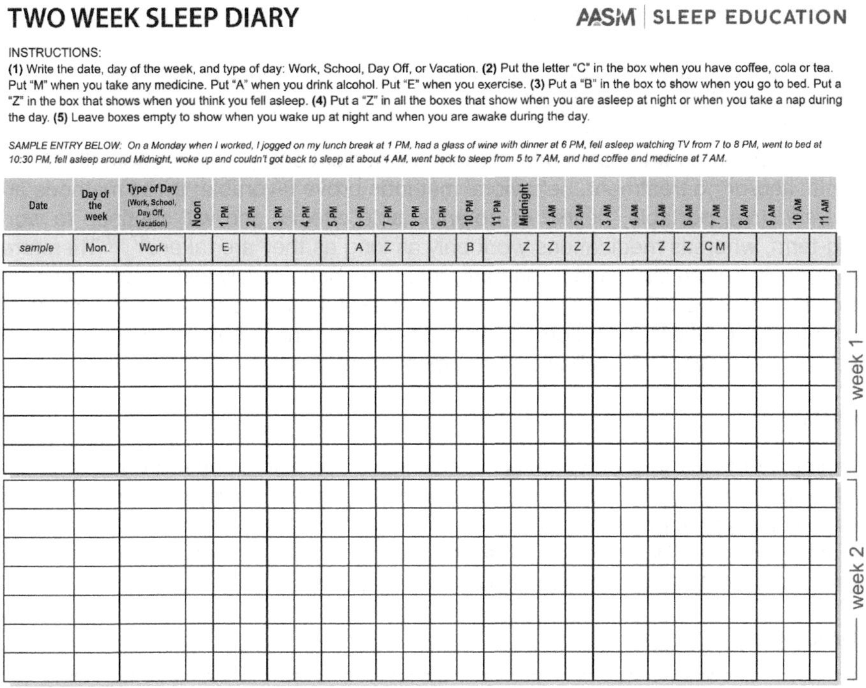

**TWO WEEK SLEEP DIARY** AASM | SLEEP EDUCATION

INSTRUCTIONS:
**(1)** Write the date, day of the week, and type of day: Work, School, Day Off, or Vacation. **(2)** Put the letter "C" in the box when you have coffee, cola or tea. Put "M" when you take any medicine. Put "A" when you drink alcohol. Put "E" when you exercise. **(3)** Put a "B" in the box to show when you go to bed. Put a "Z" in the box that shows when you think you fell asleep. **(4)** Put a "Z" in all the boxes that show when you are asleep at night or when you take a nap during the day. **(5)** Leave boxes empty to show when you wake up at night and when you are awake during the day.

*SAMPLE ENTRY BELOW: On a Monday when I worked, I jogged on my lunch break at 1 PM, had a glass of wine with dinner at 6 PM, fell asleep watching TV from 7 to 8 PM, went to bed at 10:30 PM, fell asleep around Midnight, woke up and couldn't got back to sleep at about 4 AM, went back to sleep from 5 to 7 AM, and had coffee and medicine at 7 AM.*

| Date | Day of the week | Type of Day (Work, School, Day Off, Vacation) | Noon | 1 PM | 2 PM | 3 PM | 4 PM | 5 PM | 6 PM | 7 PM | 8 PM | 9 PM | 10 PM | 11 PM | Midnight | 1 AM | 2 AM | 3 AM | 4 AM | 5 AM | 6 AM | 7 AM | 8 AM | 9 AM | 10 AM | 11 AM |
|---|---|---|---|---|---|---|---|---|---|---|---|---|---|---|---|---|---|---|---|---|---|---|---|---|---|---|
| *sample* | Mon. | Work | | E | | | | | A | Z | | | B | | Z | Z | Z | Z | | Z | Z | C M | | | | |



**Fig. 2.** Sleep diary example, American Academy of Sleep Medicine. (*From* American Academy of Sleep Medicine. Two week sleep diary. Available at: https://sleepeducation.org/resources/sleep-diary/; with permission.)

**Table 2**
**Components of Cognitive Behavioral Therapy for Insomnia**

| Therapy Component | Description |
|---|---|
| Stimulus control | Aims to break conditioned arousal between the bed and wakefulness/worry, and rather strengthen the association between the bed and sleep. |
| Sleep restriction | Limits the time allowed in bed to the patient's average reported actual sleep time, and subsequently and slowly increases the time allowed in bed as sleep improves. |
| Cognitive therapy | Targets beliefs and thoughts that directly interfere with sleep by increasing arousal in bed, or indirectly by interfering with adherence to stimulus control and sleep restriction. |
| Sleep hygiene education | Teaches patients about sleep and encourages them to limit caffeine intake, avoid alcohol prior to bedtime, incorporate daily exercise, and keep the bedroom quiet, dark, and at a comfortable temperature. |
| Relaxation techniques | Incorporates techniques such as diaphragmatic breathing, progressive muscle relaxation, and visual imagery to reduce psychic and somatic anxiety related to sleep. |

*From* Siebern AT, Manber, RM. New developments in cognitive behavioral therapy as the first-line treatment of insomnia. Psychology Research and Behavior Management 2011:4 21-28 - Originally published by and used with permission from Dove Medical Press Ltd.

it is common practice for many clinicians to prescribe medication for the management of the disorder.[61,62] Alpha-2 agonists, trazodone, and sedating antidepressants are among the most-prescribed medications; however, melatonin, a dietary supplement, has the most data supporting efficacy at this time (eg, 1 to 5 mg administered 30–60 minutes before bedtime).[62–66]

When compared with commonly prescribed medications, placebo, alternative treatments, and/or no treatment, behavioral methods prove favorable; these methods are cost-effective, portable, devoid of potential side effects, and will continue to work long-term, whereas medications work only as long as they are taken.[67,68] Therefore, we strongly advise clinicians to primarily intervene behaviorally with weekly sessions of comprehensive CBT-I. If this proves unsuccessful as a stand-alone treatment, or when treating patients with comorbid conditions, pharmacologic intervention can be used in conjunction with behavioral treatment strategies.

## SUMMARY

The impact of insomnia on youth is increasingly evident. In an ever busy, fast-paced twenty-first century society, children and adolescents are under more pressure than ever before to perform at their best, yet sleep is all too often compromised in an effort to meet these expectations. To maximize every child's potential, clinicians must assess and treat sleep disorders among their patients.

## CLINICS CARE POINTS

- Clinicians must be properly educated on the presentation of pediatric insomnia across childhood, to adequately screen for the disorder.
- All youth patients and their parents would benefit from instruction on proper sleep hygiene and the long-term consequences of poor sleep. Education on adequate sleep hygiene, notably the ramifications of excessive screen use, is critical.
- Clinicians can gather useful clinical information on the sleep of their pediatric patients by using a sleep diary and an age-appropriate screening tool.
- CBT-I is the recommended first-line treatment for pediatric insomnia, and melatonin is the most effective medication in doses of 1 to 5 mg administered 30 to 60 minutes before bedtime.

## DISCLOSURE

The authors have nothing to disclose.

## REFERENCES

1. Chattu VK, Manzar MD, Kumary S, et al. The global problem of insufficient sleep and its serious public health implications. Healthcare (Basel) 2018;7(1):1.
2. Meltzer LJ, Johnson C, Crosette J, et al. Prevalence of diagnosed sleep disorders in pediatric primary care practices. Pediatrics 2010;125(6):1410.
3. Brown KM, Malow BA. Pediatric insomnia. Chest 2016;149(5):1332–9.
4. Frank MG, Issa NP, Stryker MP. Sleep enhances plasticity in the developing visual cortex. Neuron 2001;30(1):275–87.
5. Sadeh A, Mindell J, Rivera L. "My child has a sleep problem": a cross-cultural comparison of parental definitions. Sleep Med 2011;12(5):478–82. Available at: https://doi-org.proxy.library.nyu.edu/10.1016/j.sleep.2010.10.008.

6. Owens J. Classification and epidemiology of childhood sleep disorders. Prim Care 2007;35(3):533–46.
7. Calhoun SL, Fernandez-Mendoza J, Vgontzas AN, et al. Prevalence of insomnia symptoms in a general population sample of young children and preadolescents: gender effects. Sleep Med 2014;15(1):91–5. Available at: https://doi-org.proxy. library.nyu.edu/10.1016/j.sleep.2013.08.787.
8. Johnson EO, Roth T, Schultz L, et al. Epidemiology of DSM-IV insomnia in adolescence: lifetime prevalence, chronicity, and an emergent gender difference. Pediatrics 2006;117:e247–56.
9. Symptoms. National Sleep Foundation Web site. Available at: https://www. sleepfoundation.org/insomnia/symptoms. Accessed February 20, 2020.
10. Substance Abuse and Mental Health Services Administration. Impact of the DSM-IV to DSM-5 changes on the national survey on drug use and health. Rockville (MD): Substance Abuse and Mental Health Services Administration (US); 2016. Table 3.36, DSM-IV to DSM-5 Insomnia Disorder Comparison. Available at: https://www.ncbi.nlm.nih.gov/books/NBK519704/table/ch3.t36/.
11. Nevsimalova S, Bruni O. Sleep disorders in children. Cham (Switzerland): Springer; 2017. p. 53–67. Available at: https://ebookcentral.proquest.com/lib/ [SITE_ID]/detail.action?docID=4709270. 10.1007/978-3-319-28640-2.
12. Carskadon MA. Patterns of sleep and sleepiness in adolescents. Pediatrician 1990;17(1):5–12.
13. Hysing M, Pallesen S, Stormark KM, et al. Sleep patterns and insomnia among adolescents: a population-based study. J Sleep Res 2013;22(5):549–56.
14. Pagel JF, Forister N, Kwiatkowki C. Adolescent sleep disturbance and school performance: the confounding variable of socioeconomics. J Clin Sleep Med 2007; 3(1):19–23.
15. National Sleep Foundation. Sleep in America poll. National Sleep Foundation. Oxfordshire (UK): Taylor & Francis Group; Behavioral Sleep Medicine; 2006.
16. O'Brien EM, Mindell JA. Sleep and risk-taking behavior in adolescents. Behav Sleep Med 2005;3(3):113–33.
17. Danner F, Phillips B. Adolescent sleep, school start times, and teen motor vehicle crashes. J Clin Sleep Med 2008;4(6):533–5. Available at: https://www.ncbi.nlm. nih.gov/pmc/articles/PMC2603528/.
18. Dewald JF, Meijer AM, Oort FJ, et al. The influence of sleep quality, sleep duration and sleepiness on school performance in children and adolescents: a meta-analytic review. Sleep Med Rev 2010;14(3):179–89.
19. Donskoy I, Loghmanee D. Insomnia in adolescence. Med Sci (Basel) 2018;6(3). https://doi.org/10.3390/medsci6030072. Available at: https://www.ncbi.nlm.nih. gov/pmc/articles/PMC6164454/.
20. Owens J. Insufficient sleep in adolescents and young adults: an update on causes and consequences. Pediatrics 2014;134(3):921.
21. Owens JA, Mindell JA. Pediatric insomnia. Pediatr Clin North Am 2011;58(3): 555–69.
22. Kalmbach DA, Cuamatzi-Castelan AS, Tonnu CV, et al. Hyperarousal and sleep reactivity in insomnia: current insights. Nat Sci Sleep 2018;10:193–201.
23. Bonnet MH, Arand DL. Hyperarousal and insomnia: state of the science. Sleep Med Rev 2010;14(1):9–15.
24. Riemann D, Spiegelhalder K, Feige B, et al. The hyperarousal model of insomnia: a review of the concept and its evidence. Sleep Med Rev 2010;14(1):19–31.
25. Fernandez-Mendoza J, Li Y, Vgontzas AN, et al. Insomnia is associated with cortical hyperarousal as early as adolescence. Sleep 2016;39(5):1029–36.

26. Drake CL, Cheng P, Almeida DM, et al. Familial risk for insomnia is associated with abnormal cortisol response to stress. Sleep 2017;40(10). https://doi.org/10.1093/sleep/zsx143.

27. Morin CM, Rodrigue S, Ivers H. Role of stress, arousal, and coping skills in primary insomnia. Psychosom Med 2003;65(2):259–67.

28. Britton JC, Lissek S, Grillon C, et al. Development of anxiety: the role of threat appraisal and fear learning. Depress Anxiety 2011;28(1):5–17.

29. Richdale AL, Schreck KA. Sleep problems in autism spectrum disorders: prevalence, nature, & possible biopsychosocial aetiologies. Sleep Med Rev 2009;13(6):403–11.

30. Owens JA. The ADHD and sleep conundrum: a review. J Dev Behav Pediatr 2005;26(4):312–22.

31. Corkum P, Moldofsky H, Hogg-Johnson S, et al. Sleep problems in children with attention-deficit/hyperactivity disorder: impact of subtype, comorbidity, and stimulant medication. J Am Acad Child Adolesc Psychiatry 1999;38(10):1285–93.

32. Ivanenko A, Barnes ME, Crabtree VM, et al. Psychiatric symptoms in children with insomnia referred to a pediatric sleep medicine center. Sleep Med 2004;5(3):253–9.

33. Philip P, Guilleminault C. Adult psychophysiologic insomnia and positive history of childhood insomnia. Sleep 1996;19(3 Suppl):16.

34. Merikangas KR, He J, Burstein M, et al. Lifetime prevalence of mental disorders in U.S. adolescents: results from the national comorbidity survey replication–adolescent supplement (NCS-A). J Am Acad Child Adolesc Psychiatry 2010;49(10):980–9.

35. McGlinchey EL, Courtney-Seidler EA, German M, et al. The role of sleep disturbance in suicidal and nonsuicidal self-injurious behavior among adolescents. Suicide Life Threat Behav 2017;47(1):103–11.

36. Lopes M, Boronat AC, Wang Y, et al. Sleep complaints as risk factor for suicidal behavior in severely depressed children and adolescents. CNS Neurosci Ther 2016;22(11):915–20.

37. Zullo L, Horton S, Eaddy M, et al. Adolescent insomnia, suicide risk, and the interpersonal theory of suicide. Psychiatry Res 2017;257:242–8.

38. Kemp S. Digital 2019: global Internet use accelerates. We are social Web site 2019. Available at: https://wearesocial.com/blog/2019/01/digital-2019-global-internet-use-accelerates. Accessed April 3, 2020.

39. Wang Y. More people have cell phones than toilets, U.N. study shows. 2013. Available at: https://newsfeed.time.com/2013/03/25/more-people-have-cell-phones-than-toilets-u-n-study-shows/. Accessed April 27, 2020.

40. Rideout V, Robb M B. The common sense census: media use by tweens and teens 2019. Available at: https://www.commonsensemedia.org/sites/default/files/uploads/research/2019-census-8-to-18-full-report-updated.pdf. Accessed April 3, 2020.

41. Cain N, Gradisar M. Electronic media use and sleep in school-aged children and adolescents: a review. Sleep Med 2010;11(8):735–42. Available at: http://www.sciencedirect.com/science/article/pii/S1389945710001632.

42. Fobian AD, Avis K, Schwebel DC. The impact of media use on adolescent sleep efficiency. J Dev Behav Pediatr 2016;37(1):9–14.

43. Gradisar M, Wolfson AR, Harvey AG, et al. The sleep and technology use of Americans: findings from the national sleep foundation's 2011 sleep in America poll. J Clin Sleep Med 2013;9(12):1291–9.

44. Moore RY. Circadian rhythms: basic neurobiology and clinical applications. Annu Rev Med 1997;48:253–66.

45. Moore RY. The fourth C.U. Ariëns Kappers lecture. The organization of the human circadian timing system. Prog Brain Res 1992;93:99–117.

46. Badin E, Haddad C, Shatkin JP. Insomnia: the sleeping giant of pediatric public health. Curr Psychiatry Rep 2016;18(5):47.

47. Chang A, Aeschbach D, Duffy JF, et al. Evening use of light-emitting eReaders negatively affects sleep, circadian timing, and next-morning alertness. Proc Natl Acad Sci U S A 2015;112(4):1232–7.

48. Wood B, Rea MS, Plitnick B, et al. Light level and duration of exposure determine the impact of self-luminous tablets on melatonin suppression. Appl Ergon 2013; 44(2):237–40.

49. Hysing M, Pallesen S, Stormark KM, et al. Sleep and use of electronic devices in adolescence: results from a large population-based study. BMJ Open 2015;5(1): e006748.

50. Owens JA. The practice of pediatric sleep medicine: results of a community survey. Pediatrics 2001;108(3):E51.

51. Owens JA, Dalzell V. Use of the 'BEARS' sleep screening tool in a pediatric residents' continuity clinic: a pilot study. Sleep Med 2005;6(1):63–9.

52. Carney CE, Buysse DJ, Ancoli-Israel S, et al. The consensus sleep diary: Standardizing prospective sleep self-monitoring. Sleep 2012;35(2):287–302.

53. Erwin AM, Bashore L. Subjective sleep measures in children: self-report. Front Pediatr 2017;5. https://doi.org/10.3389/fped.2017.00022.

54. Chen P, Jan Y, Yang C. Are the insomnia severity index and Pittsburgh Sleep Quality Index valid outcome measures for cognitive behavioral therapy for insomnia? Inquiry from the perspective of response shifts and longitudinal measurement invariance in their Chinese versions. Sleep Med 2017;35:35–40.

55. Smith MT, McCrae CS, Cheung J, et al. Use of actigraphy for the evaluation of sleep disorders and circadian rhythm sleep-wake disorders: an American Academy of Sleep Medicine systematic review, meta-analysis, and GRADE assessment. J Clin Sleep Med 2018;14(7):1209–30.

56. Baroni A, Bruzzese J, Di Bartolo CA, et al. Fitbit flex: an unreliable device for longitudinal sleep measures in a non-clinical population. Sleep Breath 2016;20(2): 853–4.

57. Tikotzky L, Sadeh A. Sleep medicine. Sleep Med 2010;11(7):686–91. Available at: http://www.sciencedirect.com/science/article/pii/S1389945710002200.

58. Paine S, Gradisar M. A randomised controlled trial of cognitive-behaviour therapy for behavioural insomnia of childhood in school-aged children. Behav Res Ther 2011;49(6–7):379–88.

59. de Bruin EJ, Bögels SM, Oort FJ, et al. Efficacy of cognitive behavioral therapy for insomnia in adolescents: a randomized controlled trial with internet therapy, group therapy and A waiting list condition. Sleep 2015;38(12):1913–26.

60. Stepanski EJ, Wyatt JK. Use of sleep hygiene in the treatment of insomnia. Sleep Med Rev 2003;7(3):215–25.

61. Owens JA, Rosen CL, Mindell JA. Medication use in the treatment of pediatric insomnia: results of a survey of community-based pediatricians. Pediatrics 2003;111(5 Pt 1):628.

62. Owens JA, Rosen CL, Mindell JA, et al. Use of pharmacotherapy for insomnia in child psychiatry practice: a national survey. Sleep Med 2010;11(7):692–700.

63. van Geijlswijk IM, van der Heijden, Kristiaan B, et al. Dose finding of melatonin for chronic idiopathic childhood sleep onset insomnia: an RCT. Psychopharmacology (Berl) 2010;212(3):379–91.

64. Andersen IM, Kaczmarska J, McGrew SG, et al. Melatonin for insomnia in children with autism spectrum disorders. J Child Neurol 2008;23(5):482–5.

65. Weiss MD, Wasdell MB, Bomben MM, et al. Sleep hygiene and melatonin treatment for children and adolescents with ADHD and initial insomnia. J Am Acad Child Adolesc Psychiatry 2006;45(5):512–9.

66. Smits MG, van Stel HF, van der Heijden K, et al. Melatonin improves health status and sleep in children with idiopathic chronic sleep-onset insomnia: a randomized placebo-controlled trial. J Am Acad Child Adolesc Psychiatry 2003;42(11):1286–93.

67. Mitchell MD, Gehrman P, Perlis M, et al. Comparative effectiveness of cognitive behavioral therapy for insomnia: a systematic review. BMC Fam Pract 2012; 13:40.

68. Taylor DJ, Roane BM. Treatment of insomnia in adults and children: a practice-friendly review of research. J Clin Psychol 2010;66(11):1137–47.

# The Parasomnias

Oliviero Bruni, MD[a],*, Lourdes M. DelRosso, MD[b],
Maria Grazia Melegari, MD[a], Raffaele Ferri, MD[c]

## KEYWORDS

- NREM parasomnias • Confusional arousals • Sleepwalking • Sleep terrors
- REM-related parasomnias • Sleep enuresis

## KEY POINTS

- Parasomnias affect a large proportion of children.
- Pediatricians and psychiatrists may not be aware of these sleep disorders and the implications for their patients.
- Parasomnias (especially those that are rapid eye movement related) may be associated with psychiatric comorbidities.
- Understanding of the pathogenesis and diagnostic testing for these are still being developed.

## INTRODUCTION

The International Classification of Sleep Disorder (ICSD-3) defines parasomnias as "undesirable physical events or experiences that occur during entry into sleep, within sleep, or during arousal from sleep."[1] The term parasomnia derives from the Greek word para meaning around and the Latin somnus meaning sleep.[1] The Diagnostic and Statistical Manual of Mental Disorders, Fifth Edition, defines parasomnias as recurrent episodes of incomplete awakening from sleep with usual amnesia of the episode, and little or no dream imagery and distress or social impairment.

Parasomnias include several disorders that share clinical and physiologic characteristics: (1) clear and dramatic symptoms associated with skeletal muscle activity; (2) correlation with age; (3) unassociated medical problems; (4) absence of specific polysomnographic anomalies; (5) spontaneous resolution; and (6) unknown cause.

They are classified based on the sleep stage during which they occur: non–rapid eye movement (NREM)–related parasomnias, which include disorders of arousal

This article originally appeared in *Child and Adolescent Psychiatric Clinics*, Volume 30 Issue 1, January 2021.
Funding: The authors received no funding for this article.
[a] Department of Developmental and Social Psychology, Sapienza University of Rome, Via dei Marsi 78, Rome 00185, Italy; [b] Department of Internal Medicine, University of California San Francisco, Fresno, CA, USA; [c] Department of Neurology I.C., Sleep Research Centre, Oasi Institute for Research on Mental Retardation and Brain Aging (IRCCS), Troina, Italy
* Corresponding author.
*E-mail address:* oliviero.bruni@uniroma1.it

(confusional arousals, sleepwalking, sleep terrors, and sleep-related eating disorder); rapid eye movement (REM)–related parasomnias (REM sleep behavior disorder [RBD], recurrent isolated sleep paralysis, and nightmare disorder); and other parasomnias (exploding head syndrome, sleep-related hallucinations, and sleep enuresis) (**Table 1**).

The clinical diagnosis is mainly based on description of the event by parents, but often these descriptions are inaccurate and a home video recording of the event (ie, with a smartphone) can be helpful for the diagnosis. Parents should be guided to have a better picture of the event with a set of specific questions: (1) timing of appearance of the symptom; (2) specific manifested movements and symptoms; (3) reaction to external interventions; (4) presence of stereotypies (rhythmic, repetitive movements); and (5) recall of the episode in the morning.[2]

Polysomnography(PSG), or better video-PSG (vPSG), is not always recommended for the diagnosis or evaluation of typical parasomnias, but it is indicated for injurious parasomnias and when nocturnal seizures or other comorbid sleep disorders are suspected.

Most parasomnias are associated with specific sleep stages and have a benign evolution, with spontaneous resolution during puberty.[3]

## NON–RAPID EYE MOVEMENT–RELATED PARASOMNIAS

NREM-related parasomnias, also named disorders of arousal (DoAs), are defined in the ICSD-3 as recurrent episodes of incomplete awakening from sleep, characterized by inappropriate or absent responsiveness to efforts of others to intervene or redirect the person during the episode and with limited or no associated cognition or dream imagery. Patients have partial or complete amnesia for the episode.[1]

DoAs include confusional arousals, sleep terrors, sleepwalking (also called somnambulism), and sleep-related eating disorder (SRED). There is usually only 1 event per night, which typically occurs during the first third of the major (usually nocturnal) sleep episode. The individual may continue to appear confused and disoriented for several minutes, or even longer, following the episode. DoAs are benign events, typically occurring in childhood and ceasing by adolescence. Some individuals may experience more than 1 type of arousal parasomnia.[3]

In some cases, differential diagnosis is not simple because DoAs may mimic nocturnal seizures or RBD and parents' descriptions of events may be inaccurate, especially when the events make them anxious or frightened.

### Pathophysiology

DoAs result from an NREM sleep-wake state dissociation because patients appear to be simultaneously awake (with retention of their motor and behavioral functions) and asleep (with impairment of cognition, judgment, and memory for the events).[4]

| Table 1 Classification of parasomnias based on the International Classification of Sleep Disorders, Third Edition | | |
|---|---|---|
| **NREM-Related Parasomnias** | **REM-Related Parasomnias** | **Other Parasomnias** |
| Confusional arousals | RBD | Exploding head syndrome |
| Sleepwalking | Recurrent isolated sleep paralysis | Sleep-related hallucinations |
| Sleep terrors | Nightmare disorder | Sleep enuresis |
| Sleep-related eating disorder | — | — |

A cranial single-photon emission computed tomography (SPECT) study captured a sleepwalking event in a 16-year-old boy characterized by activation (increased regional cerebral blood flow) of thalamocingulate (motor coordination) pathways, with simultaneous deactivation in the frontal lobe.[5] The stereotactic electroencephalogram (EEG) recordings of NREM parasomnias showed local activations of the motor cortex, with an EEG pattern of wakefulness in the motor and central cingulate cortices paralleled by a concomitant increase in slow waves in the dorsolateral prefrontal cortex.[6,7] This finding confirmed the coexistence of simultaneous wakelike and sleeplike activities in different brain regions during an episode, which explains the motor and emotional activation along with clumsiness, uninhibited behavior, and amnesia of the event. The variable level of awareness during an NREM parasomnia could depend on the quantity and position of the local persistence of these slow waves.[4]

EEG studies showed increased arousals and cyclic alternating pattern rate during slow wave sleep, reflecting an alteration of NREM sleep continuity and different dynamics of slow wave activity throughout the night.[8] An EEG spectral analysis study showed a significantly greater number of arousals during stage N3 in sleepwalkers, particularly during the first NREM sleep cycle.[9]

Some behaviors observed in DoAs resemble stereotyped, archaic behaviors (such as defensive postures, violent gestures, and feeding) that result from the activation of neural circuits (mainly subcortical), namely central pattern generators (CPGs). CPGs are functional neural organizations located in the spinal cord, mesencephalon, pons, and medulla regulating innate behavioral automatisms and survival behaviors.[10] Some manifestations of DoAs could result from CPG disinhibition, as a result of prefrontal cortex dysfunction, permitting the expression of complex behaviors without conscious control.[11]

NREM parasomnias can also occur or worsen when specific factors are present: (1) conditions that increase slow wave sleep, such as sleep deprivation and drugs (zolpidem, lithium, and sodium oxybate); (2) conditions that cause repeated cortical arousals determining sleep fragmentation, such as sleep disorders (obstructive sleep apnea, periodic limb movements of sleep, chronic pain, narcolepsy), noise, fever, physical activity late in the day, emotions, stress, and anxiety; and (3) impaired arousal mechanism and persistence of sleep drive resulting in a failure of the brain to fully transition into wakefulness.[3]

In addition to the precipitating factors mentioned earlier, there is a strong genetic contribution to DoAs. Positive family history is found in up to 80% of children presenting with DoA[12] (ie, precipitating factors act on an underlying genetic predisposition). The contributions of both determine the frequency and severity of the parasomnia events.

### Epidemiology

NREM parasomnias are common pediatric sleep disorders that tend to decrease across development and in adulthood, possibly because of decreased slow wave sleep with aging. Laberge and colleagues[13] found that about 17% of children between 3 and 13 years old experienced occasional or frequent episodes of confusional arousals.

Ohayon and colleagues[14] observed that confusional arousal affects 4.2% of the general population, decreasing from 6.1% among those 15 to 24 years old to 3.3% among those aged 25 to 34 years old, and stabilizing around 2% after age 35 years. The prevalence of sleepwalking in children ranges from 3% to 14.5%, and most episodes resolve after age 10 years. Sleep terrors have the greatest incidence in preschool children, with a reported overall prevalence of 17.3% in children between 3 and 13 years old. The peak prevalence of sleepwalking (13%) occurred at age 10 years. One-third of children who had sleep terrors went on to develop sleepwalking.[15]

### Clinical Features

NREM parasomnias occur along a continuum, ranging from confusional arousals with low motor and autonomic activation at the lower end of the spectrum up to night terrors characterized by intense motor activity and autonomic activation at the high end of the spectrum. There is an age-related evolution with different presentations: a child might present a sequence of confusional arousals in early childhood and sleep terrors later on, followed by sleepwalking in late childhood and adolescence. These 3 disorders show common and distinct features (**Table 2**).

### Confusional arousal

Confusional arousals are characterized by mental confusion or confused behavior that occurs while the patient is in bed, in the absence of terror or ambulation outside the bed.[1] These events often begin with the individual sitting up in bed with eyes open and staring or looking around: the child looks awake but is confused, disoriented, does not respond adequately to orders, can be engaged in conversation with slowed speech, and shows blunted response to questioning.

Episodes usually start with a moan and some movements and then progress toward crying; the expression of terror typical of pavor nocturnus is missing. The duration varies from a few minutes to 40 to 60 minutes. The exact prevalence is unknown because of the difficulty of identification, in part because symptoms can be too mild to be recognized, or because of inaccurate descriptions by distressed parents. Onset is before the child turns 5 years old.[3]

### Sleepwalking

Sleepwalking is characterized by complex behaviors that are usually initiated during arousals from slow wave sleep and culminate in leaving the bed in an altered state of consciousness. The child acts out more or less complex, automatic movements that vary from simply standing by the bed to walking around the house in an agitated manner associated with semipurposeful behaviors such as eating, drinking, or leaving home. These episodes can be concomitant with vocalization, often in an

**Table 2**
**Clinical features of disorders of arousal**

|  | Confusional Arousal | Sleepwalking | Night Terrors |
|---|---|---|---|
| Age (y) | 2–10 | 4–12 | 1.5–10 |
| Onset | First third of night | First third of night | First third of night |
| Agitation | Mild | No/poor | Marked |
| Autonomic Activity | Mild | Mild | Marked |
| Motor Activity | Low | Complex | Rarely complex |
| Ictal Behavior | Whimpering, some articulation, sitting up in bed, inconsolable | Walking around, quiet or agitated, unresponsive to verbal commands | Screaming, agitation, flushed face, sweating, inconsolable |
| Amnesia | Yes | Yes | Yes |
| Threshold of Arousal | High | High | High |
| Familiality | High | High | High |

incomprehensible language, and aggressive acts can occur, usually in relation to attempts to block or awaken the child.

The average duration is around 10 minutes. Typically, parents report that the episode ends after the child has gone to the bathroom to urinate; this has led to the supposition that bladder repletion may contribute to these episodes by triggering a partial arousal.

The age of onset is generally between 4 and 8 years, with a peak at 10 years and resolution during adolescence. Prevalence is between 15% and 30% for sporadic episodes and 3% for frequent episodes without differences between boys and girls.[13]

A positive family history was found in up to 80% of subjects; other family members might be affected by sleepwalking or other arousal disorders, with a chance of recurrence of 45% if 1 parent is affected and 60% if both parents are affected.[8]

Association with mental disorder has only been noted when sleepwalking persists into adulthood.[8]

### Sleep terrors

Sleep terrors are distinguished from other DoAs by their prominent autonomic activation and distinct expression of terror. During the episode, the child presents with a sudden onset of partial awakening, a loud cry, intense agitation, autonomic symptoms (pallor, sweating, tachycardia, tachypnea, increased arterial pressure, mydriasis) and increased muscle tone. The child is not very responsive to environmental stimulation and does not recognize those close to them; the child may seem to look beyond, appears terrified, and is inconsolable; less often, the child may also get out of bed and walk around. Some children show prolonged inconsolability without awareness. If awakened, the child will be confused and disoriented, although they usually return to sleep quickly and do not remember the episode in the morning. The episodes are short (but can range from 30 seconds to 30 minutes) and rarely occur more than once in a night.[16]

Prevalence varies between 1% and 6% and is slightly higher among boys; typical age of onset is from 2 to 4 years, with a peak between 5 and 7 years. There is a high overlap between sleep terrors and other parasomnias. Precipitating factors are stress, fever, bladder distension, and sleep deprivation, and there is no apparent relationship with mental disorder.[17]

### Differential Diagnosis

The diagnosis of DoA is mainly based on clinical descriptors; the availability of a video-recording of an episode is extremely useful. A clear clinical history can be sufficient to diagnose an NREM parasomnia in most cases, but in others only vPSG recording can clarify the nature of the disorder. Typical PSG features of sleep architecture of patients with NREM parasomnia include hypersynchronous delta waves, irregular slow wave activity, and NREM sleep instability. NREM parasomnia needs to be distinguished from other parasomnias and sleep-related seizures.[18]

Although the diagnosis can be made clinically, some situations warrant further evaluation. A sleep study (vPSG) should be ordered if a concomitant sleep disorder is suspected (obstructive sleep apnea, periodic leg movement disorder, and so forth). Consider referral to child psychiatry if posttraumatic stress disorder, anxiety, depression, or a neurodevelopmental disorder is suspected, and referral to neurology if there are frequent, stereotypic, and brief episodes suspicious for seizures.

Nightmares can resemble sleep terrors but occur during REM sleep in the second half of the night. After a nightmare, children become fully alert quickly, respond positively to comforting, may report the dream content after awakening, and show lower levels of autonomic activation and mobility. Nocturnal panic attacks are characterized by waking from sleep in a state of panic, with intense fear or discomfort, but are more frequent in adults; immediately after the episodes, children appear oriented, can vividly recall the attack, and have difficulty returning to sleep.[19]

A challenge in differential diagnosis is represented by sleep hypermotor epilepsy (SHE), previously called nocturnal frontal lobe epilepsy, in which seizures occur almost exclusively during sleep with different sleep-related motor attacks of increasing complexity and duration. Seizures are usually brief, abrupt, can occur at any time in the night (or several times), and the presentation ranges from stereotypic movements to dystonic positions and nocturnal wandering". However, there are some similarities and possible coexistence of parasomnias in children with SHE, and the differential diagnosis between these disorders can be complicated. Further evaluation by neurology and vPSG study is recommended if SHE if suspected.[20]

### Non–rapid Eye Movement Parasomnia Treatment

Parasomnia episodes are often benign and normally require no treatment. General management considerations include prevention, safety measures, and bystander intervention guidelines (**Table 3**). Relaxation techniques before sleep and hypnosis can also be helpful. Another technique is anticipatory or scheduled awakenings, which consist of awakening the child about 15 minutes before the presumed time when the episode will occur (usually within 2 hours of falling asleep). This technique may shift the child into a lighter state of sleep, thereby aborting the event. The Lully Sleep Guardian is a vibrating alarm placed under the mattress and connected to the parent's smartphone that can be set to activate at predetermined times, resulting in arousal.[21]

Pharmacotherapy should be considered only when episodes are frequent or dangerous to the patient or others, or when they cause undesirable secondary consequences, such as excessive daytime sleepiness, or distress to the patient or their family. Parents should be advised that prescribed drugs are considered off-label.[16,22] L-5-Hydroxytryptophan, a precursor of serotonin that may modify central serotoninergic system dysfunction or enhance production of sleep-promoting factors, can be effective for treating sleep terrors.[23] Melatonin has also been reported to be helpful for patients with sleepwalking and sleep terrors.[24] A referral to sleep medicine specialists may be indicated when a coexisting sleep disorder is suspected.

### Sleep-related eating disorder

SRED consists of "recurrent episodes of involuntary eating and drinking during arousals from sleep, associated with diminished levels of consciousness and

**Table 3**
**Prevention and safety approach for non–rapid eye movement parasomnias**

| Safety Measures | Prevention | Bystander Guidelines |
|---|---|---|
| Remove furniture or objects near bed | Good sleep hygiene | Silently observe |
| Lock doors and windows | Avoid sleep deprivation | Permit episodes to run course |
| Security alarm to warn family members | Avoid environmental stimulation (ie, light, sound, touch) | Intervene only to prevent injury |
| Stairwell barriers and night light to prevent falls/injuries | Address comorbid sleep disorders (obstructive sleep apnea, periodic limb movement disorder) | Avoid physically restraining the child |

subsequent recall, with problematic consequences."[1] Episodes typically occur during partial arousals from sleep during the first third of the night, with impaired subsequent recall.[25] SRED occurs predominantly in young women, with average age of onset approximately 22 to 27 years. However, this disorder is often hidden or overlooked and, on average, patients receive treatment of it after 12 to 16 years from onset.[16]

## RAPID EYE MOVEMENT–RELATED PARASOMNIAS

RBD, sleep paralysis, and nightmare disorders are the parasomnias of REM sleep, according to the ICSD-3.[1]

The main differences between NREM parasomnias and REM-related parasomnias are (1) the linkage to specific REM stage; (2) the occurrence during the second half of the night, when REM is more prevalent; (3) dream enactment behaviors; and (4) absence of mental confusion on awakening. On very rare occasions, some patients meet the diagnostic criteria for both NREM and REM parasomnia and are diagnosed with parasomnia overlap disorder.[26]

### Rapid Eye Movement Sleep Behavior Disorder

RBD is characterized by complex and violent behaviors with enactment of dreams that are often unpleasant, action-filled, and violent and that can cause sleep disruption and injuries to the patients or to their bedpartners.

Pathogenesis is linked to the absence of the typical REM elimination of muscle tone (atonia). In the absence of normal REM atonia, patients present with recurrent episodes of enacting their dreams, behaviors that can vary from small hand movements to violent activities, such as punching, kicking, or leaping out of bed.[26] The patient usually remembers the dream. For instance, patients with RBD may dream of being chased and run out of the bed, or that they are fighting and punch their bed partner.

RBD in childhood and adolescence is rare and is usually associated with narcolepsy or idiopathic hypersomnia, neurodevelopmental-neurodegenerative disorders, or structural brainstem abnormalities; it can also represent a side effect of pharmacologic agents, such as selective serotonin reuptake inhibitor agents.[27] Further evaluation is always indicated in children presenting with symptoms suspicious of RBD. Evaluation should include referral to a sleep specialist or a neurologist, vPSG, and brain imaging.

### Nightmare Disorder

Nightmare disorder is characterized by "recurrent, highly dysphoric dreams, which are disturbing mental experiences that generally occur during REM sleep and that often result in awakening."[1] On awakening from the dysphoric dreams, the person rapidly becomes oriented and alert.

Occasional nightmares are common in children, ranging from 60% to 75%, but the prevalence of nightmare disorder is estimated to be 1.8% to 6%. Nightmares can also occur more frequently in children with posttraumatic stress disorder.[28] A child with nightmare disorder may be scared but usually manages to report the dream and is well oriented, with an intact sensorium; parental intervention is accepted well. During the nightmare, there is little motor activity and the child does not move out of bed (because of REM atonia) and there is no dream enactment.

Emotional contents of nightmares are characteristically negative, with anxiety and fear but also anger, rage, embarrassment, and disgust. Exposure to violent content in electronics (television or computer programs) may contribute to nightmares and should be avoided as part of the sleep hygiene and bedtime routine education.

Monsters or other fantastical images often characterize the dreams of young children, whereas adolescents may experience more realistic images linked to daytime stressors or traumatic events.[29]

### Recurrent Isolated Sleep Paralysis

Recurrent isolated sleep paralysis is defined as a period of inability to perform voluntary movements that occurs at the beginning of sleep of a sleep period (hypnagogic) and/or after waking up (hypnopompic). Each episode lasts seconds to a few minutes and causes clinically significant distress, including bedtime anxiety or fear of sleep. The disturbance is not better explained by another sleep disorder (especially narcolepsy), mental disorder, medical condition, medication, or substance use.[30] Prevalence estimates vary widely, between 6% to 40%. Isolated episodes are exacerbated by sleep deprivation, stress, and sleep-wake rhythm irregularities.[31]

The individual experiencing sleep paralysis is conscious and alert, but feels paralyzed; all muscle groups are involved, with the exception of the diaphragm and the extrinsic muscles of the eye. The attacks usually end spontaneously, although they may occasionally be stopped intentionally if the individuals move their eyes rapidly or are administered tactile stimuli. These episodes commonly begin in adolescence, but can also appear in childhood.[32] Hallucinations can also occur during paralysis and commonly include sensing the presence of others nearby, pressure on the chest, or hearing footsteps.

The pathogenesis of this disorder is linked to the persistence of REM atonia into wakefulness, thus normal mental activity occurs in the presence of body paralysis.

First-line treatment is reassurance that the episodes are benign. Because sleep deprivation exacerbates sleep paralysis, recommendation of an adequate amount of sleep per age and education about sleep hygiene should be implemented. Pharmacologic treatment is rarely needed but may be considered in severe, debilitating cases with significant daytime consequences. REM-suppressing agents such as low doses of tricyclics, clonidine, or clonazepam could be tried.[31] Other sleep disorders that interrupt sleep (such as obstructive sleep apnea) can contribute to sleep deprivation and exacerbation of sleep paralysis. If snoring, gasping, or witnessed apneas are reported, a sleep study should be ordered. Sleep paralysis is also a symptom commonly seen in narcolepsy. If other symptoms, such as excessive daytime sleepiness, cataplexy, or hallucinations, are reported, referral to a sleep specialist or neurologist is recommended.

## SLEEP ENURESIS

Sleep enuresis (SE) is characterized by recurrent involuntary voiding that occurs during sleep. In primary SE, recurrent involuntary voiding occurs at least twice a week during sleep after 5 years of age in a patient who has never been consistently dry during sleep for 6 consecutive months. SE is considered secondary in a child or adult who had previously been dry for 6 consecutive months and then began wetting at least twice a week. Both primary and secondary enuresis must be present for a period of at least 3 months.[33]

SE is one of the most common problems in pediatrics, with a general prevalence of 3% to 15%. SE is more frequent in boys less than 11 years of age, although after 11 years of age no sex differences are reported. Spontaneous remission during childhood occurs in around 15%. There is a strong genetic predisposition for primary SE.

SE is defined as monosymptomatic when the child has no associated daytime symptoms of bladder dysfunction (such as wetting, increased voiding frequency, urgency, jiggling, squatting, and holding maneuvers).[34]

The most accepted hypothesis for the pathogenesis of SE is that it involves 3 systems: excessive nocturnal urine production, nocturnal bladder overactivity, and failure to awaken in response to bladder sensations.[35] Other pathophysiologic mechanisms are mostly related to sleep fragmentation, which can be secondary to sleep-disordered breathing[36] or periodic limb movements during sleep.[37]

From a developmental point of view, complete control of the bladder at night is usually achieved by age 5 years; thus, bed-wetting in toddlers is considered physiologic.

Children with SE are often described as deep sleepers, with higher arousal thresholds.[38] Enuretic events happen mainly during the first part of the night, and can occur in all sleep stages.[33] One study reported that patients with enuresis are subjectively sleepier than healthy controls and more difficult to awaken[39]; this was attributed to sleep fragmentation, which might be responsible for the higher arousal threshold and is consistent with a large body of research.[40]

Secondary SE is more commonly associated with urinary tract infections, malformations of the genitourinary tract, medical conditions that result in an inability to concentrate urine (diabetes mellitus or insipidus, sickle cell disease), and increased urine production secondary to excessive evening fluid intake (caffeine ingestion, diuretics, or other agents). Furthermore, neurologic diseases (spinal cord abnormalities with neurogenic bladder or seizures) and psychosocial stressors (parental divorce, neglect, physical or sexual abuse, institutionalization) should be considered.[33]

Enuresis can lead to a reduction of a child's self-esteem and to personality problems. Behavioral therapy is based on general hygiene measures (moderate restriction of evening drinks), elimination of negative family habits (eg, repeated intimate care, excessively careful attitudes toward sphincter control), sphincter conditioning exercises and bladder gymnastics training, behavioral and conditioning measures (keeping a diary, scheduled awakenings), and motivational techniques with positive reinforcement.

The most effective treatment of enuresis is a bed-wetting alarm, a system consisting of a small sensor clipped to the underwear, which is connected to a small battery-powered speaker that is activated when the sensor becomes wet. The resulting alarm awakens the wearer (or parents), alerting them that enuresis has begun. Controlled studies have shown that this approach is superior to all other methods, including pharmacologic or psychotherapeutic treatment. The drug options include desmopressin, imipramine, and oxybutynin.[41]

## SUMMARY

Pediatricians and psychiatrists have multidisciplinary tasks when managing parasomnia sleep disorders in children. Education to encourage a regular lifestyle, adequate sleep hygiene, avoid sleep deprivation, create a personalized sleep ritual with a regular bedtime even on weekends, and provide quiet sleeping conditions are the first steps in the management of these disorders.

Understanding of the pathogenesis and key diagnostic testing for parasomnias is still a work in progress; a critical step in the correct diagnosis will be to transcend phenomenological categorization of these disorders and to establish a pathophysiologically defined classification scheme. Such an approach might incorporate candidate biomarkers such as hypersynchronous slow waves and genetic links, which should provide improved ways to classify these mysterious events and to identify their precise management.

Cognitive behavior therapy or relaxation training may be helpful and possibly lead to a long-term benefit to these children or adolescents if they learn how to recognize the signs of the condition and how to cope with it. Even if benign, parasomnia events can have a substantial negative repercussion on quality of life.

Pharmacologic treatment currently focuses primarily on sedative medications, which are obviously not the first choice in children. The development of pathophysiologically based categorization is essential to support further research showing the efficacy of clinical therapies and identifying the key characteristics for optimal therapeutic outcomes, leading to tailoring treatments, whether nonpharmacologic or pharmacologic, for individual patients.[42]

## CLINICS CARE POINTS

- Parasomnias are usually benign and self-resolving.
- Parasomnias can be exacerbated by sleep deprivation or another sleep disorders, such as obstructive sleep apnea or periodic leg movements of sleep.
- Treatment options often include sleep extension, sleep hygiene, and safety measures to avoid injuries.
- Most parasomnias resolve by adulthood, but they can persist or coexist with another sleep disorder.
- If another sleep disorder is suspected, referral for vPSG is warranted.
- Stereotypic movements with repetitive, brief episodes can be suspicious of seizures and a neurology referral is recommended.

## DISCLOSURE

The authors have nothing to disclose.

## REFERENCES

1. American Academy of Sleep Medicine. International classification of Sleep Disorders, 3rd edn. American Academy of Sleep Medicine, Darien, IL, 2014.
2. Nevsimalova S, Prihodova I, Kemlink D, et al. Childhood parasomnia–a disorder of sleep maturation? Eur J Paediatr Neurol 2013;17(6):615–9.
3. Proserpio P, Nobili L. Parasomnias in children. In: Nevšímalová S, Bruni O, editors. Sleep disorders in children. Cham (Switzerland): Springer International Publishing; 2017. p. 305–35.
4. Castelnovo A, Lopez R, Proserpio P, et al. NREM sleep parasomnias as disorders of sleep-state dissociation. Nat Rev Neurol 2018;14(8):470–81.
5. Bassetti C, Vella S, Donati F, et al. SPECT during sleepwalking. Lancet 2000; 356(9228):484–5.
6. Terzaghi M, Sartori I, Tassi L, et al. Dissociated local arousal states underlying essential clinical features of non-rapid eye movement arousal parasomnia: an intracerebral stereo-electroencephalographic study. J Sleep Res 2012;21(5): 502–6.
7. Terzaghi M, Sartori I, Tassi L, et al. Evidence of dissociated arousal states during NREM parasomnia from an intracerebral neurophysiological study. Sleep 2009; 32(3):409–12.
8. Zadra A, Desautels A, Petit D, et al. Somnambulism: clinical aspects and pathophysiological hypotheses. Lancet Neurol 2013;12(3):285–94.

9. Gaudreau H, Joncas S, Zadra A, et al. Dynamics of slow-wave activity during the NREM sleep of sleepwalkers and control subjects. Sleep 2000;23(6):755–60.

10. Tassinari CA, Cantalupo G, Högl B, et al. Neuroethological approach to frontolimbic epileptic seizures and parasomnias: the same central pattern generators for the same behaviours. Rev Neurol (Paris) 2009;165(10):762–8.

11. Baldini T, Loddo G, Sessagesimi E, et al. Clinical features and pathophysiology of disorders of arousal in adults: a window into the sleeping brain. Front Neurol 2019;10:526.

12. Hublin C, Kaprio J. Genetic aspects and genetic epidemiology of parasomnias. Sleep Med Rev 2003;7(5):413–21.

13. Laberge L, Tremblay RE, Vitaro F, et al. Development of parasomnias from childhood to early adolescence. Pediatrics 2000;106(1 Pt 1):67–74.

14. Ohayon MM, Priest RG, Zulley J, et al. The place of confusional arousals in sleep and mental disorders: findings in a general population sample of 13,057 subjects. J Nerv Ment Dis 2000;188(6):340–8.

15. Petit D, Touchette E, Tremblay RE, et al. Dyssomnias and parasomnias in early childhood. Pediatrics 2007;119(5):e1016–25.

16. Howell MJ. Parasomnias: an updated review. Neurotherapeutics 2012;9(4):753–75.

17. Mason TBA, Pack AI. Sleep terrors in childhood. J Pediatr 2005;147(3):388–92.

18. Derry CP, Davey M, Johns M, et al. Distinguishing sleep disorders from seizures: diagnosing bumps in the night. Arch Neurol 2006;63(5):705–9.

19. Craske MG, Tsao JCI. Assessment and treatment of nocturnal panic attacks. Sleep Med Rev 2005;9(3):173–84.

20. Tinuper P, Bisulli F, Cross JH, et al. Definition and diagnostic criteria of sleep-related hypermotor epilepsy. Neurology 2016;86(19):1834–42.

21. Simon SL, Byars KC. Behavioral treatments for non-rapid eye movement parasomnias in children. Curr Sleep Med Rep 2016;2(3):152–7.

22. Kotagal S. Treatment of dyssomnias and parasomnias in childhood. Curr Treat Options Neurol 2012;14(6):630–49.

23. Bruni O, Ferri R, Miano S, et al. L -5-Hydroxytryptophan treatment of sleep terrors in children. Eur J Pediatr 2004;163(7):402–7.

24. Jan JE, Freeman RD, Wasdell MB, et al. A child with severe night terrors and sleep-walking responds to melatonin therapy. Dev Med Child Neurol 2004;46(11):789.

25. Howell MJ, Schenck CH, Crow SJ. A review of nighttime eating disorders. Sleep Med Rev 2009;13(1):23–34.

26. Stefani A, Holzknecht E, Högl B. Clinical neurophysiology of REM parasomnias. Handb Clin Neurol 2019;161:381–96.

27. Kotagal S. Rapid eye movement sleep behavior disorder during childhood. Sleep Med Clin 2015;10(2):163–7.

28. Zadra A, Donderi DC. Nightmares and bad dreams: their prevalence and relationship to well-being. J Abnorm Psychol 2000;109(2):273–81.

29. Sándor P, Szakadát S, Bódizs R. Ontogeny of dreaming: a review of empirical studies. Sleep Med Rev 2014;18(5):435–49.

30. Sharpless BA, Kliková M. Clinical features of isolated sleep paralysis. Sleep Med 2019;58:102–6.

31. Sharpless BA. A clinician's guide to recurrent isolated sleep paralysis. Neuropsychiatr Dis Treat 2016;12:1761–7.

32. Sharpless BA, Barber JP. Lifetime prevalence rates of sleep paralysis: a systematic review. Sleep Med Rev 2011;15(5):311–5.

33. Bruni O, Novelli L, Finotti E, Ferri R. Sleep enuresis. In: Thorpy MJ, Plazzi G, editors. The Parasomnias and Other Sleep-Related Movement Disorders. Cambridge: Cambridge University Press; 2010. p. 175–83. https://doi.org/10.1017/CBO9780511711947.020.

34. Harari MD. Nocturnal enuresis. J Paediatr Child Health 2013;49(4):264–71.

35. Butler RJ, Holland P. The three systems: a conceptual way of understanding nocturnal enuresis. Scand J Urol Nephrol 2000;34(4):270–7.

36. Alexopoulos EI, Malakasioti G, Varlami V, et al. Nocturnal enuresis is associated with moderate-to-severe obstructive sleep apnea in children with snoring. Pediatr Res 2014;76(6):555–9.

37. Dhondt K, Van Herzeele C, Roels SP, et al. Sleep fragmentation and periodic limb movements in children with monosymptomatic nocturnal enuresis and polyuria. Pediatr Nephrol 2015;30(7):1157–62.

38. Nevéus T. Sleep enuresis. Handb Clin Neurol 2011;98:363–9.

39. Wolfish NM, Pivik RT, Busby KA. Elevated sleep arousal thresholds in enuretic boys: clinical implications. Acta Paediatr 1997;86(4):381–4.

40. Soster LA, Alves RC, Fagundes SN, et al. Non-REM sleep instability in children with primary monosymptomatic sleep enuresis. J Clin Sleep Med 2017;13(10):1163–70.

41. Caldwell PHY, Deshpande AV, Von Gontard A. Management of nocturnal enuresis. BMJ 2013;347:f6259.

42. Erickson J, Vaughn BV. Non-REM parasomnia: the promise of precision medicine. Sleep Med Clin 2019;14(3):363–70.

# Restless Legs Syndrome in Children and Adolescents

Lourdes M. DelRosso, MD, MEd[a], Maria Paola Mogavero, MD[b,c],
Argelinda Baroni, MD[d], Oliviero Bruni, MD[e], Raffaele Ferri, MD[f,*]

## KEYWORDS

- Restless legs syndrome • Anxiety • Depression • ADHD • ODD • Sleep

## KEY POINTS

- Restless legs syndrome (RLS) is a common and often underdiagnosed sleep disorder in children and adolescents.
- Children with psychiatric conditions may be at higher risk of RLS, especially children with attention-deficit/hyperactivity disorder.
- Many psychotropic medications, including antidepressants, sedating antihistamines, and antipsychotics, are associated with increased RLS or restless sleep.
- Both nonpharmacologic and pharmacologic therapies can be used in children with RLS.

## RESTLESS LEGS SYNDROME

Restless legs syndrome (RLS), or Willis-Ekbom disease, is a neurologic disorder initially described by Sir Thomas Willis in 1685 and further defined by Ekbom in 1944; however, pediatric RLS was not described until 1994. Diagnostic criteria for pediatric-onset RLS, introduced in 2003 and updated in 2013, outline specific considerations for diagnosis in children and allow the use of age-related descriptive terms and words.[1] The recency of its recognition and limited education in sleep medicine by most clinicians have resulted in RLS still generally overlooked. This is true particularly in children who usually present with complaints related to bedtime refusal or insomnia, rather than with classic RLS symptoms. Additionally, children with RLS have been found to have an increased risk of comorbidities, in particular

This article originally appeared in *Child and Adolescent Psychiatric Clinics*, Volume 30 Issue 1, January 2021.

[a] Department of Internal Medicine, University of California San Francisco, Fresno, CA 93721, USA; [b] Vita-Salute San Raffaele University, Via Olgettina, 58, 20132 Milan, Italy; [c] San Raffaele Scientific Institute, Division of Neuroscience, Sleep Disorders Center, Via Stamira d'Ancona 20, 20127 Milan, Italy; [d] Department of Child and Adolescent Psychiatry, NYU Grossman School of Medicine, One Park Avenue, 7th Floor, New York, NY 10016, USA; [e] Department of Developmental and Social Psychology, Sapienza University, Via dei Marsi 78, 00185 Rome, Italy; [f] Sleep Research Centre, Oasi Research Institute – IRCCS, Via C. Ruggero 73, Troina 94018, Italy
* Corresponding author.
*E-mail address:* rferri@oasi.en.it

attention-deficit/hyperactivity disorder (ADHD). This article discusses clinical features of RLS, its treatment, and the association between RLS and ADHD and other comorbid psychiatric conditions.

## CLINICAL FEATURES

RLS is a clinical diagnosis and polysomnogram is not required for the diagnosis, although it can be useful in specific situations. The primary feature of RLS is the urge to move the legs, with or without accompanying leg sensations. If sensations are present, they invariably involve the legs, although the arms and other body parts sometimes are affected. Symptoms occur in the evening, when patients are settling for sleep and are relieved by movement. The discomfort associated with RLS can engender bedtime refusal and delayed sleep onset, which might be mistaken for behavioral insomnia in children.

RLS is relatively common in pediatrics, with an estimated prevalence of 2% to 4% in school-aged children and adolescents.[2] It often is misdiagnosed and generally is ignored by most pediatricians and general practitioners because of the mild and intermittent nature of the symptoms at younger ages or the inability of young children to characterize the sensations or discomfort in the legs. RLS is, however, usually progressive and can cause significant functional impairment.

A majority of children with RLS also report daytime leg discomfort. This differs from the typical increase during the evening or at night of adults and may be linked to the number of hours children spend sitting during the school day.[3]

The *International Classification of Sleep Disorders – Third Edition* (*ICSD-3*), states that "for children, the description of these symptoms should be in the child's own words." The interview questions should be phrased using words developmentally appropriate for the child. Language and cognitive development determine the applicability of the RLS diagnostic criteria, rather than age. As in adults, a significant impact on sleep, mood, cognition, and function is found. Impairment is manifest, however, more often in behavioral and educational domains.

Differentiating pediatric RLS from other conditions, or mimics, can be complicated.[4] Some of the common mimics of pediatric RLS are positional discomfort, sore leg muscles, ligament sprain/tendon strain, positional ischemia (numbness), dermatitis, bruises, growing pains, leg cramps, arthritis, peripheral neuropathy, radiculopathy, myelopathy, myopathy, fibromyalgia, and sickle cell disease.[5]

### *Patient Evaluation Overview*

RLS is difficult to diagnose in children. The formal evaluation of children with RLS starts with a comprehensive history and physical examination. The sleep history must include a thorough bedtime routine, with particular attention to symptoms that occur while trying to fall asleep. Sensory symptoms are difficult for children to explain, so simple descriptions, such as a funny feeling, pain, hurting, tickling, bugs, spiders, ants, and goose bumps in the legs, can be clues alerting the clinician. Children may draw pins, needles, tiny sand particles, bugs, or a saw over their legs when asked to depict their symptoms. Walters and colleagues[6] initially described the presenting symptoms of children with RLS, which included, similarly to adults, nocturnal predominance of leg paresthesia or discomfort, and relief with movement. In younger children, other symptoms, such as delayed sleep onset, bedtime struggles, and parental concern of restlessness, were included as symptoms of pediatric RLS. In qualitative interviews, children expressed their symptoms as "have to move," "need to kick," "hurts," "bugs crawling," "weird feelings," and "tingling."[7] In this study, 48% of children expressed having similar feelings in their arms in addition to their legs, and 67% described experiencing the same symptoms during the day.[7] RLS-related pain in children typically occurs from both knees down and especially involves the calves, although symmetric or asymmetric thigh pain also may occur.

Family history is of utmost importance. Most early-onset cases (by definition with onset before age 35) are familial; approximately 40% to 92% of children with RLS have affected family members.[8] Several medical conditions, however, are associated with RLS symptoms. Causes of secondary RLS include peripheral neuropathy and uremia. In patients who are thought to have secondary RLS, screening for renal disease, thyroid dysfunction, vitamin $B_{12}$, and folic acid deficiency (peripheral neuropathy) should be considered.[9]

Periodic limb movements (PLMs) occur in approximately two-thirds of children with RLS and are considered an objective motor finding in RLS and supportive of an RLS diagnosis.[10] PLMs are brief extremity jerks that can be accompanied by transient arousals from sleep that are identified and measured by polysomnography. Often, a diagnosis of PLM disorder (PLMD) precedes the diagnosis of RLS in children under 6 years of age who do not yet have sufficiently well-developed language skills to describe the sensory component of RLS.[11] For this reason, although a sleep study is not indicated for RLS, a PLM during sleep (PLMS) index greater than 5 per hour in polysomnography could aid in the diagnosis.[6]

Finally, daytime symptoms are important to evaluate RLS. Children present with cognitive and academic difficulties in approximately half of cases and mood changes, irritability, or sadness in 58% of cases.[7]

### Differential Diagnoses

Differential diagnoses should include mimics of RLS. Growing pains can occur intermittently in the evening and have a peak prevalence at 4 years to 6 years of age. Growing pains can be confused with RLS, but the urge to move the legs and the relief by movement differentiates RLS.[5] Furthermore, growing pains always are described as painful, whereas childhood RLS is considered painful only in 45% of cases.[12] In painful nocturnal leg cramps, there is no urge to move the legs and they do not necessarily occur in the evening prior to sleep.[13] Skin inspection during physical examination can rule out eczema. Examination and palpation of the legs also can exclude bruises, ligament tear, and tendon or muscle pain.

### Offending Medications

Several classes of medications and common drugs can unmask or aggravate RLS, including selective serotonin reuptake inhibitors (SSRIs), tricyclic antidepressants, metoclopramide, diphenhydramine, nicotine, caffeine, and alcohol.[9] For this reason, treating children with psychiatric disorders and RLS can be tricky. Objectively, it also has been shown that antidepressants or antipsychotics can cause an increase in PLMS, as a proxy for RLS.[14] Commonly used antidepressants, such as venlafaxine,[15] mirtazapine,[16] and tricyclic antidepressants,[17] can lead to an increase in PLMS. By contrast, drugs, such as levetiracetam, perampanel, or gabapentin, reduce PLMS[18,19]; valproic acid or carbamazepine have no effect on PLMS.[20,21] Considering the frequent association between PLMS and RLS in children[22] and the their presence since adolescence,[23,24] the choice of antidepressants for treating pediatric psychiatric disorders should seek to avoid possible drug-induced onset or worsening of PLMS.

## PRESENTATION IN CHILDREN WITH PSYCHIATRIC COMORBIDITIES

Children with RLS have a higher incidence of ADHD, oppositional defiant disorder, anxiety disorders, and depression.[25] A retrospective study of 374 children with RLS found that 64% had 1 or more comorbid psychiatric conditions. ADHD was found in 25%, mood disturbances in 29%, and anxiety in 11.5% of children.[26] Work on children with PLMS by DelRosso and colleagues[14] demonstrated that 21.6% also have a mood disorder/anxiety and 10% have ADHD. Unfortunately, there are scarce data on the link of pediatric depression and anxiety with RLS. The most commonly studied association is the one between ADHD and RLS although the directionality between the 2 conditions is unclear. Therefore, the remainder of this article discusses the link between ADHD and RLS in children.

Additionally, gender differences and possible iatrogenic factors might complicate the issue. A retrospective study showed that RLS was associated with ADHD in boys and mood disorders in girls and that there was a greater number of antidepressants prescribed in the same year of the diagnosis of RLS, possibly indicating a worsening of preexisting pathology by psychotropics.[26]

Both RLS and elevated PLMS are common in children with ADHD.[27] For instance, 93% of children with RLS and ADHD reported sleep problems whereas this concern was seen in only 56% of children without ADHD, even if the high comorbidity may be due to recruitment bias because the clinic at which the study was conducted specializes in ADHD and RLS. A study of 129 children (aged 6–17 years) with PLMS index greater than 5 per hour found that 91% were diagnosed with ADHD.[28] Other studies have shown that 26% to 64% of children with ADHD meet criteria for PLMD. Furthermore, an elevated PLMS index correlates with inattention/hyperactivity scores.[27,29] There is increased morbidity when the 2 conditions co-occur; children with PLMD and ADHD have more enuresis, nightmares, and difficulty initiating sleep than children with PLMD alone. ADHD, RLS, and PLMD have been postulated to result from reduced dopamine activity, potentially related to low iron stores, leading to the suggestion that improving ferritin levels also may improve ADHD symptoms.[27,29]

Pullen and colleagues[26] evaluated 374 children with RLS and found that 25% met criteria for ADHD; 29% had either a transient mood disturbance (eg, adjustment disorder) or a recurrent mood disturbance (ie, major depressive disorder or bipolar disorder); 11.5% had an anxiety disorder; and 11% had behavioral disturbances. Mood disturbances and anxiety disorders were more prevalent in girls and ADHD and behavioral disorders were more prevalent in boys. The study concluded that two-thirds of children with RLS had at least 1 psychiatric comorbidity, with 35% having more than 1. Picchietti and Stevens[25] studied 18 children with RLS and found that 13 had ADHD, 4 had oppositional defiant disorder, and 6 were diagnosed with anxiety and 5 with depression. Three children had both anxiety and depression. In all cases of anxiety and depression, the sleep disturbance occurred before the psychiatric diagnosis but the definite RLS diagnosis was given after the psychiatric condition was diagnosed, illustrating the common delay in RLS diagnosis. Oner and colleagues[30] studied 87 children with ADHD and found that 33% met criteria for RLS, and children with ADHD and RLS had lower ferritin levels than children without RLS. The impact of RLS on psychiatric comorbidities, however, has not been reported. The study also demonstrated that children and adolescents with RLS often present first for psychiatric evaluation rather than for sleep medicine evaluation. This dual relationship suggests both sleep-related symptoms and ADHD should be evaluated simultaneously. **Table 1** summarizes studies showing the increased prevalence of RLS in children with ADHD and the increased prevalence of ADHD symptoms in children with RLS.

**Table 1**
Studies in children with attention-deficit/hyperactivity disorder and restless legs syndrome

| Authors, Year of Publication | Method | Age (Mean [SD]), or Range | Sample Size | Findings |
| --- | --- | --- | --- | --- |
| Liu et al,[31] 2019 | AHQ | 14.5 y (1.4 y) | 11,831 | RLS (OR 1.47; 95% CI, 1.02–2.11) was associated with subsequent symptoms of ADHD. |
| Castano-De la Mota et al,[32] 2017 | SDSC questionnaire | 6–18 y | 73 | RLS prevalence of 6.8% in children with ADHD |
| Kwon et al,[33] 2014 | Questionnaire | 10.8 y (2.3 y) | 56 | Family history of RLS (12.5%); symptoms of RLS in 24 patients (42.9%); probable or definite RLS (7.2%) |
| Pullen et al,[26] 2011 | Diagnostic criteria | 0–18 y | 374 | 25% (94/374) of RLS patients met criteria for ADHD |
| Silvestri et al,[34] 2009 | SDSC, Conners, video polysomnography | 8.9 y (2.7 y) | 45 | RLS in 11.9%. IRLS severity scale average 18.6 (SD 8.6) |
| Picchietti and Stevens,[25] 2008 | DSM-IV, ICSD-3 criteria | 0.2–17 y | 18 | ADHD was diagnosed in 13/18 children with RLS. |
| Oner et al,[30] 2007 | Conners, RLS criteria | 9.4 y (2.5 y) | 87 | 33.3% of children with ADHD had RLS. Children with ADHD and RLS had lower ferritin levels. |

*Abbreviations:* AHQ, Adolescent Health Questionnaire; Conners, Conners Parent Rating Scale; *DSM-IV, Diagnostic and Statistical Manual of Mental Disorders* (Fourth Edition); SDSC, Sleep Disturbance Scale for Children.

## TREATMENT

Treating pediatric RLS is important, because the associated sleep disturbances can lead to significant developmental, behavioral, and cardiovascular morbidities as well as impact on family well-being. **Table 2** summarizes the treatment options of RLS in children with psychiatric comorbidities while **Fig. 1** displays a recommended algorithm for their evaluation and management.

### Nonpharmacologic Treatment Options

All children and parents should be educated on elements of sleep hygiene, including consistent bedtime routines, avoidance of electronics at bedtime/evening, and avoidance of caffeinated products. Caffeine consumption can exacerbate symptoms of RLS. Children should avoid not only coffee but also any other substances containing caffeine, including iced tea or chocolates.[35]

Other interventions include leg movements to alleviate the symptoms of RLS. These may include exercise in the afternoon or brief walks a few hours prior to bedtime. Similarly, stretching, rubbing, or massaging the legs may provide relief.[36] Incidentally, some children find relief using cool or heating pads or weighted blankets. Parents can try these interventions one at the time for a few days and keep a sleep diary to assess effectiveness.

Avoiding or discontinuing medications that could aggravate RLS, that is, SSRIs, tricyclic antidepressants, metoclopramide, diphenhydramine, nicotine, caffeine, and alcohol, also may help.[9]

### Pharmacologic Treatments

There currently are no Food and Drug Administration (FDA)-approved medications for RLS in children, and clinical guidelines and recommendations are sparse.

**Table 2**
**Treatment options of restless legs syndrome in children with psychiatric comorbidities**

| Intervention Modality | Recommendation | Concerning Side Effect |
|---|---|---|
| Antidepressant medication assessment | Treat underlying psychiatric condition. Consider using dopaminergic antidepressants (bupropion) when RLS present. | Worsening psychiatric symptoms if changing medications |
| Other medication assessment | Limit antihistaminic or other medications that can exacerbate RLS when possible. | |
| Avoid caffeine | Avoid chocolates, tea, coffee. | |
| Lifestyle modification | Exercise, massage, heating/ cooling pads | |
| If ferritin <50 ng/mL | Oral iron supplementation (1–6 mg/kg/d) to a maximum of 65 mg/d | Constipation, teeth staining |
| If ferritin >50 ng/mL (off-label) | Clonazepam, 0.1–1 mg, at bedtime | Drowsiness, suicidal ideation |
| | Gabapentin, 50–100 mg, at bedtime | Depression, suicidal ideation |
| | Clonidine, 0.05–0.1 mg, at bedtime | Hypotension, depression |
| | Pramipexole, 0.03–0.25 mg/d | Psychosis, impulse control disorders |

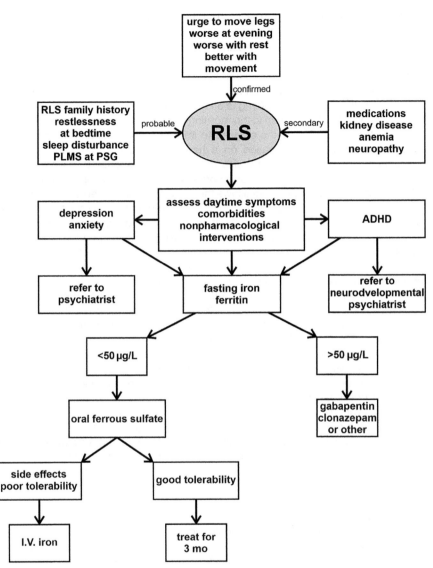

**Fig. 1.** Recommended algorithm for the evaluation and management of children with RLS and psychiatric comorbidities. I.V., intravenous.

Furthermore, the International Restless Legs Syndrome Study Group has published guidelines on treatment of RLS using iron supplementation in children, stating that evidence to recommend iron supplementation for children with RLS remains insufficient.[37] Iron supplementation, nevertheless, remains the first-line therapy for children with RLS in clinical care.[9,38]

### Iron therapy
Serum ferritin is the best indicator of early iron deficiency . Saturation of peripheral iron stores typically occurs at ferritin levels of 80 ng/mL to 100 ng/mL. Current evidence suggests that achieving and maintaining serum ferritin above 50 ng/mL can be

beneficial for RLS, PLMS, and ADHD.[39] The dopaminergic theory of RLS further supports the iron deficiency hypothesis, because iron is fundamental for the biosynthesis of dopamine and is necessary for tyrosine hydroxylation, which is the rate-limiting step for dopamine production.[40] The authors recommend checking fasting iron profile and ferritin levels prior to beginning oral iron supplementation. Iron is offered for patients with ferritin levels below 50 μg/Lng/mL, with dose ranges of 1 mg/kg/d to 6 mg/kg/d of ferrous sulfate at a dose of 50 mg to 65 mg of elemental iron.[9] To enhance absorption, iron ideally should be taken in the morning on an empty stomach with a source of vitamin C. It may take 3 months or more to improve iron levels and to demonstrate improvement of symptoms, based on a handful of studies.[35,41,42] In addition to improving symptoms, iron therapy also may improve response to psychostimulant drugs,[43,44] an important consideration if correct management of iron status in children with RLS and psychiatric disorders allows the use of a lower antidepressant dose, with a lower probability of adverse effects. The most frequent adverse effects resulting from oral iron administration are constipation, nausea, and unpleasant taste[45]; these can reduce or prevent adherence. Moreover, not all patients respond to oral iron therapy; most responders show an improvement in ferritin levels after 2 months to 3 months of supplementation, with further improvement over time, whereas nonresponders maintain a low ferritin level, despite adherence.[45] When oral iron administration is not successful due to adverse effects or poor absorption, intravenous iron supplementation might be an alternative. Intravenous iron has been shown effective and safe in adults with RLS and some data appear to prove to support its efficacy for pediatric RLS and PLMD patients who do not tolerate or do not respond to oral iron; the most common adverse events reported are difficulty in positioning the intravenous access with risk of extravasation, changes in blood pressure, skin discoloration, and transient hypophosphatemia. A careful selection of candidates is needed because of possible allergic reaction, and caution should be considered in children from families with hemochromatosis, recent infections, or malaria.[46] Although various intravenous iron preparations have been tried in adults (iron dextran, iron gluconate, iron sucrose, ferumoxytol, iron isomaltoside, and ferric carboxymaltose), a single study using iron sucrose 1.2 mg/kg to 6.6 mg/kg, infused over 2 hours in 16 children aged 2 years to 16 years, showed improvement in sleep symptoms in 62.5% of them.[46]

### Iron and psychotropic agents

Treatment of pediatric RLS always should include nonpharmacologic interventions, elimination of factors that worsen or precipitate RLS such as elimination of caffeine, and assessment of ferritin levels.[3,47] Because there are no FDA-approved medications for the management of RLS in children, any pharmacologic option used is off-label. When symptoms persist after iron supplementation, combination therapy with a second medication may be considered. In a study of 25 children with RLS and 28 controls, clonazepam (0.1–1 mg) or pramipexole (0.03–0.25 mg) was added to oral iron supplementation in children with persistent symptoms after 2 months.[48] Clonazepam is a long-acting benzodiazepine shown to improve sleep consolidation in patients with RLS albeit without reducing the motor or sensory manifestations of RLS.[49,50] Clonidine (0.05–0.1 mg) is used commonly in children to improve symptoms of insomnia. Clonidine is an $\alpha_2$-adrenergic agonist that improves sleep onset in children with RLS and has been given in combination with iron supplementation.[51] Gabapentin is used commonly in adults with RLS to improve sleep-onset latency.[52] A small cohort of children treated with gabapentin (50–100 mg at bedtime) for RLS showed resolution of symptoms.[35] Gabapentin also can be combined with iron supplementation in

**Table 3**
**Studies with treatment options for children with attention-deficit/hyperactivity disorder and restless legs syndrome**

| Authors, Year of Publication | Medication, Dose | Age (Mean [SD]) or Range | Sample Size | Conclusions |
|---|---|---|---|---|
| Baykal and Karakurt,[53] 2017 | Atomoxetine, 0.8 mg/kg/d | 9 y | 1 | Resolution of RLS symptoms |
| England et al,[54] 2011 | Carbidopa/ ʟevo-dopa, 25/100 controlled-release | 9.3 (1.3) y | 29 | ʟevo-dopa improved RLS symptoms on international RLS severity scale. ADHD symptoms were worse in the non-RLS group and did not improve after treatment (Conners Parent Rating Scale) |
| Gagliano et al,[18] 2011 | Levetiracetam, 10–20 mg/kg/d, up to 50–60 mg/kg/d | 5–12 y | 7 | All showed significant improvement in the international RLS severity scale, quality of sleep, and daytime function. Behavioral symptoms improved although not overall ADHD. |
| Konofal et al,[55] 2005 | Ferrous sulfate, 80 mg Ropinirole, 0.25 mg | 6 y | 1 | Conners Parent Rating Scale improved from 30 to 21 after 3 mo of ferrous sulfate. After ropinirole, Conners Parent Rating Scale, oppositional behavior, attention, and sleep improved. |
| Walters et al,[39] 2000 | ʟ-dopa/carbidopa, CR 75/300–150/ 600 mg Pergolide, 0.4–1 mg daily | 6–14 y | 7 | PLMS index improved from 72 to 15, the PLMS index decreased from 11.7 to 2.1. RLS symptoms improved. |

*(continued on next page)*

| Table 3 (continued) | | | | |
|---|---|---|---|---|
| Authors, Year of Publication | Medication, Dose | Age (Mean [SD]) or Range | Sample Size | Conclusions |
| | | | | Conners Parent Rating Scale from 15.1 to 6.26. Significant improvement on oppositional defiant disorder scale and on Child Behavior Checklist |

refractory cases. The use of dopaminergic agonists should be restricted to the purview of pediatric sleep specialists. Consideration of side effects, risks, and benefits of each medication needs to be discussed with the family. **Table 3** lists treatment studies on children with ADHD and RLS.

### Evaluation of Outcome and Long-Term Recommendations

Children with RLS should be evaluated periodically. If oral iron supplementation is initiated, side effects should be assessed within a couple of weeks. Side effects can be the limiting factor in treatment success for oral iron. Rapid identification of problems, such as bad taste or constipation, can delineate a strategy to address the side effects, such as switching to a more palatable preparation or a sustained-release tablet and increasing fiber and liquid intake, among others. Discussion of alternative treatments should be done early to educate the family on potential risks, side effects, and alternatives to treatment. Studies on natural progression of RLS are lacking but, based on adult studies, a waxing and waning progression, with periods of exacerbation alternating with asymptomatic periods, can be expected. Education is key in identification of symptoms and prompt evaluation.

Treatment success can be assessed clinically by symptom relief. Questionnaires developed for symptom assessment have not been validated in children. If another sleep disorder, such as obstructive sleep apnea, is suspected or if symptoms are not improved, a sleep study may be indicated.

In summary, treatment of RLS should not be delayed in children with comorbid psychiatric conditions and both should be assessed and treated simultaneously to ensure improvement in quality of life and outcomes.

### NEW DEVELOPMENTS

Recently, a new disorder has been proposed, restless sleep disorder (RSD).[40] Children with RSD do not have symptoms of RLS or leg movements on polysomnography but present with frequent movements and repositioning during sleep. The parent usually brings a child for evaluation with concerns of restless sleep and daytime symptoms which include, often, hyperactivity, daytime sleepiness, or behavioral problems. The proposed criteria include motor movements, involving large muscle groups, that occur during sleep and that persist all night and occur almost every night. The movements are evident on polysomnography and should be more than 5 per hour and cause clinically significant impairment in an area of functioning.[56] RSD has been shown to have a prevalence of 7.7% in patients referred to sleep centers and also is suspected to be associated with low iron stores in the brain.[57] Further studies are needed to assess the comorbidity of RSD with other neurodevelopmental, psychiatric, or neurologic conditions.

## SUMMARY

RLS is a common and often overlooked disorder in children and adolescents. The relationship between RLS, ADHD, and psychiatric comorbidities is complex and bidirectional. Children with RLS have a significantly increased prevalence of symptoms of ADHD, anxiety, depression, and oppositional defiant disorder. But children diagnosed with ADHD also have an increased prevalence of RLS. This association calls for awareness of sleep disorders, in particular RLS, in children with ADHD and psychiatric disorders. Furthermore, commonly used psychotropic medications can exacerbate the symptoms of RLS. Patients with RLS present with difficulty with sleep onset, nocturnal awakenings, and daytime symptoms, such as behavioral problems. These symptoms can be masked by the presence of a comorbid conditions. Children often are referred to psychiatric evaluation before they are suspected of having RLS, and psychiatrists should become familiar with clinical assessment and iron replacement therapy for RLS. The authors recommend concurrent evaluations, screening, and prompt treatment of RLS in children with ADHD or psychiatric diagnoses. The treatment of RLS improves both nighttime and daytime symptoms. Treatment options include behavioral interventions, iron supplementation, and combination therapy. For refractory cases of RLS, a referral to a pediatric sleep specialist is indicated.

Areas of future research include the impact of RLS treatment on symptoms of depression or anxiety in children and further assessment of RSD in the presence of comorbid ADHD or other psychiatric diagnoses. More studies are needed on pharmacologic treatment of RLS in children.

## CLINICS CARE POINTS

- Screening of RLS and sleep disorders is recommended for all children referred for psychiatric evaluation.
- RLS often is associated with ADHD, anxiety, and depression.
- A diagnosis of RLS often is delayed in children with RLS and psychiatric comorbidities.
- Sleep problems, such as difficulty with sleep onset, are common in children with RLS and ADHD.
- Initial evaluation of children with RLS includes a thorough sleep history and physical examination.
- Fasting ferritin and iron profile should be obtained in all children with RLS.
- Iron supplementation is the first-line treatment in children with RLS.
- Nonpharmacologic treatment options include stretching exercises, cool or warm compresses, and weighted blankets.
- Common adverse effects of oral iron can limit adherence to treatment and need to be assessed early to find alternative treatments.
- There currently are no FDA-approved drugs for treating pediatric RLS; gabapentin and clonazepam often are used off-label as second-line treatment options.
- Concurrent evaluation and treatment of RLS and psychiatric comorbidities, especially ADHD, is recommended.

## DISCLOSURE

This study was partially supported by a fund from the Italian Ministry of Health "Ricerca Corrente" (RC n. 2757319) (Dr R. Ferri). The other authors have indicated no financial conflicts of interest.

## REFERENCES

1. Picchietti DL, Bruni O, de Weerd A, et al. Pediatric restless legs syndrome diagnostic criteria: an update by the International Restless Legs Syndrome Study Group. Sleep Med 2013;14(12):1253–9.
2. Picchietti D, Allen RP, Walters AS, et al. Restless legs syndrome: prevalence and impact in children and adolescents–the Peds REST study. Pediatrics 2007;120(2):253–66.
3. Picchietti MA, Picchietti DL. Advances in pediatric restless legs syndrome: iron, genetics, diagnosis and treatment. Sleep Med 2010;11(7):643–51.
4. Benes H, Walters AS, Allen RP, et al. Definition of restless legs syndrome, how to diagnose it, and how to differentiate it from RLS mimics. Mov Disord 2007; 22(Suppl 18):S401–8.
5. Walters AS, Gabelia D, Frauscher B. Restless legs syndrome (Willis-Ekbom disease) and growing pains: are they the same thing? A side-by-side comparison of the diagnostic criteria for both and recommendations for future research. Sleep Med 2013;14(12):1247–52.
6. Walters AS, Picchietti DL, Ehrenberg BL, et al. Restless legs syndrome in childhood and adolescence. Pediatr Neurol 1994;11(3):241–5.
7. Picchietti DL, Arbuckle RA, Abetz L, et al. Pediatric restless legs syndrome: analysis of symptom descriptions and drawings. J Child Neurol 2011;26(11):1365–76.
8. Bruni O, Angriman M. Management of RLS in children (unique features). In: Manconi M, Garcia-Borreguero D, editors. Restless legs syndrome/Willis Ekbom disease. New York: Springer; 2017. p. 261–78.
9. DelRosso L, Bruni O. Treatment of pediatric restless legs syndrome. Adv Pharmacol 2019;84:237–53.
10. Picchietti DL, Rajendran RR, Wilson MP, et al. Pediatric restless legs syndrome and periodic limb movement disorder: parent–child pairs. Sleep Med 2009; 10(8):925–31.
11. Picchietti MA, Picchietti DL. Restless legs syndrome and periodic limb movement disorder in children and adolescents. Semin Pediatr Neurol 2008;15(2):91–9.
12. Hamilton-Stubbs P, Walters AS. Sleep disorders in children: simple sleep-related movement disorders. In: Nevšímalová S, Bruni O, editors. Sleep disorders in children. Cham (Switzerland): Springer; 2017. p. 227–51.
13. Chokroverty S. Differential diagnoses of restless legs syndrome/Willis-Ekbom disease: mimics and comorbidities. Sleep Med Clin 2015;10(3):249–62, xii.
14. Delrosso LM, Lockhart C, Wrede JE, et al. Comorbidities in children with elevated periodic limb movement index during sleep. Sleep 2020;43(2):zsz221.
15. Yang C, White DP, Winkelman JW. Antidepressants and periodic leg movements of sleep. Biol Psychiatry 2005;58(6):510–4.
16. Fulda S, Kloiber S, Dose T, et al. Mirtazapine provokes periodic leg movements during sleep in young healthy men. Sleep 2013;36(5):661–9.
17. Goerke M, Rodenbeck A, Cohrs S, et al. The influence of the tricyclic antidepressant amitriptyline on periodic limb movements during sleep. Pharmacopsychiatry 2013;46(3):108–13.

18. Gagliano A, Arico I, Calarese T, et al. Restless Leg Syndrome in ADHD children: levetiracetam as a reasonable therapeutic option. Brain Dev 2011;33(6):480–6.

19. Garcia-Borreguero D, Cano I, Granizo JJ. Treatment of restless legs syndrome with the selective AMPA receptor antagonist perampanel. Sleep Med 2017;34: 105–8.

20. Eisensehr I, Ehrenberg BL, Rogge Solti S, et al. Treatment of idiopathic restless legs syndrome (RLS) with slow-release valproic acid compared with slow-release levodopa/benserazid. J Neurol 2004;251(5):579–83.

21. Zucconi M, Coccagna G, Petronelli R, et al. Nocturnal myoclonus in restless legs syndrome effect of carbamazepine treatment. Funct Neurol 1989;4(3):263–71.

22. Durmer JS, Quraishi GH. Restless legs syndrome, periodic leg movements, and periodic limb movement disorder in children. Pediatr Clin North Am 2011;58(3): 591–620.

23. Ferri R, DelRosso LM, Arico D, et al. Leg movement activity during sleep in school-age children and adolescents: a detailed study in normal controls and participants with restless legs syndrome and narcolepsy type 1. Sleep 2018; 41(4):zsy010.

24. Ferri R, DelRosso LM, Silvani A, et al. Peculiar lifespan changes of periodic leg movements during sleep in restless legs syndrome. J Sleep Res 2019;29:e12896.

25. Picchietti DL, Stevens HE. Early manifestations of restless legs syndrome in childhood and adolescence. Sleep Med 2008;9(7):770–81.

26. Pullen SJ, Wall CA, Angstman ER, et al. Psychiatric comorbidity in children and adolescents with restless legs syndrome: a retrospective study. J Clin Sleep Med 2011;7(6):587–96.

27. Picchietti DL, England SJ, Walters AS, et al. Periodic limb movement disorder and restless legs syndrome in children with attention-deficit hyperactivity disorder. J Child Neurol 1998;13(12):588–94.

28. Picchietti DL, Walters AS. Moderate to severe periodic limb movement disorder in childhood and adolescence. Sleep 1999;22(3):297–300.

29. Picchietti DL, Underwood DJ, Farris WA, et al. Further studies on periodic limb movement disorder and restless legs syndrome in children with attention-deficit hyperactivity disorder. Mov Disord 1999;14(6):1000–7.

30. Oner P, Dirik EB, Taner Y, et al. Association between low serum ferritin and restless legs syndrome in patients with attention deficit hyperactivity disorder. Tohoku J Exp Med 2007;213(3):269–76.

31. Liu X, Liu ZZ, Liu BP, et al. Associations of sleep problems with ADHD symptoms: findings from the Shandong adolescent behavior and health cohort (SABHC). Sleep 2019.

32. Castano-De la Mota C, Moreno-Acero N, Losada-Del Pozo R, et al. [Restless legs syndrome in patients diagnosed with attention deficit hyperactivity disorder]. Rev Neurol 2017;64(7):299–304.

33. Kwon S, Sohn Y, Jeong SH, et al. Prevalence of restless legs syndrome and sleep problems in Korean children and adolescents with attention deficit hyperactivity disorder: a single institution study. Korean J Pediatr 2014;57(7):317–22.

34. Silvestri R, Gagliano A, Aricò I, et al. Sleep disorders in children with Attention-Deficit/Hyperactivity Disorder (ADHD) recorded overnight by video-polysomnography. Sleep Med 2009;10(10):1132–8.

35. Amos LB, Grekowicz ML, Kuhn EM, et al. Treatment of pediatric restless legs syndrome. Clin Pediatr (Phila) 2014;53(4):331–6.

36. Bega D, Malkani R. Alternative treatment of restless legs syndrome: an overview of the evidence for mind-body interventions, lifestyle interventions, and neutraceuticals. Sleep Med 2016;17:99–105.

37. Allen RP, Picchietti DL, Auerbach M, et al. Evidence-based and consensus clinical practice guidelines for the iron treatment of restless legs syndrome/Willis-Ekbom disease in adults and children: an IRLSSG task force report. Sleep Med 2018;41:27–44.

38. Earley CJ. Clinical practice. Restless legs syndrome. N Engl J Med 2003;348(21):2103–9.

39. Walters AS, Mandelbaum DE, Lewin DS, et al. Dopaminergic therapy in children with restless legs/periodic limb movements in sleep and ADHD. Dopaminergic Therapy Study Group. Pediatr Neurol 2000;22(3):182–6.

40. DelRosso LM, Bruni O, Ferri R. Restless sleep disorder in children: a pilot study on a tentative new diagnostic category. Sleep 2018;41(8):zsy102.

41. Mohri I, Kato-Nishimura K, Kagitani-Shimono K, et al. Evaluation of oral iron treatment in pediatric restless legs syndrome (RLS). Sleep Med 2012;13(4):429–32.

42. Tilma J, Tilma K, Norregaard O, et al. Early childhood-onset restless legs syndrome: symptoms and effect of oral iron treatment. Acta Paediatr 2013;102(5):e221–6.

43. Calarge C, Farmer C, DiSilvestro R, et al. Serum ferritin and amphetamine response in youth with attention-deficit/hyperactivity disorder. J Child Adolesc Psychopharmacol 2010;20(6):495–502.

44. Cortese S, Angriman M, Lecendreux M, et al. Iron and attention deficit/hyperactivity disorder: what is the empirical evidence so far? A systematic review of the literature. Expert Rev Neurother 2012;12(10):1227–40.

45. DelRosso LM, Yi T, Chan JHM, et al. Determinants of ferritin response to oral iron supplementation in children with sleep movement disorders. Sleep 2019;43(3):zsz234.

46. Grim K, Lee B, Sung AY, et al. Treatment of childhood-onset restless legs syndrome and periodic limb movement disorder using intravenous iron sucrose. Sleep Med 2013;14(11):1100–4.

47. Garcia-Borreguero D, Kohnen R, Silber MH, et al. The long-term treatment of restless legs syndrome/Willis-Ekbom disease: evidence-based guidelines and clinical consensus best practice guidance: a report from the International Restless Legs Syndrome Study Group. Sleep Med 2013;14(7):675–84.

48. Furudate N, Komada Y, Kobayashi M, et al. Daytime dysfunction in children with restless legs syndrome. J Neurol Sci 2014;336(1–2):232–6.

49. Saletu M, Anderer P, Saletu-Zyhlarz GM, et al. Comparative placebo-controlled polysomnographic and psychometric studies on the acute effects of gabapentin versus ropinirole in restless legs syndrome. J Neural Transm (Vienna) 2010;117(4):463–73.

50. Manconi M, Ferri R, Zucconi M, et al. Dissociation of periodic leg movements from arousals in restless legs syndrome. Ann Neurol 2012;71(6):834–44.

51. Dye TJ, Jain SV, Simakajornboon N. Outcomes of long-term iron supplementation in pediatric restless legs syndrome/periodic limb movement disorder (RLS/PLMD). Sleep Med 2017;32:213–9.

52. Foldvary-Schaefer N, De Leon Sanchez I, Karafa M, et al. Gabapentin increases slow-wave sleep in normal adults. Epilepsia 2002;43(12):1493–7.

53. Baykal S, Karakurt MN. The effect of atomoxetin use in the treatment of attention-deficit/hyperactivity disorder on the symptoms of restless legs syndrome: a case report. Clin Neuropharmacol 2017;40(2):93–4.

54. England SJ, Picchietti DL, Couvadelli BV, et al. L-Dopa improves Restless Legs Syndrome and periodic limb movements in sleep but not Attention-Deficit-Hyperactivity Disorder in a double-blind trial in children. Sleep Med 2011;12(5): 471–7.
55. Konofal E, Arnulf I, Lecendreux M, et al. Ropinirole in a child with attention-deficit hyperactivity disorder and restless legs syndrome. Pediatr Neurol 2005;32(5): 350–1.
56. DelRosso LM, Jackson CV, Trotter K, et al. Video-Polysomnographic character-ization of sleep movements in children with restless sleep disorder. Sleep 2019;42(4):zsy269.
57. DelRosso LM, Ferri R. The prevalence of restless sleep disorder among a clinical sample of children and adolescents referred to a sleep centre. J Sleep Res 2019; 28(6):e12870.

# Just Let Me Sleep in

## Identifying and Treating Delayed Sleep Phase Disorder in Adolescents

Michael A. Feder, PhD[a,b], Argelinda Baroni, MD[c,*]

## KEYWORDS

- Delayed sleep phase disorder • Chronotherapy • Blue light • Insomnia • Melatonin
- Adolescents

## KEY POINTS

- Delayed sleep phase disorder (DSPD) is the inability to fall asleep and awaken at conventionally appropriate times, caused by circadian misalignment with the environment.
- DSPD is common in adolescents and young adults, with a prevalence as high as 16%.
- Melatonin and appropriate bright light exposure are mainstays of treatment.
- Wind-down and wake-up routines can promote shifting sleep schedules.
- Patients must be motivated to make these changes and be prepared for relapse.

## INTRODUCTION

Delayed sleep phase disorder (DSPD) is an often-undiagnosed but common disorder that affects individuals of any age but is especially prevalent in adolescence.[1] This condition is highly associated with psychiatric comorbidity, suggesting wide-ranging negative psychological effects.[2] Moreover, DSPD entails numerous social, academic, interpersonal, and occupational negative outcomes stemming from difficulties in maintaining a socially acceptable sleep-wake schedule.[3] Despite the substantial prevalence among adolescents and the morbidity of DSPD, many clinicians are unaware of its clinical features and how it can be treated. This article provides an essential guide for child and adolescent psychiatrists and clinicians to diagnose and treat DSPD in adolescents.

## DELAYED SLEEP PHASE DISORDER SYMPTOMS

Per the Diagnostic and Statistical Manual of Mental Disorders, Fifth Edition (DSM-5), DSPD is a circadian rhythm disorder, characterized by "a pattern of delayed sleep

This article originally appeared in *Child and Adolescent Psychiatric Clinics*, Volume 30 Issue 1, January 2021.

[a] Department of Child and Adolescent Psychiatry, Hassenfeld Children's Hospital at NYU Langone, NYC H+H/Bellevue, New York, NY, USA; [b] Child Study Center, One Park Avenue, 7th Floor, New York, NY 10016, USA; [c] Department of Child and Adolescent Psychiatry, NYU Grossman School of Medicine, One Park Avenue, 7th Floor, New York, NY 10016, USA

* Corresponding author. Child Study Center, One Park Avenue, 7th Floor, New York, NY 10016.

*E-mail address:* Argelinda.Baroni@nyulangone.org

onset and awakening times, with an inability to decrease asleep and awaken at a desired or conventionally acceptable earlier time"[4] and consequent functional impairment. Although most adolescents report that socially required sleep and wake times are earlier than they would naturally choose, they are able to adapt to them with minimal to moderate difficulty and minor changes to their routines.[5] In contrast, individuals with DSPD have extreme difficulty in adapting to the usual schedules required by school and work. The core feature of DSPD is a shift of the natural sleep period to a later schedule (at least 2 hours compared with expected times), thus constituting a delayed sleep phase, rather than an inability to fall asleep tout court. DSPD is significantly more represented in adolescents and young adults. The prevalence in this age group ranges from 1% to 16%,[1] compared with general population estimates from 0.17% to 8.9% depending on the diagnostic criteria and methodologies used.[5-7]

Circadian rhythms refer to cyclic variations in sleep-wake propensity that are entrained by external cues such as light and meals and typically adhere to an approximately 24-hour period. Young adults and adolescents with DSPD tend to have circadian period lengths up to 30 minutes longer than those without DSPD (ie, longer than 24 hours).[1] This finding means that, in the absence of external cues to entrain the circadian rhythm, people with DSPD fall asleep almost a half-hour later each day. Because of their delayed sleep phase, patients with DSPD struggle to fall asleep as well as wake up at the socially expected times. The misalignment of the natural sleep-wake phase with social expectations drives most of the resulting functional impairment. When allowed to follow their natural, delayed schedule (eg, during summer vacation), these same individuals can experience good-quality sleep and feel refreshed. For this reason, individuals with DSPD would prefer to attend exclusively afternoon and evening courses in college or work afternoon shifts to follow their circadian preference.

### Challenges for Adolescents with Delayed Sleep Phase Disorder

However, in most instances, adolescents are expected to arrive at high school by 8 AM or earlier, so schedule accommodations are not possible. Thus, many of the negative sequelae patients experience from DSPD arise in the mornings (no pun intended). Adolescents with DSPD struggle to wake up to attend school and to remain awake in class, which can lead to school refusal, academic failure, or disciplinary action.[3,8,9] Adolescents with DSPD may also experience familial challenges, because their difficulty waking up may delay others in the household. Even when adolescents with DSPD are able to wake up on time during school days, because of their circadian misalignment, they are unable to fall asleep when expected, experiencing significant sleep deprivation and its negative effects.[10] In addition, the chronic sleep deprivation from DSPD usually leads to irregular sleep schedules between weekdays and weekends, with typical weekend so-called sleep marathons or daytime napping, which can worsen the sleep phase misalignment.[5,11] The term sleep jetlag refers to the difference in timing between the person's sleep on work/school days versus free days, with larger values of social jetlag being associated with higher risk of poor cardiac health and other negative physical sequelae.[12]

### Delayed Sleep Phase Disorder Versus Insomnia

Many clinicians are puzzled by the differences between insomnia and DSPD. Insomnia is a disorder characterized by difficulties initiating and maintaining sleep, usually caused by anxiety surrounding the inability to fall asleep, negative associations around sleep, hyperarousal, and poor sleep habits, rather than a circadian misalignment.[5] Because both individuals with DSPD and those with insomnia have difficulty falling asleep, it can be difficult to tease them apart. Individuals with DSPD usually sleep well when allowed to sleep following their natural schedule of late bedtime and wake-up time. In contrast, people with insomnia struggle falling asleep, independently of their bedtime, because their difficulties falling asleep are caused by negative associations around sleep that caused anxiety and hyperarousal.[5] In addition, the natural wake-up times of people with insomnia are not as consistently delayed as is observed in DSPD. In addition, people with insomnia (but not DSPD) would be able to fall asleep at socially acceptable times once their negative cognitions and associations are addressed. However, an overlap between the 2 conditions can occur, because DSPD tends to be a chronic disorder and individuals with DSPD can also develop the typical anxiety surrounding inability to fall asleep and other negative cognitions characteristic of insomnia.[13]

## COMORBIDITIES OF DELAYED SLEEP PHASE DISORDER
### Adults

Comorbidity between DSPD and other psychiatric disorders is common, even if rarely investigated.[2] In a systematic study on comorbidity in 48 adults with DSPD and 25 adults with subclinical DSPD, 70% had a lifetime axis I disorder; approximately 35% met criteria for an anxiety disorder, 15% for a mood disorder, 15% for a substance use disorder, and 3% for schizophrenia.[2] In an online survey of 979 adults, individuals with DSPD symptoms reported higher absenteeism, loss of productivity, disruption in work or school activities, and interference with home responsibilities, compared with individuals without DSPD symptoms.[3]

### Adolescents

In a sample of 63 hospitalized adolescents, approximately 15% had DSPD associated with personality disorders and mood lability.[14] A particularly close association exists between DSPD and attention-deficit/hyperactivity disorder (ADHD), because daytime sleepiness is highly associated with attentional difficulties, and sleepiness may cause the attentional difficulties that have been attributed to late-onset ADHD in adolescents.[15] DSPD is associated with hyperactivity, impulsivity, and inattentiveness; the association between DSPD and ADHD is an area of continued study because this connection suggests that the treatments outlined here for DSPD may also serve as treatments for ADHD.[16–18] In a study of nearly 1300 high school students in Norway, 8.4% self-reported significant difficulties falling asleep before 2 AM and awakening at the desired time to attend classes at least 3 days per week, which the investigators operationalized as DSPD.[19] In this sample, DSPD was associated with lower grade point average, smoking, alcohol use, and increased anxiety and depression symptoms.[19] In a sample of adolescents seeking treatment of DSPD, 16% were not attending school.[20] Taken together, DSPD is associated with poorer outcomes across multiple areas of daily functioning.

On a positive note, multiple positive health effects have been observed following the implementation of later school start times.[21] School districts that have chosen to delay start times by approximately 1 hour have been rewarded with students and faculty who report improved sleep, improved daytime functioning, and improved academic engagement.[22,23]

## BIOLOGICAL AND ENVIRONMENTAL FACTORS AFFECTING SLEEP PHASE
### Biological and Genetic Factors

Sleep-wake periods are tightly regulated processes whose regularity and stability is maintained by 2 interacting systems: the homeostatic (process S) and circadian (process C) systems.[24] The homeostatic system is based on the length of awake time, as the pressure to sleep accumulates. Biochemically, sleep pressure is regulated by extracellular adenosine concentration in the basal forebrain increasing during wakeful-ness and decreasing during sleep.[25] Caffeine decreases sleepiness by countering the effects of adenosine at one of the adenosine receptors.[26] Concurrently, the circadian system establishes an approximately 24-hour cycle of sleep and wakefulness and other physiologic functions via concerted coexpression of specific clock genes in the suprachiasmatic nucleus in the hypothalamus.[27] Presumably to handle seasonal and geographic variability, the circadian system is set, for most people, to a period length slightly longer than 24 hours (on average ~24.2 hours), which is then adjusted for individual circumstances by zeitgebers, or time cues, that entrain the rhythms to the person's individual environment.[28]

A mutated version of *CRY1*, a circadian clock gene, is associated with longer circa-dian rhythms in adults.[29] A polymorphism in another clock gene, *PER3*, has also been implicated in DSPD in a study with adults.[30] Providing psychoeducation about the bio-logical underpinnings of DSPD can alleviate the frustration and shame people with DSPD may feel when beginning treatment.

### Environmental Factors

Light is the most powerful zeitgeber and the intensity and timing of light can advance or delay sleep-wake phase.[28] One of the outputs of the circadian system is the timing of melatonin secretion, a hormone secreted by the pineal gland.[28] Exposure to bright light in the subjective morning (at, or just before, the person's natural wake-up time, not necessarily coinciding with societal morning) determines earlier secretion of mela-tonin in the evening and an earlier sleep period. In contrast, bright light before bedtime suppresses melatonin secretion. Melatonin has hypnotic properties (ie, facilitating sleep onset) as well as chronobiotic effects (ie, affecting phase adjustments in body clocks), as light does.[28]

### Social Factors

Social factors also play a role in the sleep phase. Scott and Woods[31] found that ado-lescents' fear of missing out (FOMO) on social experiences led them to delay their bedtimes to remain on social media, which also leads to increased cognitive arousal, resulting in delayed sleep onset and reduced sleep duration. Similarly, Woods and Scott[32] found that adolescents with high levels of anxiety or depression were more likely to become angry or anxious if their use of social media was restricted. Moreover, many modern video games integrate social media and chat capabilities, and are developed in consultation with researchers who provide input on how to maximize time and engagement on the games.[33]

### Developmental Factors

Developmentally, circadian rhythms naturally shift to a later cycle during puberty, which often dovetails with an increased amount of homework and evening extracur-ricular activities; these external factors can serve as zeitgebers to further delay adoles-cents' already naturally delayed circadian rhythm.[34] Increased levels of estrogen and androgen that occur in puberty may lead to increasing suprachiasmatic nucleus sensi-tivity to light, further affecting adolescents' sleep cycles.[27] This combination of factors seems to predispose adolescents to DSPD.

## ASSESSMENT OF DELAYED SLEEP PHASE DISORDER AND SLEEP CYCLES

Adolescents with suspected DSPD should be interviewed about their sleep habits, including sleep, school, and work schedules; naps; exercise time; intake and timing of caffeine or other stimulants; and bedtime routines. A useful tool to collect this information is a sleep diary (available at http://yoursleep.aasmnet.org/pdf/sleepdiary.pdf), a grid-based document in which the user shades in boxes corresponding with the approximate times they fell asleep and awoke, and in which they can note when they drank caffeinated beverages, exercised, or took medications.[35] Identification of natural sleep periods (ie, sleep-wake periods when the person sleeps naturally and unconstrained; eg, during vacation or weekends) is particularly important to determine behavioral treatment and timing of light exposure. Clinicians can also obtain corroborating sleep data from a patient's parent, roommate, or partner, if applicable. Patients may wish to use wearable technology, usually based on an accelerometer that collects data about movements and periods of stillness (a proxy for sleep). As a cautionary note, commercial wearable devices do not use a uniform method of identifying sleep patterns via movement and are not always reliable, compared with research-grade actigraphy.[36]

Although several sleep questionnaires are used for children and adolescents, few are designed to identify DSPD. The Morningness-Eveningness Questionnaire is a 19-item self-report measure assessing the sleep and wake times people would naturally use if they had no external obligations or appointments.[37] It was designed for adults but it can be used in adolescents. The 17-item Munich Chrono-Type Questionnaire identifies circadian preferences in adults and adolescents.[38] The Children's ChronoType Questionnaire (CCTQ) is a parent-report, 27-item mixed-format questionnaire resulting in multiple measures of chronotype in children 4 to 11 years old.[39] The School Sleep Habits Survey is a self-report measure that incorporates use of caffeine, alcohol, and other substances that may affect sleep-wake cycles in adolescents.[40]

In addition, adolescents should be screened for other sleep disorders before receiving a DSPD diagnosis. Obstructive sleep apnea can cause excessive daytime sleepiness and should be ruled out. Presence of chronic or loud snoring or witnessed apneas should raise suspicion for obstructive sleep apnea and determine a referral to sleep medicine specialists.

In summary, a combination of these assessment measures should be used to provide the most robust mix of objective and subjective information about a patient's sleep (See Suman K.R. Baddam and colleagues' article, "Screening and Evaluation of Sleep Disturbances and Sleep Disorders in Children and Adolescents, in this volume"). See **Table 1** for more details about assessment.

## TREATMENT
### Melatonin

To treat DSPD, the chronobiotic effects of exogenous melatonin can be maximized by administering low doses, typically ranging from 0.3 mg to 1 mg, 4 to 5 hours before the target sleep time, depending on the patient's age and difficulty falling asleep.[41] Of note, maximizing the chronobiotic effects of melatonin (ie, its ability to affect the circadian entrainment) differs from maximizing the hypnotic effects of melatonin, which is typically done through higher doses (eg, 3–5 mg) taken close to bedtime.[42] A meta-analysis revealed that, across various studies in which children and adults with DSPD were treated with exogenous melatonin alone by maximizing its chronobiotic effects, on average, participants fell asleep more than 30 minutes faster and woke up approximately 20 minutes earlier than participants who ingested a placebo.[43] In general, the chronobiotic effects of melatonin are most helpful as an adjunct to the behavioral strategies discussed later rather than as a stand-alone treatment.[44]

**Table 1**
Assessment of delayed sleep phase disorder

| | | In DSPD |
|---|---|---|
| Schedules | Bedtime and time to fall asleep on weekdays, weekends, and vacations | Individuals tend to fall asleep >2 h later than expected. If they retire at their natural sleep time (eg, 2 AM), they might experience fewer problems falling asleep<br>Assess with a sleep diary and actigraphy |
| | Wake-up time on weekdays, weekends, and vacations | Significant morning drowsiness, difficulty getting up, multiple-alarm snoozing, parental involvement needed to get up<br>During weekends or vacation, late wake-up time (>2 h from usual wake-up time), often later than 11 AM or noon<br>Always important to clarify presence of weekend/vacation activities that required early rising<br>Assess with a sleep diary and/or actigraphy |
| | Alertness in the later part of the evening | Typical of DSPD. Increased alertness, energy, and creativity later in the day, often peaking at 9–11 PM<br>Assess with interview and/or questionnaires |
| | Regularity of sleep schedule | Usually irregular, especially when there are morning demands, otherwise regular but delayed (eg, 2–10 AM daily) if no morning demands<br>Input from family and friends often helpful in this area |
| | Presence of naps, their timing and duration | Often present<br>Input from family and friends often helpful in this area |
| | Schedule of school, work, extracurricular and social activities | Understanding patient's daily schedule is key to having an open conversation how to prioritize sleep |
| Bedtime Routines and Sleep Environment | Presence of regular and calming bedtime routines | In DSPD, individuals are often energized and engaged in stimulating activities, which are not sleep conducive in the evening |
| | Exposure to electronic devices or bright light in the hour before sleep | If present, it should be discouraged. Parents should negotiate electronic curfew; adults should stop using their devices at an established time |
| | Bedroom environment (shared bed/bedroom, dark, quiet, cool) | Important to ascertain whether noise or light are affecting the person's sleep. Eye masks, silicone ear plugs, and/or white noise machine can be suggested. A fan can help with noise and increased temperature |

| Presence of Excessive Daytime Sleepiness | Inability to wake up when expected | Typical of DSPD |
| | School or work tardiness or absences | Typical of DSPD |
| | Dozing off in class or in other public spaces | Typical of DSPD |
| | Fatigue or daytime fogginess | Typical of DSPD |
| | Accidents or near misses related to sleepiness for driving teens or adults | Typical of DSPD, especially in the morning |
| | Feeling refreshed on awakening | Usually only during vacation or when allowed to follow natural schedule |
| Substances that Affect Sleep | Amount and timing of: | Important to ascertain whether substances play a role in difficulties falling asleep and suggest appropriate changes when needed |
| | Stimulants (formulation, extended vs immediate release) | |
| | Caffeine | Questionnaires can be helpful in assessing substance use |
| | Nicotine | |
| | Alcohol | |
| Other Sleep Disorders That Can Present With Difficulties Falling Asleep | Insomnia | — |
| | Restless legs syndrome | |
| | Obstructive sleep apnea | |

*Adapted from* Baroni A. Teens who can't sleep: insomnia or circadian rhythm disorder? J Am Acad Child Adolesc Psychiatry. 2019;58(3):307–12; with permission.

## Behavioral and Cognitive Interventions

Behavioral and cognitive strategies are key elements of the treatment of DSPD. Most DSPD interventions include initial psychoeducation about sleep-wake physiology, baseline assessment with a sleep diary (discussed earlier), and setting realistic treatment goals.[13,45] Next, as described later, clinicians and patients develop a wind-down routine to help induce sleepiness every evening and a wake-up routine to increase movement and appropriate light exposure every morning. In addition, patients are encouraged to reduce napping.[46] Cognitive reframing can be used to challenge negative cognitions about sleep, whereas a motivational interviewing framework can help patients stay motivated for treatment.[47]

### Strategy: wind-down routine

A robust wind-down routine includes dim lighting and engaging in relaxing activities that decrease cognitive or emotional arousal in the hours before bedtime. Dim lighting is one of the most critical elements because melatonin is only produced in the absence of light.[41,48] Melatonin secretion naturally starts later in the night as people reach puberty,[49] making it all the more important for adolescents to follow a wind-down routine that includes dim lighting as early as possible in the evening. Blue-green (shortest) wavelengths suppress melatonin production the most.[50] However, electronic screens radiate significant amounts of such wavelengths.[51] Esaki and colleagues[51] found that, when participants with DSPD were instructed to wear blue-blocking glasses starting at 9 PM each night, without requiring any reductions in electronics usage, participants' sleep onset time occurred earlier than when they did not wear the glasses. Another study found that participants who wore blue light–blocking glasses 3 hours before bedtime reported significantly improved sleep quality and mood compared with control participants who wore amber light–blocking glasses.[52] Although blue light–blocking glasses are unlikely to cure DSPD alone, they are a tool that can be used, especially if it is difficult to minimize electronics usage close to bedtime.[53] Besides reducing light exposure, tasks such as showering, drawing, reading a book, doing a puzzle, or listening to calming music and other relaxing evening tasks are appropriate for a wind-down routine. Patients should also stay out of bed until they are ready to go to sleep to avoid associating being in bed with wakefulness.[46] An evening routine can become a virtuous cycle, in which relaxing activities not only reduce arousal but also begin to act as zeitgebers that sleep is approaching, further entraining the circadian rhythm. Patients should avoid moderate-intensity or high-intensity exercise during wind-down routines, because even 20 minutes of such exercise can suppress melatonin release.[40]

As noted earlier, social media and video games often present a major challenge to developing an appropriate wind-down routine because of FOMO.[31] Discussing with patients the Web sites they visit and the video games they play can be helpful in assessing the factors motivating them to maintain a delayed sleep phase. Some adolescents report that their closest friends are peers in other time zones with whom they communicate via online platforms. If so, it is critical to problem solve with these patients how they can both achieve their sleep goals and maintain relationships with their online peers. A simple measure to address FOMO is to notify friends that notifications will not be addressed after 10 PM on schooldays. In some cases, and especially with younger patients, it is advisable that cellphones and other electronic devices be removed by parents after a certain hour. However, for young adults, the patient's input is key to developing a successful strategy to address FOMO.

### Strategy: reducing naps

Throughout the day, but especially in the afternoon, it is critical that patients with DSPD avoid naps, because they reduce sleep pressure and thus sleep propensity.[46]

Even if a patient follows a wind-down routine with dim lighting and melatonin, remaining asleep throughout the night is less likely if sleep pressure is reduced by napping. In addition, it is important that the wake-up and sleep times vary by no more than 2 hours on any day to maintain circadian stability[5]; this restriction can be especially difficult to maintain on weekends, when adolescents (and adults) can sleep in.

### Strategy: increasing morning light exposure

Just as it is critical to avoid bright light in the evening, one of the most important elements of a wake-up routine is to be exposed to light when awake, especially natural light.[54] The ideal timing of light exposure is discussed later. A secondary benefit to natural light exposure is that it can lead to engaging in outdoor activities that increase energy levels.

### A transdiagnostic approach

The strategies discussed earlier have been recently organized systematically in the Transdiagnostic Intervention for Sleep and Circadian Dysfunction (TranS-C), a modular treatment of DSPD built on cognitive behavior therapy for insomnia and motivational interviewing.[46] Of note, adolescents rating the effectiveness of the TranS-C components found the modules on avoiding naps the most effective, followed by developing a wind-down ritual.[46] Two studies have found that TranS-C reduces adolescents' daytime sleepiness (as reported by both parents and adolescents), reduces adolescents' self-reported eveningness preference, and also leads to earlier dim light melatonin onset.[55,56] Regardless of the particular treatment plan chosen by a patient, it is important to emphasize that DSPD is a chronic condition, similar to diabetes, and requires the use of multiple strategies.

## ADVANCING AND DELAYING SLEEP PHASE

Concurrent with implementing wake-up and wind-down routines, treatment of DSPD includes either delaying or advancing the sleep phase so that the sleep-wake schedule aligns with the patient's needs, be it a school or work schedule. Advancing the sleep phase refers to going to bed at progressively earlier times. Chronotherapy is the term for delaying sleep-wake periods so sleep occurs at progressively later times each day until the desired sleep-wake period is achieved.[57] It is easier to change sleep phase by delaying it rather than advancing it, especially if the person's natural sleep period is extremely delayed.[58,59] For example, if a person's natural sleep period is from 4 AM to 12 PM, but the person wants to sleep from 12 AM to 8 AM, it is generally easier to delay going to sleep by a set amount of time, usually by 3 hours every day. Using this strategy, treatment success has occurred in less than 1 week of intensive chronotherapy.[60] However, such shifts can be highly disruptive to people's schedules, especially to daily commitments. Delaying sleep phase may be most practical for students on extended summer or winter breaks when they have few, if any, responsibilities.

For these reasons, it is often more practical to advance the sleep-wake period (ie, move the sleep-wake time earlier progressively), usually by 15 to 30 minutes every few nights. In this case, the clinician works with the patient to set realistic treatment goals. For example, if the patient falls naturally asleep around 2:30 AM, a bedtime around 2 AM for few days is a realistic goal. When the patient sleeps regularly around 2 AM, the sleep time can be progressively moved earlier by another 30 minutes.

If patients wish to advance the sleep phase rather than delay it, they must be extra vigilant about modifying the environmental factors that affect sleep to overcome the natural resistance to advancing sleep phase. For example, as described later, at the beginning of a sleep-advancing protocol, patients should expose themselves to light

**Table 2**
Treatment of delayed sleep phase disorder

### Psychoeducation and Goal-setting

| | |
|---|---|
| Education about dual-process model, circadian rhythms, and light's effect are fundamental for patients' adherence. Goals need to be reasonable and ideally incremental | Use motivational interviewing to emphasize that adherence to DSPD treatment is hard, and assess the patient's motivation to engage |
| Assessment should include social elements such as FOMO | Adequate rewards need to be set for adolescents, and adults should create their own reward systems too |

### Melatonin

| | |
|---|---|
| Low-dose melatonin (0.3—1 mg) can be administered 4–6 h before target bedtime | Safe, usually well tolerated to maximize chronobiotic effects |
| | Liquid or dissolvable formulations are often preferred and easier to use at lower doses |

### Routines

| | |
|---|---|
| Create evening wind-down routine, including dim light and rote, relaxing activities while avoiding exercise and cognitively taxing or emotionally charged activities | Patients' engagement is key and often parental supervision is needed. For adult patients, collaboration with partners or spouses is often crucial as well |
| Appropriate activities include showering, tidying up, drawing, reading a book, doing a puzzle, stretching, or listening to calming music or an audiobook | |
| Consider blue-blocking glasses after 8–9 PM if evening use of electronic devices is necessary (homework, work) | |
| Address FOMO by informing friends which notifications will not be addressed after a certain time (eg, 10 PM). | |
| Avoid being in bed awake for more than 20–30 min | |
| Create morning wake-up routine including exposure to light and exercise after the subjective wake-up time | |

### Sleep-Wake Schedule

| | |
|---|---|
| Maintenance of regular sleep-wake schedule with no more than 2-h variation from weekdays to weekend. No sleeping in even during weekends or vacations | Patients' engagement is key, and often parental supervision is needed. For adult patients, collaboration with partners or spouses is often crucial as well |

| | |
|---|---|
| Limit naps to 30 min, never later than 4 PM | Many patients experience significant sleep deprivation during schedule adjustments. Patients should be aware of possible sleep-deprivation impairment, especially if they drive or perform other alertness-requiring activities |
| If sleep-wake advance strategy is chosen, initial bedtime should be approximately set at the time of natural sleep onset, as observed from sleep diary, or 30 min earlier, to minimize time in bed awake | |
| Bedtime can be set progressively earlier (15–30 min every 3–7 d) until target bedtime is reached | |
| Wake-up time should be established based on required or appropriate wake-up time on week/school days ± 2 h | |

*Chronotherapy*

| | |
|---|---|
| In chronotherapy, bedtime is progressively delayed (ie, moved later daily) by 2–3 h, until the desired sleep schedule is reached (eg, sleep time will be first day at 6 AM, the second at 9 AM, the third at noon, and so on until target bedtime is reached) | Indicated for severe phase shift |
| | More rapid resetting of internal clock |
| | Difficult to implement because requires missing day activities and close family supervision around the clock |
| | Bedtimes can instead be advanced, but it is more difficult for the body to adapt to advancing bedtimes, so environmental factors to help with sleep should be maximized |
| | Caution should be used in patients with bipolar disorder |

*Light Treatment*

| | |
|---|---|
| Exposure to 2000–10,000 lux for 30–60 min 2 h after natural sleep midpoint or 1–2 h before natural wake-up time (subjective morning). Bright light is progressively administered 15–30 min earlier until target wake-up time is achieved and sustained | Safe, usually well tolerated, but often not covered by insurance |
| | Requires days to weeks to reach desired goal |
| | Most treatment lamps are portable and battery operated. Adolescents are often reluctant to use it in school |
| Dawn simulators might be an easy-to-administer alternative to classic light boxes and increase compliance | IEP/504 accommodations to receive treatment in nursing office might increase compliance |
| Walking to school/work for 20–30 min can be a good alternative when timing is appropriate | Light therapy should be used cautiously in patients with bipolar disorder |
| | Safe |
| Avoidance of intense light before subjective morning (ie, 2 h after sleep midpoint) | No electronic devices 1–2 h before scheduled sleep time. Otherwise, patients might have to use blue light–blocking glasses or sunglasses fin the evening 1–2 hours prior to bedtime. |

*Abbreviation:* IEP, Individualized Educational Plan.
*Adapted from* Baroni A. Teens who can't sleep: insomnia or circadian rhythm disorder? J Am Acad Child Adolesc Psychiatry. 2019;58(3):307–12; with permission.

after their natural wake-up times and gradually shift the exposure timing earlier as they advance the sleep phase over the following weeks.

## LIGHT EXPOSURE AND LIGHTBOXES

As noted earlier, light effects depend critically on time of exposure, and specifically on the subjective circadian time for each patient.[61] Initial ideal time of bright light exposure differs between a patient waking up naturally at 10 AM versus one waking up at 2 PM Notably, clinicians should assess sleep-wake periods occurring naturally during vacations or weekends, rather than when curtailed by daily commitments. Optimal time of light exposure should be in the subjective morning of the treated individual, which usually occurs 1 to 2 hours after the sleep midpoint (ie, the time that divides the physiologic sleep period in 2).[61] For example, if a teen's sleep period is 6 AM to 2 PM, the sleep midpoint occurs at 10 AM and subjective morning starts after 12 PM, so the teen should receive bright light after 12 PM and avoid bright light before then. Progressively, light exposure can be moved earlier by 15 to 30 minutes every other day until the desired natural wake-up time is reached.[5] A simpler alternative is to start light treatment after the patient's natural wake-up time. (See Baroni[5] (2019) for a detailed illustrative example.)

New forms of technological aids can assist with behavioral strategies for increasing morning light exposure. For example, if exposure to natural sunlight as part of a wake-up routine is not possible, a lightbox may be a viable alternative. Lightboxes with 10,000 lux light capacity are affordable and commercially available. Such boxes, which include a broad light spectrum, are effective in helping shift sleep-wake cycles in adults and adolescents.[20] However, they are not particularly portable, which means that the patient must be willing to stay in close proximity to the lightbox for the duration of use (approximately 30 min/d) to gain the sleep cycle–altering effect; remaining close to the light may inhibit the patient from engaging in activities that require exertion and increase energy level. However, lightboxes can be used at breakfast or during some morning routines, such as makeup time. Similarly, if a patient would already be sitting at home or in an office, the use of a lightbox can be a simple, low-effort method to improve the sleep cycle. A commercially available wake-up light (also known as a dawn simulator) is similar to a lightbox but operates on a preset clock, gradually turning on and becoming brighter for 30 minutes before the target wake-up time; initial evaluations with adolescents with an eveningness preference indicate that the use of a wake-up light alone can lead to earlier wake-up times and self-reported increases in alertness.[62]

One promising extension of the lightbox is a mask worn before going to bed with built-in light-emitting diode bulbs that automatically turn on to provide bright light exposure at progressively earlier times in the morning. This option provides bright light in a manner that does not affect the sleep of the patient's partner and does not require much effort from the wearer. Initial results indicate that this mask helped patients with DSPD advance their sleep phases more easily than a placebo version of the mask providing dim red light.[63] **Table 2** provides a summary of these treatment options.

## SUMMARY

DSPD is a chronic condition that can contribute to lifelong difficulties in maintaining a socially acceptable schedule, academic failure, social isolation, poor physical health, and various psychiatric illnesses. However, it is treatable and there are multiple therapeutic options to address it. Clinicians should be familiar with DSPD assessment and its treatment modalities. Long-term monitoring is often required to prevent relapses.

## FUTURE DIRECTIONS

Why are some individuals predisposed to later sleep-wake cycles than most of the population? This question is still largely unanswered. The study of DSPD is still in its infancy, and further research is needed to better understand how the homeostatic and circadian systems interact. Similarly, the connection between DSPD and insomnia is not fully understood. Given the overlap between the two disorders, are there similar genetic contributors to both disorders? Why might some people develop DSPD but not insomnia, even if they have trouble falling asleep at conventional times? The long-term effects of extended blue light exposure from ever-present screens on adolescents' sleep patterns also deserves further study.[64] The study of DSPD also raises the question of whether clinicians should take a stronger role in advocating for later school start times. As discussed, delayed school start times are associated with improvements in both student and staff functioning in school.[22] More broadly, a robust understanding of the nuances of the natural sleep-wake mechanisms may allow more effective, targeted treatments that reduce relapse.[65]

## CLINICS CARE POINTS

- Treatment of DSPD requires significant effort and motivation from the patients to make lifestyle changes.
- It is often most practical to gradually shift the sleep and wake times earlier until the patients reach their target sleep-wake times, but this requires many environmental and behavior changes.
- Environmental and behavior changes include strict wind-down routines, consisting of minimizing light exposure and maximizing the use of relaxing, routine tasks.
- Similarly, a strict wake-up routine in which the patient gets out of bed at the chosen wake-up time and engages in activities with exposure to light is crucial.
- Evening melatonin, prevention of daytime napping, and use of blue light–blocking glasses before sleep also help establish a more appropriate schedule.

## DISCLOSURE

The authors have nothing to disclose.

## REFERENCES

1. Gradisar M, Crowley SJ. Delayed sleep phase disorder in youth. Curr Opin Psychiatry 2013;26(6):580–5.
2. Reid KJ, Jaksa AA, Eisengart JB, et al. Systematic evaluation of Axis-I DSM diagnoses in delayed sleep phase disorder and evening-type circadian preference. Sleep Med 2012;13(9):1171–7.
3. Rajaratnam SM, Licamele L, Birznieks G. Delayed sleep phase disorder risk is associated with absenteeism and impaired functioning. Sleep Health 2015;1(2):121–7.
4. Association AP. Diagnostic and statistical manual of mental disorders (DSM-5®). Washington, DC: American Psychiatric Pub; 2013.
5. Baroni A. Teens who can't sleep: insomnia or circadian rhythm disorder? J Am Acad Child Adolesc Psychiatry 2019;58(3):307–12.

6. Saxvig IW, Pallesen S, Wilhelmsen-Langeland A, et al. Prevalence and correlates of delayed sleep phase in high school students. Sleep Med 2012;13(2):193–9.

7. Danielsson K, Markström A, Broman J-E, et al. Delayed sleep phase disorder in a Swedish cohort of adolescents and young adults: prevalence and associated factors. Chronobiol Int 2016;33(10):1331–9.

8. Sivertsen B, Glozier N, Harvey AG, et al. Academic performance in adolescents with delayed sleep phase. Sleep Med 2015;16(9):1084–90.

9. Tomoda A, Miike T, Yonamine K, et al. Disturbed circadian core body temperature rhythm and sleep disturbance in school refusal children and adolescents. Biol Psychiatry 1997;41(7):810–3.

10. Owens JA, Weiss MR. Insufficient sleep in adolescents: causes and consequences. Minerva Pediatr 2017;69(4):326–36.

11. Phillips AJ, Clerx WM, O'Brien CS, et al. Irregular sleep/wake patterns are associated with poorer academic performance and delayed circadian and sleep/wake timing. Sci Rep 2017;7(1):1–13.

12. Sűdy ÁR, Ella K, Bódizs R, et al. Association of social jetlag with sleep quality and autonomic cardiac control during sleep in young healthy men. Front Neurosci 2019;13:950.

13. Lack LC, Wright HR. Clinical management of delayed sleep phase disorder. Behav Sleep Med 2007;5(1):57–76.

14. Dagan Y, Stein D, Steinbock M, et al. Frequency of delayed sleep phase syndrome among hospitalized adolescent psychiatric patients. J Psychosom Res 1998;45(1):15–20.

15. Lunsford-Avery JR, Kollins SH. Editorial Perspective: delayed circadian rhythm phase: a cause of late-onset attention-deficit/hyperactivity disorder among adolescents? J Child Psychol Psychiatry 2018;59(12):1248–51.

16. CHIANG HL, GAU SSF, NI HC, et al. Association between symptoms and subtypes of attention-deficit hyperactivity disorder and sleep problems/disorders. J Sleep Res 2010;19(4):535–45.

17. Coogan AN, McGowan NM. A systematic review of circadian function, chronotype and chronotherapy in attention deficit hyperactivity disorder. Atten Defic Hyperact Disord 2017;9(3):129–47.

18. Sivertsen B, Harvey AG, Pallesen S, et al. Mental health problems in adolescents with delayed sleep phase: results from a large population-based study in Norway. J Sleep Res 2015;24(1):11–8.

19. Hysing M, Pallesen S, Stormark KM, et al. Sleep patterns and insomnia among adolescents: a population-based study. J Sleep Res 2013;22(5):549–56.

20. Gradisar M, Dohnt H, Gardner G, et al. A randomized controlled trial of cognitive-behavior therapy plus bright light therapy for adolescent delayed sleep phase disorder. Sleep 2011;34(12):1671–80.

21. Marx R, Tanner-Smith EE, Davison CM, et al. Later school start times for supporting the education, health, and well-being of high school students: a systematic review. Campbell Systematic Reviews 2017;13(1):1–99.

22. Meltzer LJ, McNally J, Wahlstrom KL, et al. 0819 impact of changing middle and high school start times on sleep, extracurricular activities, homework, and academic engagement. Sleep 2019;42(Supplement_1):A328–9.

23. Plog AE, McNally J, Wahlstrom KL, et al. 0207 impact of changing school start times on teachers/staff. Sleep 2019;42(Supplement_1):A85–6.

24. Borbély AA, Daan S, Wirz-Justice A, et al. The two-process model of sleep regulation: a reappraisal. J Sleep Res 2016;25(2):131–43.

25. Huang Z-L, Zhang Z, Qu W-M. Roles of adenosine and its receptors in sleep–wake regulation. Int Rev Neurobiol 2014;119:349–71.

26. Roehrs T, Roth T. Caffeine: sleep and daytime sleepiness. Sleep Med Rev 2008; 12(2):153–62.

27. Moore RY. Suprachiasmatic nucleus in sleep–wake regulation. Sleep Med 2007; 8:27–33.

28. Emens JS, Burgess HJ. Effect of light and melatonin and other melatonin receptor agonists on human circadian physiology. Sleep Med Clin 2015;10(4):435–53.

29. Patke A, Murphy PJ, Onat OE, et al. Mutation of the human circadian clock gene CRY1 in familial delayed sleep phase disorder. Cell 2017;169(2):203–15.e3.

30. Archer SN, Carpen JD, Gibson M, et al. Polymorphism in the PER3 promoter associates with diurnal preference and delayed sleep phase disorder. Sleep 2010; 33(5):695–701.

31. Scott H, Woods HC. Fear of missing out and sleep: cognitive behavioural factors in adolescents' nighttime social media use. J Adolesc 2018;68:61–5.

32. Woods HC, Scott H. # Sleepyteens: social media use in adolescence is associated with poor sleep quality, anxiety, depression and low self-esteem. J Adolesc 2016;51:41–9.

33. Clay RA. Video game design and development. Gradpsych 2012;1:14–6.

34. Robillard R, Naismith SL, Rogers NL, et al. Delayed sleep phase in young people with unipolar or bipolar affective disorders. J Affect Disord 2013;145(2):260–3.

35. Rogers AE, Caruso CC, Aldrich MS. Reliability of sleep diaries for assessment of sleep/wake patterns. Nurs Res 1993;42(6):368–72.

36. Baroni A, Bruzzese J-M, Di Bartolo CA, et al. Fitbit Flex: an unreliable device for longitudinal sleep measures in a non-clinical population. Sleep Breath 2016; 20(2):853–4.

37. Horne JA, Östberg O. A self-assessment questionnaire to determine morningness-eveningness in human circadian rhythms. Int J Chronobiol 1976; 4(2):97–110.

38. Roenneberg T, Keller LK, Fischer D, et al. Human activity and rest in situ. Methods Enzymol 2015;552:257–83.

39. Werner H, LeBourgeois MK, Geiger A, et al. Assessment of chronotype in four-to eleven-year-old children: reliability and validity of the Children's Chronotype Questionnaire (CCTQ). Chronobiol Int 2009;26(5):992–1014.

40. Richardson CE, Gradisar M, Short MA, et al. Can exercise regulate the circadian system of adolescents? Novel implications for the treatment of delayed sleep-wake phase disorder. Sleep Med Rev 2017;34:122–9.

41. Bruni O, Alonso-Alconada D, Besag F, et al. Current role of melatonin in pediatric neurology: clinical recommendations. Eur J Paediatr Neurol 2015;19(2):122–33.

42. Mundey K, Benloucif S, Harsanyi K, et al. Phase-dependent treatment of delayed sleep phase syndrome with melatonin. Sleep 2005;28(10):1271–8.

43. van Geijlswijk IM, Korzilius HPLM, Smits MG. The use of exogenous melatonin in delayed sleep phase disorder: a meta-analysis. Sleep 2010;33(12):1605–14.

44. Wasdell MB, Jan JE, Bomben MM, et al. A randomized, placebo-controlled trial of controlled release melatonin treatment of delayed sleep phase syndrome and impaired sleep maintenance in children with neurodevelopmental disabilities. J Pineal Res 2008;44(1):57–64.

45. Gumport NB, Dolsen MR, Harvey AG. Usefulness and utilization of treatment elements from the Transdiagnostic Sleep and Circadian Intervention for adolescents with an evening circadian preference. Behav Res Ther 2019;123:103504.

46. Harvey AG, Buysse DJ. Treating sleep problems: a transdiagnostic approach. New York: Guilford Publications; 2017.
47. Rollnick S, Miller WR. What is motivational interviewing? Behav Cogn Psychother 1995;23(4):325–34.
48. Pullman RE, Roepke SE, Duffy JF. Laboratory validation of an in-home method for assessing circadian phase using dim light melatonin onset (DLMO). Sleep Med 2012;13(6):703–6.
49. Micic G, De Bruyn A, Lovato N, et al. The endogenous circadian temperature period length (tau) in delayed sleep phase disorder compared to good sleepers. J Sleep Res 2013;22(6):617–24.
50. Wright HR, Lack LC. Effect of light wavelength on suppression and phase delay of the melatonin rhythm. Chronobiol Int 2001;18(5):801–8.
51. Esaki Y, Kitajima T, Ito Y, et al. Wearing blue light-blocking glasses in the evening advances circadian rhythms in the patients with delayed sleep phase disorder: an open-label trial. Chronobiol Int 2016;33(8):1037–44.
52. Kimberly B, James RP. Amber lenses to block blue light and improve sleep: a randomized trial. Chronobiol Int 2009;26(8):1602–12.
53. Chang A-M, Aeschbach D, Duffy JF, et al. Evening use of light-emitting eReaders negatively affects sleep, circadian timing, and next-morning alertness. Proc Natl Acad Sci U S A 2015;112(4):1232–7.
54. Arendt J, Broadway J. Light and melatonin as zeitgebers in man. Chronobiol Int 1987;4(2):273–82.
55. Dong L, Gumport NB, Martinez AJ, et al. Is improving sleep and circadian problems in adolescence a pathway to improved health? A mediation analysis. J Consult Clin Psychol 2019;87(9):757–71.
56. Harvey AG, Hein K, Dolsen MR, et al. Modifying the impact of eveningness chronotype ("night-owls") in youth: a randomized controlled trial. J Am Acad Child Adolesc Psychiatry 2018;57(10):742–54.
57. Czeisler CA, Richardson GS, Coleman RM, et al. Chronotherapy: resetting the circadian clocks of patients with delayed sleep phase insomnia. Sleep 1981;4(1):1–21.
58. Wilhelmsen-Langeland A, Dundas I, Saxvig IW, et al. Psychosocial challenges related to delayed sleep phase disorder. Delayed Sleep Phase Disorder in Adolescence and Young Adulthood Patients experiences, personality and treatment effects on daytime function. 2012.
59. Wyatt JK. Delayed sleep phase syndrome: pathophysiology and treatment options. Sleep 2004;27(6):1195–203.
60. Smith MR, Revell VL, Eastman CI. Phase advancing the human circadian clock with blue-enriched polychromatic light. Sleep Med 2009;10(3):287–94.
61. Lovato N, Micic G, Gradisar M, et al. Can the circadian phase be estimated from self-reported sleep timing in patients with Delayed Sleep Wake Phase Disorder to guide timing of chronobiologic treatment? Chronobiol Int 2016;33(10):1376–90.
62. Fromm E, Horlebein C, Meergans A, et al. Evaluation of a dawn simulator in children and adolescents. Biol Rhythm Res 2011;42(5):417–25.
63. Cole RJ, Smith JS, Alcal YC, et al. Bright-light mask treatment of delayed sleep phase syndrome. J Biol Rhythms 2002;17(1):89–101.
64. Van der Lely S, Frey S, Garbazza C, et al. Blue blocker glasses as a countermeasure for alerting effects of evening light-emitting diode screen exposure in male teenagers. J Adolesc Health 2015;56(1):113–9.
65. Fuller PM, Gooley JJ, Saper CB. Neurobiology of the sleep-wake cycle: sleep architecture, circadian regulation, and regulatory feedback. J Biol rhythms 2006; 21(6):482–93.

# The Associations Between Sleep and Externalizing and Internalizing Problems in Children and Adolescents with Attention-Deficit/Hyperactivity Disorder

## Empirical Findings, Clinical Implications, and Future Research Directions

Jenny Dimakos, BSc[a], Gabrielle Gauthier-Gagné, BA[b],
Lanyi Lin, BSc[b], Samantha Scholes, BA[b,c], Reut Gruber, PhD[b,d],*

## KEYWORDS

- Sleep • ADHD • Externalizing • Internalizing • Youth • Children • Adolescents

## KEY POINTS

- Attention-deficit/hyperactivity disorder is associated with comorbid sleep disturbances.
- Sleep problems are associated with internalizing and externalizing symptoms in youth with ADHD.
- Sleep problems precede, predict, and significantly contribute to the manifestation of internalizing and externalizing behavior problems; this association is bidirectional with regards to associations between sleep disturbances and internalizing symptoms.
- Clinicians should assess sleep and integrate sleep intervention into the management of youth with ADHD.
- Future research is needed to examine the mechanisms underlying the associations between sleep and internalizing and externalizing problems in youth with ADHD.

This article originally appeared in *Child and Adolescent Psychiatric Clinics*, Volume 30 Issue 1, January 2021.
[a] Faculty of Medicine, McGill University, Montreal, Quebec, Canada; [b] Attention Behavior and Sleep Lab, Douglas Mental Health University Institute, Montréal, Quebec H4H 1R3, Canada; [c] Department of Educational and Counselling Psychology, McGill University, Montréal, Quebec, Canada; [d] Department of Psychiatry, Faculty of Medicine, McGill University, Montréal, Quebec, Canada
* Corresponding author. Attention Behavior and Sleep Lab, Douglas Mental Health University Institute, Montréal, Quebec, Canada.
*E-mail address:* reut.gruber@douglas.mcgill.ca

Psychiatr Clin N Am 47 (2024) 179–197
https://doi.org/10.1016/j.psc.2023.06.012
0193-953X/24/© 2023 Elsevier Inc. All rights reserved.

## INTRODUCTION

Attention-deficit/hyperactivity disorder (ADHD) is a neurodevelopmental disorder characterized by symptoms of inattention, impulsivity, and/or hyperactivity that affects 5% to 7% of school-age children and adolescents.[1,2] Early deficits in executive functions (EFs), a set of cognitive abilities responsible for goal-directed behavior, have been identified as an etiologic risk factor for ADHD,[3] as has decreased activation in the frontoparietal networks and ventral attentional network, which are brain systems known to be involved in EF.[4] In addition to the core symptoms listed above, emotional symptoms and poor self-regulation are increasingly considered core features of ADHD. Low frustration tolerance, irritability, ease of negative emotional experience, and emotional lability are frequent in children and adolescents with ADHD.[5–8] These challenges can result in internalizing (eg, anxious, depressed mood) and/or externalizing (eg, oppositional/defiance, poor conduct, irritability) behavioral problems, which are major contributors to the social, occupational, educational, and relational impairments seen in individuals with ADHD. Because the outcomes of such problems are often severe, it is important that we understand the upstream pathways and seek to identify innovative, treatable intervention goals.

Inadequate sleep has been reported in up to 70% of children with ADHD,[9–17] compared with 20% to 30% of children in the general population.[18] The sleep problems experienced by children with ADHD include unhealthy lifestyle choices, such as excessive evening screen use or insufficient sleep,[19–21] behavioral problems (eg, difficulties initiating and/or maintaining sleep),[22,23] and primary sleep disorders, such as sleep-disordered breathing (SDB), sleep apnea, restless leg syndrome (RLS), delayed sleep phase syndrome (DSPS), insomnia, and narcolepsy.[24–30]

The neural areas that govern self-regulation and EF (eg, the dorsolateral prefrontal, anterior cingulate, and parietal cortices) are sensitive to sleep deprivation.[31–35] Sleep loss acutely impairs the EF necessary for effective behavioral or self-regulation, especially in the face of frustration.[36–38] The brain regions responsible for exerting top-down control are particularly sensitive to sleep deprivation. For example, the connectivity between the amygdala and medial prefrontal cortex is reduced under sleep deprivation, leading to greater amygdala activation in response to negative emotional stimuli.[39–41] In children, impairments in these cognitive processes manifest as irritability and behavioral outbursts corresponding to internalizing or externalizing behaviors.[42]

The behaviors and self-regulatory processes that are affected by inadequate sleep, namely EF and externalizing/internalizing behaviors, are also key domains of dysfunction in youth with ADHD.[36,43] Among children predisposed to behavioral difficulties, such as those with ADHD, the impact of disrupted sleep may be amplified.[28,44] Hence, the characteristics of ADHD may increase both the risk for and the vulnerability to insufficient sleep. There are documented associations between various domains of sleep and both internalizing/externalizing symptoms and the negative impacts of these symptoms on youth with ADHD.[45–48] However, we know little about the nature of the associations between sleep and these symptoms in youth with ADHD.

Addressing this knowledge gap is important as it could provide valuable intervention targets that could be used to reduce daytime impairments among youth with ADHD. If inadequate sleep predicts, causes, or worsens internalizing and externalizing problems over time, then improved sleep could be a way to reduce the burden of such mental health problems among children with ADHD. The objectives of this article are to: (1) integrate the up-to-date empirical evidence; (2) extract clinical implications; and (3) identify future research directions regarding the associations between sleep and externalizing or internalizing problems in youth with ADHD.

## METHODS

This narrative review identifies and synthesizes empirical studies that examined the associations between sleep and internalizing or externalizing problems in youth with ADHD. Three electronic databases were searched in March 2020 (Embase, PsycINFO, and PubMed) for studies published in the previous 5 years. Additional records were identified by searching the references of the selected original research papers and review articles.

Ultimately, 11 studies were identified (see **Fig. 1** for detailed information regarding the literature search, numbers of papers identified, and inclusion and exclusion of identified studies) and divided into 3 age groups: preschool (3–5 years), school-age (6–12 years), and adolescents (13–18 years). Sleep measures were identified as subjective or objective. Subjective sleep measures refer to questionnaires filled out by the patient or a parent regarding the child's sleep behavior or symptoms. Objective measures included polysomnography (PSG) and actigraphy. PSG refers to a sleep assessment during which multiple physiologic parameters are continuously and simultaneously recorded across a sleep period to characterize sleep and identify sleep disorders.[49] Actigraphy is a method of measuring sleep parameters and average motor activity over a period of days to weeks using a noninvasive accelerometer, which is housed in a small device worn like a wristwatch.[50–52]

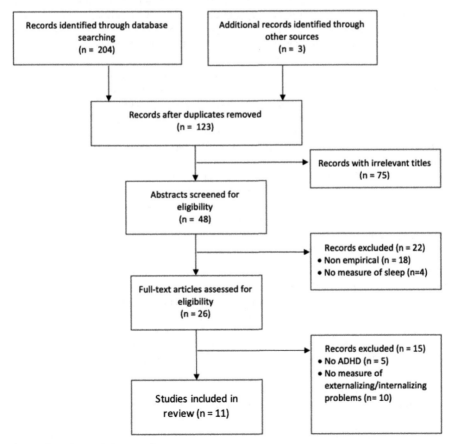

**Fig. 1.** Flowchart of the search.

Externalizing behaviors, including oppositionality, aggression, irritability, and conduct problems were assessed using only parent-reported measures. Internalizing behaviors, including symptoms of anxiety and depression were assessed using both self- and parent-report measures.

The dimensions of sleep assessed included: sleep duration; sleep continuity; and reported sleep disturbances (see **Table 1** for a summary of studies).

## RESULTS
### Key Findings

#### Sleep and externalizing problems in children and adolescents with attention-deficit/hyperactivity disorder

**Preschool children.** One cross-sectional study was conducted to examine the associations between sleep and externalizing problems in preschool children. It used concurrent subjective measures of sleep and behavior in preschool-aged children at risk for or with a clinical diagnosis of externalizing problems. This study revealed that children described by their parents as being more oppositional were reported to have poorer habits near bedtime and more night wakings.[53]

**School-age children.** In school-age children, a cross-sectional study grouped participants according to ADHD presentation and the presence of comorbidity. Sleep and daily functioning were measured using parental reports. Sleep problems were associated with impairment in daily functioning regardless of diagnostic status, but the correlation was stronger in the group of children with ADHD and internalizing comorbidity, and highest in children with ADHD and externalizing comorbidity compared with all other comorbid conditions or controls.[54] Another cross-sectional study examined the associations between objective and subjective sleep measures and irritable-angry mood and temper outbursts in children with and without ADHD.[55] Significant associations were found between the objective PSG parameters and disruptive mood dysregulation disorder (DMDD) in children in the control group. In addition, children with increased sleep problems had significantly higher levels of DMDD symptoms than children without sleep problems.[55] Of the 2 longitudinal studies conducted with school-age children to examine casual and bidirectional associations between sleep problems and externalizing problems, 1 study failed to find a bidirectional relationship between reported sleep problems and externalizing problems.[56] However, the other longitudinal study revealed that children with ADHD and transient or persistent reported sleep problems had higher behavioral and conduct problems compared with children with ADHD without sleep problems over a 12-month period.[57]

**Adolescents.** Three studies have been conducted to examine if shortened sleep duration is a causal contributor to daytime behavior and self-regulation in adolescents with ADHD. Of them, 1 study used a within-subject, crossover design, sleep restriction/extension protocol over 3 weeks to examine if sleep duration is a causal contributor to poorer/improved daytime functioning.[58] The protocol included 1 stabilization week, 1 sleep extension (SE) week in which participants obtained 9 hours of nightly sleep, and 1 sleep restriction (SR) week during which participants obtained 6.5 hours of nightly sleep. All adolescents participated in both the SR and SE conditions, with the order of conditions randomly counterbalanced across participants. Sleep information was obtained using actigraphy and daily diaries, and behavioral information was obtained using parent- and self-reported daily ratings of inattention, hyperactivity/impulsivity, and oppositionality on a 4-point scale. Across both daily and weekly measures, parents reported significantly greater inattention and oppositional behaviors during SR

**Table 1**
Summary of studies

| Author and Year | Study Design | Sample | Age Range (Mean ± SD) | Comorbid Disorders | ADHD Diagnosis | Sleep Measures (Informant; Reliability) | Sleep Dimension(s) | Symptoms Measures | | Results Associations Between Sleep and Internalizing or Externalizing Symptoms |
| --- | --- | --- | --- | --- | --- | --- | --- | --- | --- | --- |
| | | | | | | | | Externalizing (Informant; Construct Measured) | Internalizing (Informant; Construct Measured) | |
| Coto et al,[53] 2018 | Cross-sectional | 148 (82% male) | 3–6 (5.06 ± N/A) | ODD (46%) | C-DISC-IV or K-DBDS | Abbreviated CSHQ (parent; $\alpha$ = .68–.73) | Reported sleep disturbances | DBRS-PV (parent; oppositionality/ aggression) | N/A | Higher scores on parent-reported oppositionality/ aggression were positively correlated with higher levels of sleep problem scores ($r$ = .27, $P<.01$) |
| Virring et al,[54] 2017 | Cross-sectional | 188 control (52% male); 209 ADHD (79% male) | 6–13 (controls (9.7 ± 1.5); ADHD (9.6 ± 1.9) | Externalizing disorders (57%); internalizing disorders (24%); ASD (8%); tics and Tourette syndrome (11%) | DAWBA | CSHQ (parent; $\alpha$ = .62–.73) | Reported sleep disturbances | WFIRS (parent; daily functioning) | N/A | Higher sleep problem scores on the CSHQ were associated with externalizing problems in children with ADHD ($r$ = .50 [0.38, 0.60]) and in the control group ($r$ = .46 [0.31, 0.57]) |
| Waxmonsky et al,[55] 2017 | Cross-sectional | 665 control (53% male); 784 ADHD (68% male) | 6–12 (typically developing 8.7 ± 1.7; ADHD 8.3 ± 1.8) | ODD; CD; anxiety; and depression | Psychological evaluation (child, parent, teacher) and psychological testing | Sleep problems subscale PBS (parent; $\alpha$ = .45); PSG for controls | Reported sleep disturbances | PBS (parent; irritable-angry mood) | N/A | In children with ADHD, higher levels of DMDD symptoms were positively correlated with higher sleep problem scores ($r$ = .28, $P<.05$); children with ADHD and |

(continued on next page)

**Table 1**
*(continued)*

| Author and Year | Study Design | Sample | Age Range (Mean ± SD) | Comorbid Disorders | ADHD Diagnosis | Sleep Measures (Informant; Reliability) | Sleep Dimension(s) | Symptoms Measures | | Results |
|---|---|---|---|---|---|---|---|---|---|---|
| | | | | | | | | Externalizing (Informant; Construct Measured) | Internalizing (Informant; Construct Measured) | Associations Between Sleep and Internalizing or Externalizing Symptoms |
| | | | | | | | | | | increased sleep problem scores had significantly higher DMDD symptoms than children with ADHD without elevated sleep problems scores ($t = 5.4$, $P<.0001$) |
| Mulraney et al,[56] 2016 | Longitudinal | 270 (86% male) | 5–13 (10.1 ± 1.9) | ASD (24%) | Previous diagnosis by a pediatrician | CSHQ (parent; $\alpha = .62–.73$) | Reported sleep disturbances | SDQ (caregiver; conduct problems) | SDQ (caregiver; emotional problems) | Higher sleep problem scores on the CSHQ at baseline in children aged 5–13 predicted internalizing problems 6 mo later ($\beta = .17$, $P<.01$) and internalizing problems at baseline predicted sleep problems 6 mo later ($\beta = .07$, $P<.05$) in children aged 5–13; no predictive relationship between sleep problem scores and internalizing problems between 6 and |

| Study | Design | Sample | Age | Comorbidity | ADHD Diagnosis | Sleep Measure | Sleep Variable | Externalizing | Internalizing | Results |
|---|---|---|---|---|---|---|---|---|---|---|
| Lycett et al,[57] 2016 | Longitudinal | 186 (87% male) | 5–13 (10.1 ± 1.8) | Externalizing and internalizing (36%) | Previous ADHD diagnosis | Caregiver report (not standardized) | Reported sleep disturbances | SDQ (caregiver; conduct problems) | SDQ (caregiver; emotional problems) | 12 mo; no bidirectional relationship found between externalizing problems and sleep problem scores on the CSHQ; Children with ADHD and transient or persistent reported sleep problems had higher conduct problem subscale scores ($P<.001$ and $P<.04$, respectively) and higher emotional problem subscale scores ($P<.001$ and $P<.02$, respectively) compared with children with ADHD without sleep problems over a 12-mo period |
| Becker et al,[58] 2019 | Experimental | 48 (75% male) | 14–17 (5.21 ± 1.15) | Depression (2%); GAD (8%); ODD (4%); any comorbidity (12%) | K-SADS | Actigraphy; SD | Duration | VADRS (parent, ODD symptoms), IOWA-10 (parent; ODD symptoms) | N/A | Paired samples t test revealed higher levels of oppositional behaviors on the daily ($t = 2.99$, $P = .004$) and weekly ($t = 2.24$, $P = .03$) measures during sleep restriction compared with sleep extension condition |
| Becker et al,[46] 2015 | Longitudinal | 81 (75% male) | 10–14 (12.2 ± .95) | N/A | P-ChIPS | CBCL (parent; $\alpha = .61$) | Reported sleep disturbances | DBD (parent; ODD symptoms); SSIS (parent; externalizing behaviors) | RADS-2 (self; depressive symptoms); MASC (self; anxiety symptoms) | Regression analyses revealed that higher sleep problem scores at T1 in children aged 10–14 years significantly predicted higher levels of ODD symptoms ($\beta = .26$, $P = .008$), higher levels of externalizing problems ($\beta = .26$, $P = .01$), and higher levels of depressive symptoms ($\beta = .23$, $P = .045$) at T2 1 year later. Sleep problem scores at T1 did not significantly predict anxiety symptoms 1 year later |

(continued on next page)

**Table 1**
*(continued)*

| Author and Year | Study Design | Sample | Age Range (Mean ± SD) | Comorbid Disorders | ADHD Diagnosis | Sleep Measures (Informant; Reliability) | Sleep Dimension(s) | Symptoms Measures Externalizing (Informant; Construct Measured) | Symptoms Measures Internalizing (Informant; Construct Measured) | Results Associations Between Sleep and Internalizing or Externalizing Symptoms |
|---|---|---|---|---|---|---|---|---|---|---|
| Mulraney et al,[59] 2017 | Longitudinal | 140 (89% male) | 5–13 (10.2 ± 1.9) | Internalizing (60%); externalizing (56%); internalizing and externalizing (39%) | Previous diagnosis by pediatrician and ADHD rating scale IV | DIMS subscale of SDSC (parent; $\alpha$ = .79) | Continuity | ARI (parent; irritability) | N/A | Univariate linear regressions revealed higher levels of sleep problem scores were associated with greater parent-reported irritability scores ($\beta$ = .28, $P$ = .002) |
| Bar et al,[60] 2015 | Cross-sectional | 62 (68% male) | 6–17 (10.09 ± 2.68 for clinical sleep disturbance and 9.80 ± 2.41 for nonclinical sleep disturbance) | Any psychiatric diagnosis (34%); anxiety (16%); LD (17%); tic disorder (2%); CD (11%) | Previous diagnosis by a psychiatrist | CSHQ (parent; $\alpha$ = .62–.73) | Reported sleep disturbances | N/A | SCARED (parent; anxiety) | Regression analysis revealed that higher levels of parent-reported anxiety were significantly associated with higher sleep problem scores ($\beta$ = .27, $P<.05$) |
| Becker et al,[61] 2016 | Cross-sectional | 147 (59% male) | 7–11 (8.62 ± 1.17) | Internalizing; ODD; SCT | K-SADS | Parent inventory of children's sleep habits | Duration; continuity; reported sleep disturbances | CSI-4 (parent; ODD symptoms) | CSI-4 (parent; anxiety and depression symptoms) | Associations between ODD symptom scores and sleep functioning domain scores were not significant. Higher levels of anxiety symptom scores were associated with shorter sleep duration ($r$ = −.19, $P<.05$), being a poor sleeper ($r$ = .33, $P<.001$), and more frequent night wakings ($r$ = .22 $P<.01$); higher levels of depressive symptoms were positively correlated with weekend catch up sleep ($r$ = .22, $P<.01$) |

| Becker et al,[62] 2020 | Experimental | 48 (75% male) | 14–17 (15.21 ± 1.15) | Depression (2%); GAD (8%); ODD (4%); any comorbidity (12%) | K-SADS | Actigraphy; SD | Duration | N/A | RCADS (self and parent; anxiety and depression symptoms); depressed mood Subscale of SHS (self; depressive symptoms); PANAS (self and parent; affect) | Paired samples *t* test revealed higher levels of parent- and self-reported depressive symptoms (t = −5.80, P<.001 and t = −2.16, P = .36, respectively), lower levels of positive affect (t = 4.96, P<.001), and higher levels of negative affect (t = −3.05, P = .004) during the sleep restriction condition compared with the sleep extension condition |
|---|---|---|---|---|---|---|---|---|---|---|

*Abbreviations:* ADHD, attention-deficit/hyperactivity disorder; ARI, affective reactivity index; ASD, autism spectrum disorder; CBCL, child behavior checklist; CD, conduct disorder; C-DISC-IV, Diagnostic Interview Schedule for Children computerized version IV; CSHQ, Children's Sleep Habit Questionnaire; CSI-4, Child Symptom Inventory-4; DAWBA, Development and Well-Being Assessment; DBD, disruptive behavior disorders; DBRS-PV, Disruptive Behavior Disorders Rating Scale—Parent Version; DIMS, Disorders in Initiating and Maintaining Sleep); DMDD, disruptive mood dysregulation disorder; GAD, generalized anxiety disorder; IOWA-10, IOWA Conners Rating Scale; K-DBDS, Kiddie-Disruptive Behavior Disorder Schedule; K-SADS, Kiddie Schedule for Affective Disorders and Schizophrenia for School-Age Children; LD, learning disorder; MASC, multidimensional anxiety scale for children; N/A, not applicable; ODD, oppositional defiant disorder; PANAS, positive and negative affect scale; PBS, pediatric behavior scale; P-ChIPS, Children's Interview for Psychiatric Syndromes—Parent Version; PSG, polysomnography; RADS-2, Reynolds Adolescent Depression Scale, Second Edition; RCADS, Revised Child Anxiety and Depression Scales; SCARED, screen for child anxiety related disorders; SCT, sluggish cognitive tempo; SD, sleep diaries; SDQ, strength and difficulties questionnaire; SDSC, Sleep Disturbance Scale for Children; SHS, sleep habits survey; SSIS, social skills improvement system; VADRS, Vanderbilt ADHD Diagnostic Rating Scale—Parent Version; WFIRS, Weiss Functional Impairment Rating Scale.

compared with SE. Parents did not report greater hyperactivity/impulsivity during restriction compared with extension, but adolescents reported less hyperactivity/impulsivity during restriction compared with extension.[58] The other studies used a longitudinal design to examine the role of sleep in the development of externalizing behaviors in adolescents with ADHD. In the study by Becker and colleagues,[46] sleep problems were found to account for 5% of the variance in predicting youths' oppositional defiant disorder/externalizing behaviors and an additional 4% of the variance in predicting youths' depressive symptoms after accounting for youth characteristics and the stability of psychopathology over a 1-year period.[46] Mulraney and colleagues,[59] followed children with externalizing problems from age 10 to 14 years; they found that these children had higher parent-reported irritability at the follow-up assessment in adolescence, and that this was associated with sleep problems.

### Sleep and internalizing problems in children and adolescents with attention-deficit/hyperactivity disorder

**Preschool children.** No study has examined the interplay between internalizing problems and sleep in preschool children with ADHD.

**School-age children.** In school-age children, a cross-sectional study revealed that children with clinical sleep problems and ADHD reported higher levels of anxiety compared with children with ADHD and no or subclinical sleep problems.[60] Children's anxiety level and medication status were significantly associated with their sleep score, whereas ADHD symptom severity did not significantly correlate with the sleep score.[60] Another large cross-sectional study with school-age children with ADHD-inattentive presentation revealed significant associations between anxiety, shorter sleep duration, and poorer sleep.[61] In addition, this study found an association between depressive symptoms and children's need to catch up on sleep on the weekends. A longitudinal study conducted at 3 time points with school-age children over a 12-month period found a bidirectional relationship between parent-reported sleep problems and internalizing difficulties; sleep problems at baseline predicted internalizing difficulties 6 months later, and internalizing difficulties at baseline predicted sleep problems 6 months later.[56] Another longitudinal study revealed that children with ADHD and transient or persistent reported sleep problems had higher emotional problems compared with children with ADHD without sleep problems over a 12-month period.[57]

**Adolescents.** Compared with studies in school-age children, contrasting results were obtained in an experimental sleep restriction/extension protocol that examined the impact of shortened sleep duration on internalizing symptoms, emotional regulation, and affect valence in adolescents with ADHD[62] (for protocol information see Becker and colleagues[58]). This study found significantly greater parent- and adolescent-reported depressive symptoms during SR compared with SE, and less positive affect and more negative affect during SR compared with extension across both daily diary and laboratory-visit measures. However, no significant difference was found for parent- or adolescent-reported anxiety. In addition, 1 longitudinal study failed to find an association between baseline sleep problems and anxiety symptoms 1 year later.[46]

### Methodological Characteristics of the Included Studies

Of the 11 studies included in this review, 5 were cross-sectional studies that concurrently examined sleep behavior or problems and the extent to which youth with ADHD exhibited internalizing or externalizing behavior problems[53–55,60,61]; 4 used longitudinal designs examining the predictive role of sleep problems in the development of externalizing or internalizing behavioral problems in youth with ADHD and assessing the bidirectional associations between sleep problems and behavioral problems in youth with ADHD[46,56,57,59]; and 2 were experimental studies in which sleep duration was manipulated to test its impact on youth daytime behaviors.[58,62] The total number of youth with ADHD examined across all the studies was 2123; the smallest study included 48 participants with ADHD and the largest included 784. All of the studies included more boys than girls, with ratios ranging from 59% to 89% boys. The studies used objective sleep measures in addition to using subjective parental reports and/or child self-reports regarding sleep disorders, behavior, and/or patterns. The utilized scales had moderate reliability ($\alpha$ = .45–.79). Three studies used a measure that was not designed for the age group in which it was applied.[54,56,60] The measured aspects of sleep included a range of proxies for sleep disorders, disturbances, and sleep duration. Eight studies used the same informants to obtain information regarding the child's sleep and daytime behavior,[53–57,59–61] and 3 studies used different informants for sleep versus daytime behavior.[46,58,62] Eight studies measured and controlled for confounding variables (eg, sex, age, socioeconomic status, medication status, or comorbid conditions) in their analyses.[46,53,54,56,59–61]

## DISCUSSION

Externalizing and internalizing problems are common in youth with ADHD, resulting in suffering and impaired daytime functioning. Sleep plays a central role in regulating emotions and behavior, such that daytime functioning is benefited by healthy sleep but impaired by inadequate or disturbed sleep. Sleep problems are common in youth with ADHD. Despite the importance of healthy and adequate sleep to behavior and self-regulation, there has been no comprehensive review of the interplay between sleep and internalizing and externalizing problems in youth with ADHD. The primary goal of this review was to address this gap and integrate available evidence regarding how and to what extent sleep disturbances or patterns are associated with internalizing and externalizing symptoms in youth with ADHD. The results of the review reveal that: (1) sleep problems are associated with internalizing and externalizing symptoms in youth with ADHD; (2) sleep problems precede, predict, and significantly contribute to the manifestation of internalizing and externalizing behavior problems; (3) this association is bidirectional with regards to associations between sleep disturbances and internalizing symptoms; and (4) SR is causally associated with internalizing and externalizing symptoms in adolescents with ADHD.

The current review drew on a small body of evidence from 11 studies with 2123 participants. Cross-sectional studies across different age groups, from preschool to adolescence, showed significant, positive, and small- to medium-size associations between reported sleep problems and both internalizing and externalizing symptoms. The significance was held in the studies that controlled for sex, parental education or income, and/or comorbid psychiatric conditions. Longitudinal studies revealed similar results, with small associations found between sleep problems reported at an earlier time point and internalizing or externalizing symptoms at a later time point. The nature of the co-occurring internalizing problems differed across studies. One found that sleep problems longitudinally or experimentally predicted increases in depressive symptoms in adolescents with ADHD, but were not associated with anxiety.[46,62] However, other studies found that sleep problems in youth with ADHD were associated with anxiety but not depression.[60,61] Future research should seek to further differentiate the impact of sleep disturbances on depression and anxiety in youth with ADHD, as these symptoms might require different intervention strategies.[63,64]

An experimental study revealed the existence of causal associations between shorter sleep duration and oppositional behavior, inattention, and depressive symptoms in adolescents diagnosed with ADHD.[58] This was consistent with previous work demonstrating that cumulative SR caused deterioration of neurobehavioral functioning from subclinical to clinical values in children with ADHD.[14] It is also consistent with recent work,[65] showing an association between short sleep duration and increased risk of future occurrence of behavioral disorder symptoms in children with ADHD.

### Clinical Implications

Because sleep disturbances are so closely associated with internalizing and externalizing problems in youth with ADHD, they may be considered important modifiable risk factors. Hence, improving the sleep of youth with ADHD and internalizing and/or externalizing problems during developmental periods of neuromaturation could powerfully affect their emotional and behavioral health. Sleep improvement may be obtained in several steps. First, sleep assessment should be integrated into the evaluation process of youth with ADHD on a routine basis.[66] Initial distinction should be made as to the nature of the sleep issue(s). If a child/adolescent presents with unhealthy sleep patterns, such as insufficient sleep, inconsistent sleep patterns, and/or excessive screen time use, an intervention that seeks to promote the adoption of health behaviors conducive to good sleep may offer providers a relatively modifiable target to reduce the emotional and behavioral problems of youth. Simple behavioral sleep recommendations could include limiting screen time, large meals, and physical activity undertaken in the final hour before bed; keeping a consistent bedtime routine and sleep schedule; avoiding caffeine; and using the bed only for sleep.[67]

Second, if a clinical sleep disorder is suspected, it is important to take a detailed clinical history and use objective sleep measures as recommended in the International Classification of Sleep Disorders (ICSD-3).[68] This is essential to obtain an accurate diagnosis for 1 or more concomitant sleep disorders that might be comorbid with ADHD.

Third, the treatment must be selected based on the identified sleep disorder(s). For children with ADHD and SDB, surgical removal of the adenoids or tonsils is a first-line treatment.[69,70] For individuals with ADHD and RLS, behavioral interventions could include modifying the sleep environment; and treatment with iron supplementation (eg, ferrous sulfate) or gabapentin could be considered.[71,72] For individuals with ADHD and DSPS, treatment with light therapy,[73] chronotherapy,[74] and the use of timed melatonin treatment could be helpful.[75] Treatment for individuals with ADHD and insomnia will vary according to the age group, and a clear distinction must be made between insomnia and DSPS, as their treatments will differ. For children with ADHD and insomnia, behavioral treatments, such as positive reinforcement, scheduled awakenings, unmodified extinction, and faded bedtime could be starting options.[76] For adolescents with ADHD and insomnia, recent studies have demonstrated that cognitive behavioral therapy for insomnia should be considered as the first line of treatment.[77–79] For individuals with ADHD and narcolepsy, treatment with modafinil, sodium oxybate, or psychostimulants is indicated, and this treatment can be supplemented with education on sleep hygiene.[80]

## LIMITATIONS AND FUTURE RESEARCH DIRECTIONS

Clear evidence has been found for significant associations between sleep problems and symptoms of internalizing and externalizing psychopathology in youth with

ADHD, yet most of the reports have noted the presence of multiple weaknesses. Progress in the field is needed for both conceptualization and methodology.

Conceptually, little is known about the mechanisms underlying the associations between youth sleep and internalizing and externalizing problems. Impaired sleep leads to deficits in EF, which have been consistently associated with internalizing/externalizing problems and poor self-regulation in youth.[46,47,81] Future research is needed to examine if an EF deficit is a common mechanism underlying the associations between sleep and internalizing and externalizing problems in youth with ADHD. A growing body of evidence indicates that individuals with ADHD are likely prone to having an evening chronotype and disturbed circadian mechanisms.[82] Individuals with evening preferences have been shown to be more likely to present behavioral problems and psychopathology.[83] Therefore, it is possible that circadian abnormality underlies the associations between sleep disturbances and internalizing/externalizing behavior problems. Each of these possibilities is a fruitful avenue for investigations into mechanisms that might underlie the associations between sleep, internalizing or externalizing problem behaviors, and ADHD.

Multiple methodological weaknesses limit the contributions of the reviewed studies. First, the utilized measures provided limited information about the aspects of sleep that are specifically associated with externalizing or internalizing symptoms. Some of the studies used a single-item measure of sleep problems, and thus were not specific in identifying the particular sleep behaviors that contributed most to the manifestation of internalizing or externalizing symptoms. Most of the other studies used scales that were general and lumped multiple observed symptoms of sleep disturbances. Therefore, it is not known which aspects of sleep (ie, duration, continuity, timing, or consistency) cause or contribute to behavioral problems. This limits our ability to identify what aspect(s) of sleep could be associated with daytime symptoms and renders it impossible to generate specific clinical recommendations pertaining to the sleep dimensions likely to have the most clinical impact.

A second methodological limitation is the common sole use of parent-report measures to determine youth sleep problems in preschool and school-age children. This method of subjective report is prone to bias and does not allow for a complete understanding of sleep functioning. In addition, the studies did not include other relevant domains, such as circadian preferences (chronotype), even though such domains are known to have relationships with youth self-regulation abilities.[84] Future studies would benefit from using both subjective and objective sleep measures to better understand the relationships among distinct sleep-related domains and determine where intervention efforts would best be placed. For example, actigraphy can capture actual behavioral sleep patterns, and questionnaires about chronotype can reveal behavioral preferences for sleep. In addition, future research would benefit from obtaining both parent and youth reports of these domains and using objective measurements of behavior.

A third limitation is the heterogeneity of the study designs. Some excluded participants with comorbidities, some included these individuals to better reflect clinical practice and improve generalizability, and others did not report or control for these participants. Control of medication use, particularly psychostimulants, was also inconsistent. Future studies should investigate whether implementing a sleep problem intervention can decrease the occurrence of both externalizing and internalizing difficulties. Studies seeking to further elucidate the longitudinal and bidirectional associations between sleep and internalizing and externalizing difficulties examined at multiple time points over regular intervals and using consistent measures will inform the focus and timing of intervention efforts. Concerning demographic factors, there were significantly lower rates of girls than boys. This is consistent with the idea that ADHD may be less frequently identified in girls than in boys,[85] but the discrepancy could have biased the findings.

Finally, all studies failed to include multiple other factors that are likely to influence sleep and behavior, including parental mental health,[86] physical aspects of the environment, and/or school start time,[87–89] and only a few studies controlled for socioeconomic status. Future research should aim to investigate the longitudinal and likely reciprocal relations among these factors and children's sleep and self-regulatory functioning in both clinical and nonclinical populations.

## CLINICS CARE POINTS

- Conduct a baseline sleep evaluation during the initial assessment of problems to determine habitual sleep duration, identify poor sleep hygiene, and screen for a potential sleep disorder/s
- Include sleep improvement in your treatment plan
- Include sleep health monitoring as part of your ongoing clinical management
- Collaborate with a sleep specialist when conducting assessment or planning treatment of a comorbid sleep disorder
- Assess the extent to which a sleep problem could cause or contribute to daytime behavioral, emotional, or cognitive impairments
- Reassess daytime impairment/s once sleep habits or disorder/s have been treated
- When considering psychotropic medication/s take into consideration potential benefits/adverse effects on sleep and daytime alertness

## DISCLOSURE

Dr. Gruber receives CIHR grant#365284.

## REFERENCES

1. Polanczyk GV, Willcutt EG, Salum GA, et al. ADHD prevalence estimates across three decades: an updated systematic review and meta-regression analysis. Int J Epidemiol 2014;43(2):434–42.
2. American Psychiatric Association. Diagnostic and statistical manual of mental disorders (DSM-5®). Philadelphia: American Psychiatric Association; 2013.
3. Nigg JT, Goldsmith HH, Sachek J. Temperament and attention deficit hyperactivity disorder: the development of a multiple pathway model. J Clin Child Adolesc Psychol 2004;33(1):42–53.
4. Cortese S, Kelly C, Chabernaud C, et al. Toward systems neuroscience of ADHD: a meta-analysis of 55 fMRI studies. Am J Psychiatry 2012;169(10):1038–55.
5. Skirrow C, Asherson P. Emotional lability, comorbidity and impairment in adults with attention-deficit hyperactivity disorder. J Affect Disord 2013;147(1–3):80–6.
6. Graziano PA, Garcia A. Attention-deficit hyperactivity disorder and children's emotion dysregulation: a meta-analysis. Clin Psychol Rev 2016;46:106–23.
7. Martel MM. Research review: a new perspective on attention-deficit/hyperactivity disorder: emotion dysregulation and trait models. J Child Psychol Psychiatry 2009;50(9):1042–51.
8. Ramsay JR, Rostain AL. Adult ADHD research: current status and future directions. J Atten Disord 2008;11(6):624–7.

9. Yoon SY, Jain U, Shapiro C. Sleep in attention-deficit/hyperactivity disorder in children and adults: past, present, and future. Sleep Med Rev 2012;16(4): 371–88.
10. Sung V, Hiscock H, Sciberras E, et al. Sleep problems in children with attention-deficit/hyperactivity disorder: prevalence and the effect on the child and family. Arch Pediatr Adolesc Med 2008;162(4):336–42.
11. Kirov R, Kinkelbur J, Banaschewski T, et al. Sleep patterns in children with attention-deficit/hyperactivity disorder, tic disorder, and comorbidity. J Child Psychol Psychiatry 2007;48(6):561–70.
12. Kirov R, Brand S, Kolev V, et al. The sleeping brain and the neural basis of emotions. Behav Brain Sci 2012;35(3):155–6.
13. Gruber R. Sleep characteristics of children and adolescents with attention deficit-hyperactivity disorder. Child Adolesc Psychiatr Clin N Am 2009;18(4):863–76.
14. Gruber R, Wiebe S, Montecalvo L, et al. Impact of sleep restriction on neurobehavioral functioning of children with attention deficit hyperactivity disorder. Sleep 2011;34(3):315–23.
15. Konofal E, Lecendreux M, Cortese S. Sleep and ADHD. Sleep Med 2010;11(7): 652–8.
16. Cortese S, Brown TE, Corkum P, et al. Assessment and management of sleep problems in youths with attention-deficit/hyperactivity disorder. J Am Acad Child Adolesc Psychiatry 2013;52(8):784–96.
17. Owens J, Gruber R, Brown T, et al. Future research directions in sleep and ADHD: report of a consensus working group. J Atten Disord 2013;17(7):550–64.
18. Quach J, Hiscock H, Wake M. Sleep problems and mental health in primary school new entrants: cross-sectional community-based study. J Paediatr Child Health 2012;48(12):1076–81.
19. Becker SP, Lienesch JA. Nighttime media use in adolescents with ADHD: links to sleep problems and internalizing symptoms. Sleep Med 2018;51:171–8.
20. Bourchtein E, Langberg JM, Cusick CN, et al. Featured article: technology use and sleep in adolescents with and without attention-deficit/hyperactivity disorder. J Pediatr Psychol 2019;44(5):517–26.
21. Engelhardt CR, Mazurek MO, Sohl K. Media use and sleep among boys with autism spectrum disorder, ADHD, or typical development. Pediatrics 2013; 132(6):1081–9.
22. Owens JA, Spirito A, McGuinn M, et al. Sleep habits and sleep disturbance in elementary school-aged children. J Dev Behav Pediatr 2000;21(1):27–36.
23. Ball JD, Tiernan M, Janusz J, et al. Sleep patterns among children with attention-deficit hyperactivity disorder: a reexamination of parent perceptions. J Pediatr Psychol 1997;22(3):389–98.
24. Golan N, Shahar E, Ravid S, et al. Sleep disorders and daytime sleepiness in children with attention-deficit/hyperactive disorder. Sleep 2004;27(2):261–6.
25. Gamble KL, May RS, Besing RC, et al. Delayed sleep timing and symptoms in adults with attention-deficit/hyperactivity disorder: a controlled actigraphy study. Chronobiol Int 2013;30(4):598–606.
26. O'Brien LM, Holbrook CR, Mervis CB, et al. Sleep and neurobehavioral characteristics of 5- to 7-year-old children with parentally reported symptoms of attention-deficit/hyperactivity disorder. Pediatrics 2003;111(3):554–63.
27. Vélez-Galarraga R, Guillén-Grima F, Crespo-Eguílaz N, et al. Prevalence of sleep disorders and their relationship with core symptoms of inattention and hyperactivity in children with attention-deficit/hyperactivity disorder. Eur J Paediatr Neurol 2016;20(6):925–37.

28. Moreau V, Rouleau N, Morin CM. Sleep of children with attention deficit hyperactivity disorder: actigraphic and parental reports. Behav Sleep Med 2014;12(1): 69–83.

29. Wynchank D, Ten Have M, Bijlenga D, et al. The association between insomnia and sleep duration in adults with attention-deficit hyperactivity disorder: results from a general population study. J Clin Sleep Med 2018;14(3):349–57.

30. Rocca FL, Finotti E, Pizza F, et al. Psychosocial profile and quality of life in children with type 1 narcolepsy: a case-control study. Sleep 2016;39(7):1389–98.

31. Rubia K. Cognitive neuroscience of attention deficit hyperactivity disorder (ADHD) and its clinical translation. Front Hum Neurosci 2018;12:100.

32. Shao Y, Wang L, Ye E, et al. Decreased thalamocortical functional connectivity after 36 hours of total sleep deprivation: evidence from resting state FMRI. PLoS One 2013;8(10):e78830.

33. Tomasi D, Wang RL, Telang F, et al. Impairment of attentional networks after 1 night of sleep deprivation. Cereb Cortex 2009;19(1):233–40.

34. Chee MW, Chuah LY, Venkatraman V, et al. Functional imaging of working memory following normal sleep and after 24 and 35 h of sleep deprivation: correlations of fronto-parietal activation with performance. Neuroimage 2006;31(1):419–28.

35. Chee MW, Chuah YM. Functional neuroimaging and behavioral correlates of capacity decline in visual short-term memory after sleep deprivation. Proc Natl Acad Sci U S A 2007;104(22):9487–92.

36. Turnbull K, Reid GJ, Morton JB. Behavioral sleep problems and their potential impact on developing executive function in children. Sleep 2013;36(7):1077–84.

37. Bernier A, Carlson SM, Bordeleau S, et al. Relations between physiological and cognitive regulatory systems: infant sleep regulation and subsequent executive functioning. Child Dev 2010;81(6):1739–52.

38. Jan JE, Reiter RJ, Bax MC, et al. Long-term sleep disturbances in children: a cause of neuronal loss. Eur J Paediatr Neurol 2010;14(5):380–90.

39. Shao Y, Lei Y, Wang L, et al. Altered resting-state amygdala functional connectivity after 36 hours of total sleep deprivation. PLoS One 2014;9(11):e112222.

40. Yoo SS, Gujar N, Hu P, et al. The human emotional brain without sleep—a prefrontal amygdala disconnect. Curr Biol 2007;17(20):R877–8.

41. Sotres-Bayon F, Bush DE, LeDoux JE. Emotional perseveration: an update on prefrontal-amygdala interactions in fear extinction. Learn Mem 2004;11(5): 525–35.

42. Lawson RA, Papadakis AA, Higginson CI, et al. Everyday executive function impairments predict comorbid psychopathology in autism spectrum and attention deficit hyperactivity disorders. Neuropsychology 2015;29(3):445–53.

43. Connor DF, Ford JD. Comorbid symptom severity in attention-deficit/hyperactivity disorder: a clinical study. J Clin Psychiatry 2012;73(5):711–7.

44. Hansen BH, Skirbekk B, Oerbeck B, et al. Associations between sleep problems and attentional and behavioral functioning in children with anxiety disorders and ADHD. Behav Sleep Med 2014;12(1):53–68.

45. Rubens SL, Evans SC, Becker SP, et al. Self-reported time in bed and sleep quality in association with internalizing and externalizing symptoms in school-age youth. Child Psychiatry Hum Dev 2017;48(3):455–67.

46. Becker SP, Langberg JM, Evans SW. Sleep problems predict comorbid externalizing behaviors and depression in young adolescents with attention-deficit/hyperactivity disorder. Eur Child Adolesc Psychiatry 2015;24(8):897–907.

47. Quach JL, Nguyen CD, Williams KE, et al. Bidirectional associations between child sleep problems and internalizing and externalizing difficulties from preschool to early adolescence. JAMA Pediatr 2018;172(2):e174363.

48. Kang NR, Kwack YS. Temperament and character profiles associated with internalizing and externalizing problems in children with attention deficit hyperactivity disorder. Psychiatry Investig 2019;16(3):206–12.

49. Jafari B, Mohsenin V. Polysomnography. Clin Chest Med 2010;31(2):287–97.

50. Morgenthaler T, Alessi C, Friedman L, et al. Practice parameters for the use of actigraphy in the assessment of sleep and sleep disorders: an update for 2007. Sleep 2007;30(4):519–29.

51. Marino M, Li Y, Rueschman MN, et al. Measuring sleep: accuracy, sensitivity, and specificity of wrist actigraphy compared to polysomnography. Sleep 2013;36(11): 1747–55.

52. Sadeh A. The role and validity of actigraphy in sleep medicine: an update. Sleep Med Rev 2011;15(4):259–67.

53. Coto J, Garcia A, Hart KC, et al. Associations between disruptive behavior problems, parenting factors, and sleep problems among young children. J Dev Behav Pediatr 2018;39(8):610–20.

54. Virring A, Lambek R, Jennum PJ, et al. Sleep problems and daily functioning in children with ADHD: an investigation of the role of impairment, ADHD presentations, and psychiatric comorbidity. J Atten Disord 2017;21(9):731–40.

55. Waxmonsky JG, Mayes SD, Calhoun SL, et al. The association between disruptive mood dysregulation disorder symptoms and sleep problems in children with and without ADHD. Sleep Med 2017;37:180–6.

56. Mulraney M, Giallo R, Lycett K, et al. The bidirectional relationship between sleep problems and internalizing and externalizing problems in children with ADHD: a prospective cohort study. Sleep Med 2016;17:45–51.

57. Lycett K, Sciberras E, Hiscock H, et al. Sleep problem trajectories and well-being in children with attention-deficit hyperactivity disorder: a prospective cohort study. J Dev Behav Pediatr 2016;37(5):405–14.

58. Becker SP, Epstein JN, Tamm L, et al. Shortened sleep duration causes sleepiness, inattention, and oppositionality in adolescents with attention-deficit/ hyperactivity disorder: findings from a crossover sleep restriction/extension study. J Am Acad Child Adolesc Psychiatry 2019;58(4):433–42.

59. Mulraney M, Zendarski N, Mensah F, et al. Do early internalizing and externalizing problems predict later irritability in adolescents with attention-deficit/hyperactivity disorder? Aust N Z J Psychiatry 2017;51(4):393–402.

60. Bar M, Efron M, Gothelf D, et al. The link between parent and child sleep disturbances in children with attention deficit/hyperactivity disorder. Sleep Med 2016; 21:160–4.

61. Becker SP, Pfiffner LJ, Stein MA, et al. Sleep habits in children with attention-deficit/hyperactivity disorder predominantly inattentive type and associations with comorbid psychopathology symptoms. Sleep Med 2016;21:151–9.

62. Becker SP, Tamm L, Epstein JN, et al. Impact of sleep restriction on affective functioning in adolescents with attention-deficit/hyperactivity disorder. J Child Psychol Psychiatry 2020. https://doi.org/10.1111/jcpp.13235.

63. Balazs J, Kereszteny A. Attention-deficit/hyperactivity disorder and suicide: a systematic review. World J Psychiatry 2017;7(1):44–59.

64. Daviss WB. A review of co-morbid depression in pediatric ADHD: etiology, phenomenology, and treatment. J Child Adolesc Psychopharmacol 2008;18(6): 565–71.

65. Ranum BM, Wichstrøm L, Pallesen S, et al. Association between objectively measured sleep duration and symptoms of psychiatric disorders in middle childhood. JAMA Netw Open 2019;2(12):e1918281.

66. Gruber R, Carrey N, Weiss SK, et al. Position statement on pediatric sleep for psychiatrists. J Can Acad Child Adolesc Psychiatry 2014;23(3):174–95.

67. Hale L, Kirschen GW, LeBourgeois MK, et al. Youth screen media habits and sleep: sleep-friendly screen behavior recommendations for clinicians, educators, and parents. Child Adolesc Psychiatr Clin N Am 2018;27(2):229–45.

68. Kjeldsen JS, Hjorth MF, Andersen R, et al. Short sleep duration and large variability in sleep duration are independently associated with dietary risk factors for obesity in Danish school children. Int J Obes 2014;38(1):32–9.

69. Marcus CL, Brooks LJ, Draper KA, et al. Diagnosis and management of childhood obstructive sleep apnea syndrome. Pediatrics 2012;130(3):e714–55.

70. Kaditis AG, Alonso Alvarez ML, Boudewyns A, et al. Obstructive sleep disordered breathing in 2- to 18-year-old children: diagnosis and management. Eur Respir J 2016;47(1):69–94.

71. Mohri I, Kato-Nishimura K, Kagitani-Shimono K, et al. Evaluation of oral iron treatment in pediatric restless legs syndrome (RLS). Sleep Med 2012;13(4):429–32.

72. Garcia-Borreguero D, Larrosa O, de la Llave Y, et al. Treatment of restless legs syndrome with gabapentin: a double-blind, cross-over study. Neurology 2002; 59(10):1573–9.

73. Lack L, Wright H, Kemp K, et al. The treatment of early-morning awakening insomnia with 2 evenings of bright light. Sleep 2005;28(5):616–23.

74. Weitzman ED, Czeisler CA, Coleman RM, et al. Delayed sleep phase syndrome. A chronobiological disorder with sleep-onset insomnia. Arch Gen Psychiatry 1981;38(7):737–46.

75. Auger RR, Burgess HJ, Emens JS, et al. Clinical practice guideline for the treatment of intrinsic circadian rhythm sleep-wake disorders: advanced sleep-wake phase disorder (ASWPD), delayed sleep-wake phase disorder (DSWPD), non-24-hour sleep-wake rhythm disorder (N24SWD), and irregular sleep-wake rhythm disorder (ISWRD). An update for 2015: an American Academy of Sleep Medicine Clinical practice guideline. J Clin Sleep Med 2015;11(10):1199–236.

76. Morgenthaler TI, Owens J, Alessi C, et al. Practice parameters for behavioral treatment of bedtime problems and night wakings in infants and young children. Sleep 2006;29(10):1277–81.

77. de Bruin EJ, Bögels SM, Oort FJ, et al. Improvements of adolescent psychopathology after insomnia treatment: results from a randomized controlled trial over 1 year. J Child Psychol Psychiatry 2018;59(5):509–22.

78. de Bruin EJ, Bögels SM, Oort FJ, et al. Efficacy of cognitive behavioral therapy for insomnia in adolescents: a randomized controlled trial with internet therapy, group therapy and a waiting list condition. Sleep 2015;38(12):1913–26.

79. Gradisar M, Dohnt H, Gardner G, et al. A randomized controlled trial of cognitive-behavior therapy plus bright light therapy for adolescent delayed sleep phase disorder. Sleep 2011;34(12):1671–80.

80. Wise MS, Arand DL, Auger RR, et al. Treatment of narcolepsy and other hypersomnias of central origin. Sleep 2007;30(12):1712–27.

81. van Stralen J. Emotional dysregulation in children with attention-deficit/hyperactivity disorder. Atten Defic Hyperact Disord 2016;8(4):175–87.

82. Carpena MX, Hutz MH, Salatino-Oliveira A, et al. CLOCK polymorphisms in attention-deficit/hyperactivity disorder (ADHD): further evidence linking sleep and circadian disturbances and ADHD. Genes (Basel) 2019;10(2):88.

83. Li SX, Chan NY, Man Yu MW, et al. Eveningness chronotype, insomnia symptoms, and emotional and behavioural problems in adolescents. Sleep Med 2018; 47:93–9.
84. Curtis J, Burkley E, Burkley M. The rhythm is gonna get you: the influence of circadian rhythm synchrony on self-control outcomes. Soc Personal Psychol Compass 2014;8(11):609–25.
85. Rucklidge JJ. Gender differences in ADHD: implications for psychosocial treatments. Expert Rev Neurother 2008;8(4):643–55.
86. El-Sheikh M, Kelly RJ, Bagley EJ, et al. Parental depressive symptoms and children's sleep: the role of family conflict. J Child Psychol Psychiatry 2012;53(7): 806–14.
87. Johnson DA, Billings ME, Hale L. Environmental determinants of insufficient sleep and sleep disorders: implications for population health. Curr Epidemiol Rep 2018; 5(2):61–9.
88. Adolescent Sleep Working Group; Committee on Adolescence; Council on School Health. School start times for adolescents. Pediatrics 2014;134(3):642–9.
89. Owens J, Troxel W, Wahlstrom K. Commentary on healthy school start times. J Clin Sleep Med 2017;13(5):761.

# Autism Spectrum Disorder and Sleep

Kyle P. Johnson, MD*, Paria Zarrinnegar, MD

## KEYWORDS

- Autism • Sleep • Melatonin • Behavioral • Insomnia • Pediatric • Children

## KEY POINTS

- Children with autism spectrum disorder (ASD) frequently have sleep problems, most commonly insomnia.
- Sleep problems suffered by children with ASD are associated with daytime struggles.
- Parental education and behavioral interventions are effective in ameliorating the insomnia experienced by children with ASD.
- There is growing evidence that melatonin is an effective treatment of the insomnia suffered by children with ASD.

## INTRODUCTION

Autism spectrum disorder (ASD) is a neurodevelopmental disability defined by developmental deficits in 2 domains: social interaction and communication; repetitive, restricted patterns of interests, behavior, or activities (American Psychiatric Association's The Diagnostic and Statistical Manual of Mental Disorders Fifth Edition).[1] The estimated prevalence rate of ASD in the United States is now estimated to range from 1 in 59 to 1 in 40, reflecting more than a double of prevalence between 2000 to 2002 and 2010 to 2012.[2,3] ASD is thought to result from altered early brain development and circuitry formation influenced by genetics and the prenatal environment.[4,5] The disorder can be associated with genetic conditions such as Angelman syndrome, intellectual disability, and other neuropsychiatric disorders, including epilepsy, mood disorders, anxiety disorders, and attention-deficit/hyperactivity disorder (ADHD). In approximately 20% to 30% of children, ASD becomes apparent after previously acquired skills are lost, a phenomenon known as "autistic regression."[6] The cause of early developmental regression remains unclear, with recent research

This article originally appeared in *Child and Adolescent Psychiatric Clinics*, Volume 30 Issue 1, January 2021.

Division of Child & Adolescent Psychiatry, Oregon Health & Science University, Mailcode: DC-7P, 3181 Southwest Sam Jackson Park Road, Portland, OR 97239, USA

* Corresponding author.

*E-mail address:* johnsoky@ohsu.edu

Psychiatr Clin N Am 47 (2024) 199–212
https://doi.org/10.1016/j.psc.2023.06.013

focusing on genetic and immunologic causes.[7] The brain regions and neurotransmitter systems thought to be involved in the development of ASD also regulate sleep and wake.[8] Sleep disturbances are one of the biggest challenges faced by youth with ASD and often by extension, the family members taking care of them. Approximately 50% to 80% of children and adolescents diagnosed with ASD suffer sleep problems.[9–14] The most common sleep problems experienced by this population include struggles initiating and maintaining sleep, frequent and often prolonged night awakenings, early morning waking, and irregular-sleep wake schedules.[15] Problems initiating and maintaining sleep rank as one the most common concurrent clinical disorders and are less likely to diminish with age compared with peers who do not have ASD.[16,17]

## SUBJECTIVE AND OBJECTIVE FEATURES OF SLEEP PROBLEMS IN CHILDREN AND ADOLESCENTS WITH AUTISM SPECTRUM DISORDER

The high rates of sleep disturbances experienced by children with ASD initially documented in relatively small studies have been confirmed in larger studies. Malow and colleagues[18] investigated the prevalence of sleep difficulties in 1518 children aged 4 to 10 years diagnosed with ASD and enrolled in the Autism Speaks Autism Treatment Network Registry. The investigators found that 71% of the children experienced sleep disturbances although only 30% had been diagnosed with a sleep disorder. Another large study demonstrated that sleep problems that develop in early childhood often persist into adolescence although the types of sleep problems typically change with age.[19] In this study of parent-reported sleep disturbances, the younger children experienced bedtime resistance, frequent awakenings, parasomnias, and sleep anxiety, whereas the adolescents struggled with sleep onset insomnia, short sleep duration, and daytime sleepiness.

Objectively, compared with neurotypical subjects, individuals with ASD have abnormal sleep architecture as measured by polysomnography (PSG). Anomalies observed include prolonged sleep latency, reduced total sleep time, lower sleep efficiency, reductions in both rapid eye movement (REM) sleep and non-REM sleep, and a lower number of REMs during REM density.[20–22] A more recent study demonstrates that even children with ASD not complaining of sleep problems experience poor objective sleep.[23] Children with ASD who experienced regression with loss of previously acquired abilities experienced more severe alterations than those with nonregressed ASD.[24]

## NEUROBIOLOGY OF AUTISM SPECTRUM DISORDER AND SLEEP

The neurobiological factors implicated in ASD and regulating sleep and wake overlap. This intersection involves the neurotransmitters gamma-aminobutyric acid (GABA) and serotonin as well as the neurohormone melatonin. Moreover, the disrupted sleep architecture noted in individuals with ASD suggests neurobiological anomalies.

GABA, a central nervous system inhibitory neurotransmitter, is involved in a sleep-promoting system with projections from the hypothalamus to the brainstem. GABA inhibits brainstem neurons active in arousal, which in turn facilitates sleep. Children with ASD show a disruption of GABA interneurons with some demonstrating a mutation in chromosome 15q, which contains GABA genes.[25,26] The identification of an autism-susceptibility region carrying GABA-related genes suggests that altered gene expression in this region could interfere in the inhibitory function of GABA resulting in hyperarousal and insomnia.[8]

Serotonin is a wake-promoting neurotransmitter, which also inhibits REM sleep. Elevated whole blood serotonin was the first biomarker identified in patients with

ASD. Hyperserotonemia is present in more than 25% of children with ASD and often their first-degree relatives.[27,28] ASD studies have also demonstrated genetic variations related to serotonin transport and degradation.[29,30] Abnormal serotonin function may negatively affect sleep through effects on melatonin.

Melatonin is a hormone produced by the pineal gland and is critical in regulating sleep-wake schedules. It is suppressed by bright light and released in response to darkness. Melatonin is synthesized from serotonin by means of the enzyme acetylserotonin O-methyltransferase (ASMT).

Melke and colleagues have postulated that melatonin may influence the synaptic plasticity contributing to the ASD phenotype (2008); this is intriguing in light of the evidence of abnormal melatonin regulation in ASD. Several early studies found lower levels of melatonin in children with ASD compared with controls but recent studies have not found such abnormalities.[31–35] Variations in melatonin have been observed in parents of children with ASD.[36,37] Given low to normal levels of melatonin in individuals with ASD despite elevated blood serotonin, the precursor to melatonin, attention has turned to the gene involved in ASMT production. In fact, polymorphisms in the ASMT gene are associated with low melatonin levels in subjects with ASD and autistic-like traits in a general population.[36,38] Genetic variation in ASMT and another melatonin pathway enzyme, cytochrome P450 1A2 (CYP1A2), were identified in individuals with ASD and comorbid sleep onset delay.[39] Differences in sleep architecture measured by PSG provide further evidence of biological roots to many of the sleep problems experienced by individuals with ASD.[15]

## IMPACT OF SLEEP DISORDERS ON DAYTIME BEHAVIOR AND PARENTAL STRESS

It is now clear that poor sleep in children with ASD is associated with problematic daytime behavior. Children with ASD and poor sleep quality experience higher rates of aggression, self-injury, anxiety, hyperactivity, and inattention.[40–43] In addition, core symptoms of ASD such as repetitive behaviors and difficulty in social reciprocity are increased in poorly sleeping children with ASD.[44,45] Greater variation in sleep duration and timing have been found to predict subsequent disruptive, daytime behavior.[46] In another study, sleep disturbances at baseline predicted the later development of significant anxiety.[47] Sleep disturbances in children with ASD increase parenting burden and family stress, often directly affecting the parent's own sleep.[48,49] Addressing sleep problems in children with ASD may improve not only the child's daytime behavior but also parental functioning.

## ASSESSMENT

Given the high rate of sleep problems, all youth with ASD should be screened for sleep disturbances by incorporating sleep questionnaires in the assessment process. The Modified Simonds and Parraga Sleep Questionnaire and the Children's Sleep Habits Questionnaire have been validated for youth with ASD.[50] A newer clinician-rated tool, the Pediatric Sleep Clinical Global Impressions Scale, shows promise in measuring insomnia and response to treatment in ASD.[51] It is critical that the questionnaire used screen for obstructive sleep apnea (OSA). If symptoms and signs of OSA are discovered, the youth should be referred to a sleep specialist, as an overnight PSG may be indicated. Although ASD in and of itself is not a risk factor for OSA, some children with ASD have other risk factors such as obesity, hypertrophy of the adenoids and tonsils, or craniofacial abnormalities. If restless legs syndrome (RLS) or excessive movements while asleep are suspected, one should consider referral to a sleep specialist while assessing for iron deficiency, given the association between this condition and RLS (see DelRosso and colleagues' article, "Restless Legs Syndrome in Children and Adolescents," in this issue). Unusual behaviors that suggest a parasomnia such as sleep terrors or sleepwalking may also warrant a referral to a sleep specialist, particularly if the behavior is potentially dangerous to the child or disturbs the sleep of family members. Nocturnal seizures must be considered when a child with ASD engages in unusual behavior when asleep given the increased risk of epilepsy in ASD.

Insomnia will be the identified sleep problem in most of the cases. The clinician must obtain a complete history regarding the sleep environment, what occurs at sleep onset, and what family and child behaviors are engaged in after sustained, middle-of-the-night awakenings. This is necessary because insomnia is so often behavioral in origin even in ASD. Although the PSG is considered the gold standard for assessing sleep, it is not indicated when assessing uncomplicated insomnia. Sleep diaries and actigraphy are useful for this purpose.

A PSG is indicated when assessing for OSA, narcolepsy, and parasomnias not improving with supportive care. The assessment of narcolepsy requires a multiple sleep latency test following a PSG. However, these procedures are often difficult for children with ASD to tolerate, given their tactile sensitivity and anxiety in unfamiliar situations.

## TREATMENT

The treatment of sleep problems experienced by youth with ASD is multidimensional given the multitude of causative factors at play. Environmental and behavioral causes are particularly relevant to insomnia. Several environmental challenges negatively affect the sleep of any child, not just those with ASD, whereas others are more specific to youth with ASD, including intrinsic factors, common comorbid psychiatric and medical conditions, and side effects of medicines used to treat problematic daytime behaviors. As demonstrated in a recent systematic review and meta-analysis, evidence-based, behavioral interventions are feasible and efficacious in ASD.[52]

### Behavioral Interventions

Parent education in behavioral treatments is the first-line approach to improving the insomnia so commonly experienced by children and adolescents diagnosed with ASD.[53] The behavioral interventions to treat insomnia in children with ASD are essentially the same as those used to treat other children (**Table 1**). The techniques aim to correct problematic behaviors and promote good sleep habits. Positive bedtime routines and graduated extinction have been particularly helpful in combating tantrums associated with bedtime and night awakenings in young children with ASD.[54] Evidence from case series reveals that sleep restriction with bedtime fading (making bedtime gradually earlier as sleep consolidation improves) is also a powerful intervention.[55] A visual schedule of the bedtime routine is helpful for many children (**Fig. 1**).

Significant benefit comes from educating parents regarding sleep and instructing them how to institute behavioral interventions at home. Such parent training is effective whether provided in a group format or workshop.[56,57] Several randomized-controlled trials demonstrate the efficacy of parent training in ASD.[58,59] A recent systematic review of 11 studies using behavioral sleep interventions to treat sleep problems experienced by individuals with ASD and/or intellectual disability found trainings acceptable by parents who judged them to be beneficial.[60] An advantage of this model is the individualization of treatment, because parents can pick and choose which interventions may be most effective for their child and feasible in their home.

**Table 1**
Behavioral interventions to treat insomnia in children with autism spectrum disorder

| Behavioral Intervention | Brief Description of the Intervention | Areas of Impact; Special Considerations |
|---|---|---|
| Parent education | Teaching parents the basics of childhood sleep, sleep hygiene, how to establish consistent and sleep-inducing bedtime, and how to implement behavioral interventions | Sleep latency, child and family functioning; individual, group, or workshop format |
| Positive bedtime routines | Implementation of consistent series of activities that help the child with transition to sleep (ie, clean up toys, brush teeth, go potty, put pajamas on, read books, get in bed, lights off) | Bedtime difficulties, settling problems; usually combined with other techniques |
| Extinction (planned ignoring) | *Standard* withholding rewards (such as TV) and ignoring sleep-disruptive behavior<br>*Graduated* gradually increasing the time before the child is attended | Settling problems; "extinction burst," a temporary increase in target behaviors, is common with standard extinction |
| Gradual distancing (stimulus fading) | Parent gradually increases the distance to the child | Settling problems, night waking |
| Sleep restriction | Reducing total sleep time to 90% of average night-time sleep while keeping a consistent schedule. Once behaviors improve, fade back total amount of sleep to age-appropriate level | Bedtime disturbance, night waking |
| Bedtime fading | Bedtime is moved to 30 min after average sleep time at baseline. If a child falls asleep within 15–20 min of this new bedtime for 2 consecutive nights, bedtime is moved to 30 min earlier (fading). If the child does not initiate sleep within that interval, the bedtime is moved to 15 min later the subsequent night. | Bedtime disturbances and long sleep latency; can be combined with response cost (remove the child from bed if not falling asleep within the interval, keep them awake for a specified time and then return them to bed) and positive reinforcement |
| Scheduled awakening | Parents wake up the child 30 min before the time he/she usually awakens spontaneously | Night waking and night terrors |
| Chronotherapy | Moving bedtime and rise time later and later each day until the child is sleeping on a normal schedule | Circadian rhythm sleep-wake disorder (delayed phase type) |

(continued on next page)

**Table 1**
*(continued)*

| Behavioral Intervention | Brief Description of the Intervention | Areas of Impact; Special Considerations |
|---|---|---|
| Bed pass | The child is given a special card good for one free trip out of their room each night or one visit from a parent. Keep the bedtime consistent but making sure the pass is close at hand. When the child uses the pass, the card is surrendered for the rest of the night and if they leave the room again that night, they are walked back to their room with no words or attention. The child can trade unused passes for a reward at the end of the week. | Night waking; useful for verbal and higher functioning patients |

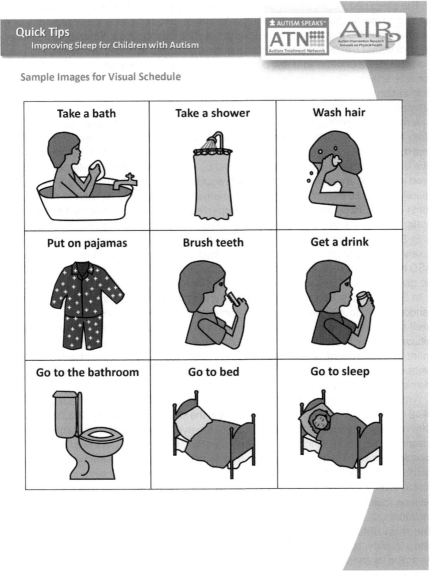

**Fig. 1.** Sample images for visual schedule. (*Courtesy of* Autism Treatment Network.)

## *Pharmacologic Interventions*

In youth with ASD experiencing sleep disturbances, pharmacologic agents are often prescribed, especially when behavioral interventions have been ineffective. Medications are used to treat sleep initiation and/or maintenance insomnia resulting in longer sleep duration even though there are no Food and Drug Administration (FDA)-approved medicines for this indication in children and adolescents.[61,62] In the Autism Speaks Treatment Network Registry, medications for sleep were prescribed to 46% of 4- to 10-year-old children given a sleep diagnosis; melatonin was the most commonly used followed by alpha-agonists such as clonidine.[18]

The sleep disturbance must be well defined with potential causes considered before turning to medication treatment. This information and the presence or absence of co-morbid conditions will inform the choice of medication used. Whenever possible, a medicine that treats the sleep disturbance while also improving the coexisting condition should be chosen with low doses initiated and titrated gradually while monitoring for side effects. This "start low and go slow" approach is important because children with autism are often sensitive to medications and have limited ability to communicate adverse effects.

A recent systematic review of pharmacologic treatments of sleep disorders in children found the evidence limited primarily to melatonin with little randomized control trial data for other drugs.[63] There is now considerable evidence that melatonin is effective in treating the insomnia often suffered by children with ASD. Melatonin is considered a nutritional supplement and is not regulated by the FDA. As a result, melatonin is readily available over the counter and relatively inexpensive. Related to sleep, melatonin has hypnotic and chronobiotic properties. When used solely as a chronobiotic, melatonin should be dosed 2 to 3 hours before the dim light melatonin onset or roughly 4 to 5 hours before habitual sleep onset time. Practically, melatonin is rarely used solely as a chronobiotic, especially for ASD. Instead, clinical trials of melatonin in ASD have dosed melatonin close to bedtime. Typically, melatonin is used as a hypnotic given about 30 to 45 minutes before desired sleep onset time.

In 2011, Rossignol and Frye published a systematic review and meta-analysis of 5 randomized, double-blind, placebo-controlled, crossover trials using melatonin to treat the insomnia experienced by children with ASD. This analysis demonstrated significant improvements in sleep-onset latency and sleep duration with melatonin treatment although night awakenings did not improve.[64] No significant adverse events were reported in these 5 trials. Following this initial evidence of efficacy, several randomized controlled trials (RCTs) have since been completed.

A multisite trial across England and Wales using immediate release melatonin (half-life of 40 minutes) demonstrated improvement in the sleep onset latency of subjects treated with melatonin compared with controls.[65] However, waking times became earlier with melatonin, negating an impact on sleep duration. As a result, the investigators recommended future trials of slow release melatonin. Cortesi and colleagues[66] studied 160 children with ASD, aged 4 to 10 years, struggling with sleep onset and sleep maintenance insomnia, randomly assigning them to 1 of 4 arms: combination of controlled-release melatonin, 3 mg, and cognitive behavioral therapy (CBT); controlled-release melatonin, 3 mg, alone; 4 sessions of CBT alone; or placebo drug treatment alone. The main outcome measures for this 12-week trial included actigraphically derived sleep latency, total sleep time, and number of awakenings, and wake after sleep onset. All active treatment groups improved, and the controlled release melatonin formulation was well tolerated with no adverse effects reported or observed.

A more recent study used pediatric-appropriate, prolonged-release melatonin formulated as easily swallowed, minitablets (PedPRM[67]; a total of 95 subjects completed the 13-week double-blind phase). Doses of PedPRM were from 2 to 5 mg/d. At the completion of 13 weeks, per sleep diaries completed by caregivers, children taking PedPRM slept on average 57.5 minutes longer compared with 9.4 minutes longer sleep in the placebo group ($P = .034$). Sleep latency also improved significantly ($P = .011$) in the PedPRM group (decreased 39.6 minutes on average compared with a decrease of 12.5 minutes in participants treated with placebo). These differences were significant as early as 3 weeks into the controlled trial. Children with and without comorbid ADHD benefited similarly to PedPRM. Headache and somnolence were more commonly reported in the PedPRM group. Daytime externalizing behaviors improved with melatonin treatment as did caregivers' quality of life.[68] Compliance with the minitablet was excellent with no need to dissolve or crush the formulation. This RCT was followed by a 39-week, open-label study in which subjects took either 2 mg, 5 mg, or 10 mg doses of PedPRM.[69] The benefits of PedPRM observed in the RCT persisted, with the most common side effect being fatigue. After 2 years of treatment with PedPRM, no detrimental effects on children's growth or pubertal development was found, and the medicine was able to be discontinued without safety or withdrawal issues.[70]

Given these recent studies, melatonin is now considered a first-line treatment when a pharmacologic agent is deemed necessary. Melatonin is effective in improving insomnia and is well tolerated with limited side effects.

Although minimal data support their use, medicines beyond melatonin may be considered in the treatment of insomnia, particularly when safety is an issue. Children with insomnia comorbid with irritability, aggression, or self-injurious behavior may benefit from treatment with second-generation antipsychotics. Risperidone and aripiprazole are FDA approved for treating aggression and severe irritability in children and adolescents with ASD. Dosing these medicines in the evening or at least giving most a twice daily dose at night may treat the insomnia and disruptive daytime behaviors. Insomnia associated with a comorbid anxiety disorder or major depressive disorder may improve with treatment with a serotonin reuptake inhibitor. Alpha-agonists such as clonidine may be an option when there is comorbid ADHD or Tourette syndrome. A recent practical review of this issue suggested sedating antidepressants such as trazodone and mirtazapine as options while noting studies of safety and efficacy are needed.[71]

When patients with ASD have certain sleep disorders beyond insomnia, other medicines are options. Clonazepam and tricyclic antidepressants may be effective treatments of non-REM arousal disorders such as sleep terrors and sleep walking, although their use should be limited to situations where injury is a possibility. REM sleep behavior disorder may also respond to clonazepam. There are no FDA-approved medicines for pediatric RLS but this condition can be treated with dopaminergic agents, gabapentin, or clonidine. Given the association between iron deficiency and RLS, ferritin levels should be determined with iron supplementation prescribed if indicated. See Vijayabharathi Ekambaram and Judith Owens' article, "Medications Used for Pediatric Insomnia," in this issue.

## SUMMARY

Youth diagnosed with ASD experience more sleep problems than their peers whether or not the peers have intellectual developmental disabilities. Although the most common sleep problem experienced by patients with ASD is insomnia, other sleep disturbances can also occur. Given the high prevalence of sleep problems and disorders in this population, all youth with ASD should be screened for sleep problems. Polysomnography is not indicated to assess uncomplicated insomnia but may be indicated when assessing unusual behaviors while sleeping, excessive movements in sleep, symptoms and signs that suggest OSA, and persistent daytime sleepiness. Behavioral treatments including parent training are effective in ASD. There is growing evidence for the utility of melatonin when treating insomnia refractory to behavioral interventions. There are no FDA-approved medicines to treat pediatric insomnia.

## CLINICS CARE POINTS

- Most of the youth diagnosed with ASD experience significant sleep problems.

- Nighttime sleeping difficulties negatively affect daytime behavior and are associated with parental stress.
- All youth diagnosed with ASD should be screened for sleep problems and disorders.
- Behavioral interventions and parent training are the first line of treatment.
- Melatonin is the first-line pharmacologic agent to address insomnia in ASD, as its efficacy has been documented in multiple clinical trials.

## DISCLOSURE

The authors have nothing to disclose.

## REFERENCES

1. American Psychiatric Association. Diagnostic and statistical manual of mental disorders. 5th edition. Washington, DC: American Psychiatric Association; 2013.
2. Baio J, Wiggins L, Christensen DL, et al. Prevalence of autism spectrum disorder among children aged 8 years—autism and developmental disabilities monitoring network, 11 sites, United States, 2014. MMWR Surveill Summ 2018;67(6):1–23.
3. Kogan MD, Vladutiu LA, Schieve LA, et al. The prevalence of parent-reported autism spectrum disorder among US children. Pediatrics 2018;142(6): e20174161.
4. O'Reilly C, Lewis JD, Elsabbagh M. Is functional brain connectivity atypical in autism? A systematic review of EEG and MEG studies. PLoS One 2017; 12(5):1–28.
5. Muhle RA, Reed HE, Stratigos KA, et al. The emerging clinical neuroscience of autism spectrum disorder: a review. JAMA Psychiatry 2018;75(5):514–23.
6. Parr JR, Le Couteur A, Baird G, et al. Early developmental regression in autism spectrum disorder: evidence from an international multiplex sample. J Autism Dev Disord 2011;41:332–40.
7. Scott O, Shi D, Andriashek D, et al. Clinical clues for autoimmunity and neuroin-flammation in patients with autistic regression. Dev Med Child Neurol 2017;59: 947–51.
8. Inui T, Kumagaya S, Myowa-Yamakoshi M. Neurodevelopmental hypothesis about the etiology of autism spectrum disorders. Front Hum Neurosci 2017; 11:354.
9. Polimeni MA, Richdale AL, Francis AJP. A survey of sleep problems in autism, Asperger's disorder and typically developing children. J Intellect Disabil Res 2005; 49(4):260–8.
10. Liu X, Hubbard JA, Fabes RA, et al. Sleep disturbances and correlates of children with autism spectrum disorders. Child Psychiatry Hum Dev 2006;37:179–91.
11. Malow BA, Marzec ML, McGrew SG, et al. Characterizing sleep in children with autism spectrum disorders: a multidimensional approach. Sleep 2006;29(12): 1563–71.
12. Richdale AL, Schreck KA. Sleep problems in autism spectrum disorders: prevalence, nature, & possible biopsychosocial aetiologies. Sleep Med Rev 2009; 13(6):403–11.
13. Fadini CC, Lamonica DA, Fett-Conte AC, et al. Influence of sleep disorders on the behavior of individuals with autism spectrum disorder. Front Hum Neurosci 2015; 9:347.

14. Elrod MG, Nylund CM, Susi AL, et al. Prevalence of diagnosed sleep disorders and related diagnostic and surgical procedures in children with autism spectrum disorders. J Dev Behav Pediatr 2016;37(5):377–84.

15. Buckley AW, Hirtz D, Oskoui M, et al. Practice guideline: treatment for insomnia and disrupted sleep behavior in children and adolescents with autism spectrum disorder. Neurology 2020;94(9):392–404.

16. Ming X, Brimacombe M, Chaaban J, et al. Autism spectrum disorders: concurrent clinical disorders. J Child Neurol 2008;23(1):6–13.

17. Hodge D, Carollo TM, Lewin M, et al. Sleep patterns in children with and without autism spectrum disorders: developmental comparisons. Res Dev Disabil 2014; 35:1631–8.

18. Malow BE, Katz T, Reynolds AM, et al. Sleep difficulties and medications in children with autism spectrum disorders: a registry study. Pediatrics 2016;137: S98–104.

19. Goldman SE, Richdale AL, Clemons T, Malow B A. Parental sleep concerns in autism spectrum disorders: variations from childhood to adolescence. J Autism Dev Disord 2012;42(4):531–8.

20. Lambert A, Tessier S, Chevrier E, et al. Sleep in children with high functioning autism: polysomnography, questionnaires and diaries in a non-complaining sample. Sleep Med 2013;14(suppl 1):e137–8.

21. Miano S, Bruni O, Elia M, et al. Sleep in children with autistic spectrum disorder: a questionnaire and polysomnographic study. Sleep Med 2007;9(1):64–70.

22. Goldman SE, Surdyka K, Cuevas R, et al. Defining the sleep phenotype in children with autism. Dev Neuropsychol 2009;34:560–73.

23. Lambert A, Tessier S, Rochette AC, et al. Poor sleep affects daytime functioning in typically developing and autistic children not complaining of sleep problems: a questionnaire-based and polysomnographic study. Res Autism Spectr Disord 2016;23:94–106.

24. Giannotti F, Cortesi F, Cerquiglini A, et al. Sleep in children with autism with and without regression. J Sleep Res 2011;20(2):338–47.

25. Nelson KB, Grether JK, Croen LA, et al. Neuropeptides and neurotrophins in neonatal blood of children with autism or mental retardation. Ann Neurol 2001; 49:597–606.

26. McCauley JL, Olson LM, Delahanty R, et al. A linkage disequilibrium may of the 1-Mb 15q12 GABA(A) receptor subunit cluster and association to autism. Am J Med Genet B Neuropsychiatr Genet 2004;131B(1):51–9.

27. Gabrielle S, Sacco R, Persico AM. Blood serotonin levels in autism spectrum disorder: a systematic review and meta-analysis. Eur Neuropsychopharmacol 2014; 24(6):919–29.

28. Piven J, Tsai GC, Nehme E, et al. Platelet serotonin, a possible marker for familial autism. J Autism Dev Disord 1991;21:51–9.

29. Prasad HC, Steiner JA, Sutcliffe JS, et al. Enhanced activity of human serotonin transporter variants associated with autism. Philos Trans R Soc Lond B Biol Sci 2009;364:163–73.

30. Verma D, Chakraborti B, Karmaker A, et al. Sexual dismorphic effect in the genetic association of monoamine oxidase A (MAOA) markers with autism spectrum disorder. Prog Neuropsychopharmacol Biol Psychiatry 2014;50:11–20.

31. Nir I, Meir D, Zilber N, et al. Brief report: Circadian melatonin, thyroid-stimulating hormone, prolactin, and cortisol levels in serum of young adults with autism. J Autism Dev Disord 1995;25:641–54.

32. Kulman G, Lissoni P, Rovelli, et al. Evidence of pineal endocrine hypofunction in autistic children. Neuro Endocrinol Lett 2000;21:31–4.
33. Tordjman S, Anderson GM, Pichard N, et al. Nocturnal excretion of 6-sulphatox-ymelatonin in children and adolescents with autistic disorder. Biol Psychiatry 2005;57:134–8.
34. Goldman SE, Adkins KW, Calcutt MW, et al. Melatonin in children with autism spectrum disorders: Endogenous and pharmacokinetic profiles in relation to sleep. J Autism Dev Disord 2014;51:30–8.
35. Goldman SE, Alder ML, Burgess HJ, et al. Characterizing sleep in adolescents and adults with autism spectrum disorders. J Autism Dev Disord 2017;47:1682–95.
36. Melke J, Goubran Botros H, Chaste P, et al. Abnormal melatonin synthesis in autism spectrum disorders. Mol Psychiatry 2008;13:90–8.
37. Braam W, Ehrhart F, Maas A, et al. Low maternal melatonin level increases autism spectrum disorder risk in children. Res Dev Disabil 2018;82:79–89.
38. Jonsson L, Anckarsater H, Zettergren A, et al. Association between ASMT and autistic-like traits in children from a Swedish nationwide cohort. Psychiatr Genet 2014;24(1):21–7.
39. Veatch OJ, Pendergast JS, Allen MJ, et al. Genetic variation in melatonin pathway enzymes in children with autism spectrum disorder and comorbid sleep onset delay. J Autism Dev Disord 2015;45:100–10.
40. Goldman SE, McGrew S, Johnson KP, et al. Sleep is associated with problem behaviors in children and adolescents with autism spectrum disorders. Res Autism Spectr Disord 2011;5(3):1223–9.
41. Sikora DM, Johnson K, Clemons T, et al. The relationship between sleep problems and daytime behavior in children of different ages with autism spectrum disorders. Pediatrics 2012;130:S83–90.
42. Mazurek MO, Sohl K. Sleep and behavioral problems in children with autism spectrum disorder. J Autism Dev Disord 2016;46(6):1906–15.
43. Johnson CR, Smith T, DeMand A, et al. Exploring sleep quality of young children with autism spectrum disorder and disruptive behaviors. Sleep Med 2018;44:61–6.
44. Gabriels RL, Cuccaro ML, Hill DE, et al. Repetitive behaviors in autism: relationships with associated clinical features. Res Dev Disabil 2005;26(2):169–81.
45. Schreck KA, Mulick JA, Smith AF. Sleep problems as possible predictors of intensified symptoms of autism. Res Dev Disabil 2004;25(1):57–66.
46. Cohen S, Fulcher BD, Rajaratnam SMW, et al. Sleep patterns predictive of daytime challenging behavior in individuals with low-functioning autism. Autism Res 2018;11(2):391–403.
47. May T, Cornish K, Conduit R, et al. Sleep in high-functioning children with autism: longitudinal developmental change and associations with behavioral problems. Behav Sleep Med 2015;13(1):2–18.
48. Meltzer LJ. Brief report: sleep in parents of children with autism spectrum disorders. J Pediatr Psychol 2008;33(4):380–6.
49. Levin A, Scher A. Sleep problems in young children with autism spectrum disorders: a study of parenting stress, mothers' sleep-related cognitions, and bedtime behaviors. CNS Neurosci Ther 2016;22:921–7.
50. Johnson CR, Turner KS, Foldes EL, et al. Comparison of sleep questionnaires in the assessment of sleep disturbances in children with autism spectrum disorders. Sleep Med 2012;13:795–801.

51. Malow BA, Connolly HV, Weiss SK, et al. The Pediatric Sleep Clinical Global Impressions Scale – a new tool to measure pediatric insomnia in autism spectrum disorders. J Dev Behav Pediatr 2016;37(5):370–6.
52. Keogh S, Bridle C, Siriwardena NA, et al. Effectiveness of non-pharmacological interventions for insomnia in children with autism spectrum disorder: a systematic review and meta-analysis. PLoS One 2019;14(8):e0221428.
53. Malow BA, Byars K, Johnson K, et al. A practice pathway for the identification, evaluation, and management of insomnia in children and adolescents with autism spectrum disorders. Pediatrics 2012;130(Suppl 2):S106–24.
54. Knight RM, Johnson CM. Using a behavioral treatment package for sleep problems in children with autism spectrum disorders. Child Fam Behav Ther 2014;36:204–21.
55. Moon E, Corkhum P, Smith I. A case series evaluation of a behavioral sleep intervention for three children with autism and primary insomnia. J Pediatr Psychol 2011;36:47–54.
56. Reed H, McGrew S, Artibee K, et al. Parent-based sleep education workshops in autism. J Child Neurol 2009;24:936–45.
57. Malow BA, Adkins KW, Reynolds A, et al. Parent-based sleep education for children with autism spectrum disorders. J Autism Dev Disord 2014;44:216–28.
58. Johnson CR, Turner KS, Foldes E, et al. Behavioral parent training to address sleep disturbances in young children with autism spectrum disorder: a pilot trial. Sleep Med 2013;14:994–1004.
59. Papadopoulos N, Sciberras E, Hiscock H, et al. The efficacy of a brief behavioral sleep intervention in school-aged children with ADHD and comorbid autism spectrum disorder. J Atten Disord 2019;23(4):341–50.
60. Kirkpatrick B, Louw JS, Leader G. Efficacy of parent training incorporated in behavioral sleep interventions for children with autism spectrum disorder and/or intellectual disabilities: a systematic review. Sleep Med 2019;53:141–52.
61. Mindell JA, Emslie G, Blumer J, et al. Pharmacological management of insomnia in children and adolescents: Consensus statement. Pediatrics 2006;117:e1223–32.
62. Hollway JA, Aman MG. Pharmacological treatment of sleep disturbance in developmental disabilities: a review of the literature. Res Dev Disabil 2011;32:939–62.
63. McDonagh MS, Holmes R, Hsu F. Pharmacologic treatments for sleep disorders in children: a systematic review. J Child Neurol 2019;34(5):237–47.
64. Rossignol DA, Frye RE. Melatonin in autism spectrum disorders: a systematic review and meta-analysis. Dev Med Child Neurol 2011;53(9):783–92.
65. Gringras P, Gamble C, Jones AP, et al. Melatonin for sleep problems in children with neurodevelopmental disorders: randomized double masked placebo controlled trial. BMJ 2012;345:e6664.
66. Cortesi F, Giannotti F, Sebastiani T, et al. Controlled-release melatonin, singly or combined with cognitive behavioural therapy, for persistent insomnia in children with autism spectrum disorders: a randomized placebo-controlled trial. J Sleep Res 2012;21(6):700–9.
67. Gringras P, Nir T, Breddy J, et al. Efficacy and safety of pediatric prolonged-release melatonin for insomnia in children with autism spectrum disorder. J Am Acad Child Adolesc Psychiatry 2017;56(11):948–57.
68. Schroder CM, Malow BA, Athanasios M, et al. Pediatric prolonged-release melatonin for sleep in children with autism spectrum disorder: impact on child behavior and caregivers' quality of life. J Autism Dev Disord 2019;49:3218–30.

69. Maras A, Schroder CM, Malow BA, et al. Long-term efficacy and safety of pediatric prolonged-release melatonin for insomnia in children with autism spectrum disorder. J Child Adolesc Psychopharmacol 2018;28(10):699–710.

70. Malow BA, Findling RL, Schroder CM, et al. Sleep, growth, and puberty after 2 years of prolonged-release melatonin in children with autism spectrum disorder. J Am Acad Child Adolesc Psychiatry 2020. https://doi.org/10.1016/j.jaac.2019.12.007.

71. Bruni O, Angriman M, Calisti F, et al. Practitioner review: treatment of chronic insomnia in children and adolescents with neurodevelopmental disabilities. J Child Psychol Psychiatry 2018;59(5):489–508.

# Sleep-Related Problems and Pediatric Anxiety Disorders

Katherine Crowe, PhD[a],*, Carolyn Spiro-Levitt, PhD[b]

## KEYWORDS

• Sleep • Anxiety • Youth • Child • Adolescent • Intervention

## KEY POINTS

- Anxiety disorders are highly prevalent in youth, and there is growing evidence that the majority of anxious children experience at least 1 sleep-related problem.
- There is more research to support the notion that sleep-related problems are a risk factor for the development of anxiety than the converse.
- Sleep needs and patterns change across development; anxiety can interact with these developmental shifts to create general and age-specific sleep-related problems.
- Interventions such as cognitive behavioral therapy and psychopharmacology have demonstrated efficacy in the treatment of anxiety disorders, and there is growing evidence that both treatments may also improve sleep-related problems in youth with anxiety.

| Abbreviations | |
|---|---|
| DSM-5 | Diagnostic and Statistical Manual of Mental Disorders, Fifth Edition |
| GAD | generalized anxiety disorder |
| OCD | obsessive–compulsive disorder |
| SAD | separation anxiety disorder |
| SoP | social phobia |
| SRPs | Sleep-related problems |

This article originally appeared in *Child and Adolescent Psychiatric Clinics*, Volume 30 Issue 1, January 2021.

Disclosure Statement: The authors have nothing to disclose.

[a] Home for Anxiety, Repetitive Behaviors, OCD, and Related Disorders (HARBOR), 1518 Walnut Street, Suite 1506, Philadelphia, PA 19102, USA; [b] Department of Child and Adolescent Psychiatry at Hassenfeld Children's Hospital at New York University (NYU) Langone, 1 Park Avenue, Seventh Floor, New York, NY 10016, USA

[a] If the nature of fears seems to be related to a realistic threat in the environment (eg, high rates of crime in the neighborhood), an intervention should address ways to help the child and parent to communicate more effectively around this issue so that the child can understand ways that their family can help keep them safe.

* Corresponding author.

*E-mail address:* kcrowe@harborpa.com

Psychiatr Clin N Am 47 (2024) 213–228
https://doi.org/10.1016/j.psc.2023.06.014
0193-953X/24/© 2023 Elsevier Inc. All rights reserved.

## INTRODUCTION

Anxiety disorders are among the most prevalent psychopathologies in childhood and adolescence—research with youth samples estimates that the lifetime prevalence of an anxiety disorder is 15% to 20%.[1] Sleep-related problems (SRPs) represent commonly observed phenomena, but are a traditionally understudied area of childhood anxiety. SRPs refer to a heterogeneous set of challenges that occur in the context of sleep. These challenges can include behavioral problems during bedtime routines, subjective and objective difficulties with falling and staying asleep, abnormal behaviors during the sleep period such as parasomnias, and daytime sleepiness or fatigue.

Surveys of the prevalence of SRPs in clinically anxious youth have shown that 85% to 90% experience at least 1 type of sleep problem, with the majority of youth experiencing multiple.[2–4] The effects of sleep disturbance are well-documented in children and are linked to impairment in behavior and emotion regulation, worse academic and cognitive functioning, and physical health problems.[5] Nonetheless, despite its importance, sleep is often excluded as a direct target of intervention in evidence-based treatment approaches for child anxiety.[6]

This review aims to summarize the empirical literature regarding SRPs in child and adolescent anxiety, with particular attention paid to the nature of the relationship between sleep and anxiety and previous intervention efforts to ameliorate SRPs in this population. The focus is on conditions in the anxiety disorders category in the *Diagnostic and Statistical Manual of Mental Disorders, Fifth Edition* (DSM-5)[7]—separation anxiety disorder (SAD), generalized anxiety disorder (GAD), specific phobia, social phobia (SoP), and panic disorder with and without agoraphobia. Although obsessive–compulsive disorder (OCD) was removed from this category in DSM-5, OCD is included in this review given that many of the studies conducted on this topic have included children with OCD in their samples.

## ASSESSMENT

There are many ways to assess SRPs in individuals with and without anxiety disorders, including both subjective and objective measures. Methods used depend on a variety of factors, including the child's age, resources available, and the goals of the assessment. Information about the nature, purpose, benefits, and limitations of these methods are described in **Table 1**.

## ASSOCIATIONS BETWEEN SLEEP-RELATED PROBLEMS AND ANXIETY

At an overarching level, there seem to be positive relationships between the presence of sleep difficulties and anxiety symptoms. Having more SRPs is associated with greater anxiety symptom severity in both clinical samples[2,4] and community samples.[8–10] The presence of more than 1 anxiety disorder may confer additional risk for sleep challenges.[4] Research has investigated the association between particular SRPs and anxiety symptoms or disorders.

### Behavioral Problems Around Bedtime

Nighttime behavioral challenges are common among anxious youth, particularly younger children. Many behaviors are driven by nighttime fears, including fear of the dark, intruders, fantastical creatures, and being separated from a caregiver. Estimates suggest that approximately 60% of typically developing 4- to 6-year-old children and approximately 80% of school-age children experience nighttime fears, with the

**Table 1**
**Assessment methods for SRPs in youth**

| Assessment Type | Function | Benefits and Limitations |
|---|---|---|
| **Subjective measures** | | |
| Child/parent self-report measures | Most typical format for assessing SRPs; collect retrospective report on sleep-wake patterns and related issues.<br>Examples include: Children's Sleep Habit Questionnaire[76] and the Sleep Disturbance Scale for Children.[77] | Easily accessible, requiring few resources to administer.<br>Limited by self-reported and retrospective nature of the data. |
| Sleep diaries | Often used as diagnostic tool; used to record typically at least 1 week of sleep data.[78]<br>Patients record their sleep–wake times, number/duration of awakenings, and perception of sleep quality. | Easily accessible, requiring few resources to administer.<br>Limited by self-reported and retrospective nature of the data. |
| **Objective measures** | | |
| Polysomnography | Often used for screening and diagnosis of sleep disturbance.[78]<br>Typically performed in a laboratory setting.<br>Polysomnography uses electrodes for the measurement of electroencephalography to record brain activity, electrooculography to assess eye movements, and electromyography to assess changes in muscle tone.[43] | Polysomnography provides the most detailed information on an individual's sleep.<br>High cost and resources required so not typically recommended for routine assessment.<br>Typically only used to capture one night of sleep. |
| Actigraphy | Measurement of physical movement using motion sensors; used to measure sleep patterns.[78] | Well-validated as an assessment tool in youth.[43]<br>Does not measure breathing or specific behaviors, only physical activity.[79]<br>More resource intensive than subjective measures. |

prevalence of certain types of fears changing over the course of development (eg, fantastical fears becoming less common and fears of intruders increasing).[11] For approximately 10% to 20% of these children, such fears are associated with clinical levels of anxiety.[11,12] Accompanying interfering behaviors are often directly related to avoiding aspects of the sleep process, such as refusal to sleep alone or sleep outside the house, refusal to get ready for or get into bed, and ritualizing during bedtime (eg, checking under the bed, requiring parents to extend bedtime routines).[2,13,14] Anxious behaviors can also interfere with sleep, even if they are not directly intended to do so. Examples include spending excessive time at night completing homework (as driven by perfectionism), engaging in extended interactions online with peers (as driven by social anxiety), and completing ritualized behaviors in preparation for sleep such as those related to grooming (as driven by obsessions).

### Sleep Duration and Timing

Some evidence suggests that anxious youth are more likely to obtain an insufficient amount of sleep compared with their nonanxious peers.[15] Researchers have observed a small but significant delay in the time that anxious children and adolescents go to bed, equating to about half an hour of less total sleep; this difference seems to be particularly relevant on school nights.[15,16] Despite this delay, children did not report increased sleepiness the next day. As theorized by the authors, this may be due to a baseline level of hyperarousal owing to their anxiety, which serves to counteract sleepiness.[15] Still, other research has shown that, when insufficient sleep has been obtained, anxiety symptoms and an anxiety disorder are more likely to be present: adolescents who obtain an average of less than 7.0 to 7.5 hours of sleep per night seem to be at greater risk for anxiety compared with peers who sleep more.[17,18] The amount of time spent in bed also seems to be relevant to anxiety: youth who spend either significantly less or more time in bed than recommended for their age group tend to have more severe anxiety symptoms.[19] Finally, variability in sleep–wake times is likely associated with greater anxiety as well.[16,17] As discussed in greater detail elsewhere in this article, variability in sleep–wake times across days (and especially between weekdays vs weekends) is particularly relevant and problematic for adolescents.

### Difficulties Falling and Staying Asleep

Anxious children may have mild problems with sleep onset latency. This difficulty could be due to preoccupation with anxious thoughts, physiologic activation, or mental or behavioral ritualizing, among many factors. Sleep onset delays of up to 15 minutes have been found for youth with GAD compared with unaffected peers, as captured by both subjective and objective measures.[20,21] More significant difficulties with falling asleep are not common, but when present are impactful. Insomnia likely has a negative effect on anxiety symptoms as children age, predicting symptoms of GAD and SoP as youth transition from early to middle childhood[22] and again to adolescence.[23] Of note, it is important for clinicians to be mindful of how such problems with sleep onset and maintenance can elicit greater parental involvement and accommodation, which have the potential to maintain and exacerbate these sleep challenges.

### Sleep Quality

Anxiety symptoms seem to be negatively associated with ratings of sleep quality.[19] Sleep quality can be defined as the degree to which one's sleep experience is satisfying and restorative, based on factors such as sleep duration, sleep initiation and maintenance, and feeling rested upon waking.[24] Sleep quality can be impacted by other variables as well, including the amount of time in various stages of sleep and the presence of parasomnias. Results have been mixed as to whether anxious youth have more awakenings during sleep than nonanxious peers.[15,25] Some research suggests that anxious youth self-report poorer quality of sleep compared with their unaffected peers.[21] While this can be difficult to explain by examining objective measures of sleep (eg, actigraphy reports), these authors theorize that this may be due to self-report bias as influenced by general negative affect, or possibly that an overactive sympathetic nervous system during the day makes these youth more tired and sleep less restorative. This may become particularly true as youth enter adolescence.[26]

### Parasomnias

Parasomnias are a group of sleep disorders characterized by abnormal, unwanted events, including behaviors, movements, dreams, and affective or perceptual experiences. Parasomnias may arise in the context of sleep-wake transitions or during sleep, with some occurring during non-REM sleep (eg, sleepwalking and night terrors) and others occurring during REM sleep (eg, nightmares). Nightmares are experienced by the majority of anxious children and are among the most commonly reported SRPs,[2,4,27] particularly among preschool and school-aged anxious children, when nightmares tend to peak.[28] Previous research has noted a specific association between nightmares and GAD[29,30] and a higher prevalence of nightmares among anxious girls.[31] Although often neglected for their clinical impact, nightmares seem to play an important role in children's sleep experience and functioning. Anxiety is associated with greater nightmare distress.[32] Nightmares can also lead to other SRPs, because they likely elicit greater family involvement and specifically parental accommodation behaviors (eg, delayed bedtimes, cosleeping) among anxious youth.[29,33] Aside from nightmares, parasomnias are present but less common among anxious children compared with behavioral problems associated with going to sleep.[5] Sleepwalking may have particular relevance to separation anxiety—it is positively associated with separation anxiety symptoms,[34] and sleepwalking in early childhood predicts later separation anxiety.[22] Adolescents with a history of sleep walking or night terrors are more likely to have an anxiety disorder compared with unaffected peers and are also more likely to report a history of sleep talking and nightmares.[35]

### Case Illustration

The following deidentified case description is illustrative of ways in which SRPs can co-occur and interact with youth anxiety. Trevor is a 9-year-old boy with longstanding fears of being separated from his parents. He has become intrigued by the idea of attending sleepaway camp with his friends and states that he is capable of going, although as summer approaches, his sleep patterns have become increasingly disrupted. Trevor describes worries that someone will break into his room as the reason for such sleep difficulties. Parents observe numerous behavioral problems at night, including trying to stay physically close to parents before and during his bedtime routine, delaying during bedtime routine tasks, and requiring parents to engage in extensive bedtime rituals, such as checking multiple times that his windows are locked and staying in his room after the lights are turned off. Trevor experiences challenges with falling and staying asleep owing to a combination of worry thoughts and hypervigilance: he reports listening carefully for any sign of intruder and feeling his heart race in response to sounds from outside. This often delays sleep onset for 30 to 40 minutes, and he typically wakes up 3 or more times per night. On each occasion of waking, he seeks out his parents for comfort. Sometimes his parents will allow him to sleep in their bed or else they will walk him back to his room and stay with him until he falls back asleep. Although Trevor denies feeling tired the next day, his parents generally observe more irritability and anxiety on days after particularly disrupted sleep.

## ASSOCIATIONS WITH SPECIFIC ANXIETY DISORDERS

A subset of research has examined SRPs in the context of particular anxiety disorders. In GAD and SAD, sleep-related challenges are also part of the DSM-5 diagnostic criteria for the disorder. GAD criteria include the possibility that persistent worry is associated with "sleep disturbance (difficulty falling or staying asleep, or restless, unsatisfying sleep)."[7] SAD criteria include "persistent reluctance or refusal to sleep away from home or to go to sleep without being near a major attachment figure" as well as "repeated nightmares involving the theme of separation."[7]

### Generalized Anxiety Disorder

GAD is an anxiety disorder marked by pervasive, difficult to control worries about a variety of domains, such as school performance, social functioning, and small mistakes. A broad range of SRPs have been observed among children and adolescents with GAD. Compared with anxious youth without GAD, they have more sleep problems overall, more general self-reported difficulty sleeping, and a greater likelihood of insomnia and parasomnias.[2,3] In comparison with nonanxious children, they have greater sleep onset delays and more variability in their sleep schedules.[10,21,36] They also self-report lower satisfaction with their sleep.[21] As noted elsewhere in this article, these authors report that chronic overactivation of the sympathetic nervous system during the day may make these youth more tired and sleep less restorative. Some research on sleep architecture in this population supports the hypothesis that their sleep is less restorative, demonstrating that they spend less time in slow wave sleep compared with nonanxious peers.[25]

### Separation Anxiety Disorder

SAD is characterized by excessive anxiety about separation from a caregiver or attachment figure beyond a developmentally appropriate age. It is often associated with refusal to separate or significant difficulty separating from this figure. SAD is associated with a range of sleep challenges, in part owing to the fact that bedtime is key point of separation for children. For children with SAD, bedtime has the potential to trigger a variety of behaviors to avoid or delay separation (eg, asking for another person to sleep with them, refusing to sleep alone, refusing to sleep away from home), which can consequently interfere with bedtime, sleep onset, and sleep maintenance. Further, the point of separation from the caregiver can increase perceptions of threat, acutely increasing arousal and thus interfering with sleep initiation.[37] Research demonstrates that children with SAD are more likely to have insomnia in particular as well as and parasomnias, especially sleepwalking, sleep talking, and nightmares.[2-4,36] Compared with anxious children without SAD, those with SAD also have a greater number of SRPs overall.[2,4]

### Social Phobia

SoP is an anxiety disorder in which the individual has a disproportionate degree of anxiety about social situations that could lead them to feel scrutinized or judged by others. Individuals with SoP frequently avoid or attempt to avoid these feared situations. SoP has been the focus of comparatively less sleep research. The limited body of empirical data makes it difficult to draw conclusions about SRPs among socially anxious youth, and reports are equivocal as to whether these children demonstrate greater, fewer, or equivalent numbers of SRPs compared with youth with other types of anxiety.[2,4] SoP symptoms may be associated with poorer quality of sleep and restless sleep.[36,38] This factor may help to explain why socially phobic youth also report greater fatigue.[4]

### Obsessive Compulsive Disorder

OCD is a disorder characterized by the presence of intrusive and unwanted thoughts, images, or urges (obsessions) as well as ritualized behaviors (compulsions) that the individual often feels compelled to perform in response to the obsessions. Similar to those with other anxiety conditions, the vast majority of youth with OCD experience SRPs,[39,40] and SRPs are significantly more common in children with OCD versus their unaffected peers.[41] Frequent SRPs include needing to sleep next to someone, nightmares, fatigue, overtiredness, and poor sleep quality.[39–41] Poor sleep quality has been corroborated by objective measures—Alfano and Kim[42] found evidence for less total sleep time and more time awake after sleep onset compared with controls.

## DIRECTIONALITY OF THE RELATIONSHIPS BETWEEN SLEEP AND ANXIETY

Because the majority of research conducted in this area has been cross-sectional, the directionality of the effects is still not well-understood. However, this has been an area of increasing interest which is the subject of several recent reviews.[37,43,44] Evidence has been found for the bidirectional relationship between sleep and anxiety, with more robust data to support the impact of sleep problems on the later development of anxiety as compared with the reverse. Longitudinal studies of children as early as preschool age have demonstrated support for a range of different SRPs increasing risk for anxiety over multiyear periods of childhood. A greater number of SRPs at ages 3 and 4 predicted higher anxiety at age 7,[45] and refusal to sleep alone and sleep-onset latency among 3- to 6-year-olds predicted greater anxiety severity at ages 9 to 13.[46] Some investigators have particularly focused on the transition to adolescence. This period represents a time when sleep and anxiety may uniquely interact to influence long-term health trajectories, given that it is typically character-ized by the onset of puberty, which includes a variety of biological changes related to sleep–wake patterns and emotion regulation.[47] For instance, Kelly and El-Sheikh[26] conducted a 5-year longitudinal study of children, assessing them at ages 8, 10, and 13 years of age. In a cross-lagged panel model, they found that self-reported sleep–wake problems predicted greater anxiety over time, but that actigraphy-measured sleep duration and sleep quality predicted anxiety only from the second to third time-point (ages 10–13) and not from the first to the second timepoint (ages 8–10).

This study, as well as a limited body of other longitudinal investigations,[36,48] also provides some evidence for possibly bidirectional effects between anxiety and sleep over time. Kelly and El-Sheikh[26] note that effects were less robust in the opposite di-rection and were limited to the effect that anxiety has on sleep quality, as opposed to other aspects of sleep. As indicated by the findings of Shanahan and colleagues,[36] it may be that the long-term effects of anxiety on sleep are especially pronounced in youth with clinically significant GAD, a disorder marked by high negative affect that may, importantly, impact one's ability to fall asleep. Ecological momentary assess-ment research lends support to this notion: Cousins and colleagues[49] found that among anxious youth, daytime negative affect, and more time awake at night exerted bidirectional influences on one another.

## ANXIETY AND SLEEP ACROSS DEVELOPMENTAL STAGES

Anxiety is associated with sleep problems across development,[8] and SRPs overall may not be more prevalent at one stage than another.[4] Although some problems in-crease as youth age, others tend to recede.[50] Awareness of normative changes in sleep patterns aids in distinguishing typical from anxiety-related sleep challenges. For infants and young children, sleep loss and late bedtimes have a more substantial impact on anxiety symptoms than fragmented sleep.[51] Preschool age is frequently the age of onset for separation anxiety fears, which often precipitate a number of behav-ioral problems at bedtime, including a refusal to sleep alone.[2,13,14] Increasing cognitive abilities also provide greater imaginative capacity, but young children have difficulty separating fantasy from reality[52]; thus, fear of the dark and nightmares are com-mon.[2,53] Some SRPs from early childhood can persist into the middle childhood period for anxious youth, including bedtime resistance, nighttime fears, and nightmares.[3,40] Cognitive and emotional maturation mean that the nature of nighttime anxiety usually changes, such that worries become focused on more real-life events and bedtime provides an extended opportunity for worry. The end of this period and the entry into adolescence coincides with typical onset of puberty, which—as noted elsewhere in this article—has been pointed to as a sensitive developmental period for the onset of problematic connections between sleep and affective challenges.[26] Owing to further biological (eg, shift in circadian preference) and environmental changes (eg, increased academic and social obligations, increased screen time), insufficient sleep typically becomes a more substantial problem in adolescence,[54,55] and a shorter sleep duration among adolescents has been linked to increases in anxiety.[17,18] Greater variability in bedtime also becomes more problematic and is associated with greater anxiety.[16,17] Social jet lag—attempting to make up sleep on the weekends—tends to emerge during this developmental period.[56] Some research has shown that it can be helpful for adolescents to recapture some lost sleep (1–2 hours) to decrease the cumulative effects of sleep loss during the week; however, more than this modest amount creates more irregular sleep–wake patterns and is associated with a greater risk for an anxiety disorder.[18] Some factors thought to contribute to SRPs among anxious adolescents include high social media use and negative cognitive processes (eg, rumination). Although these issues are often present among anxious teenagers and can be anecdotally linked to SRPs, evidence to suggest a causal link is equivocal.[57–59]

## INTERVENTIONS

Any intervention to address comorbid anxiety and sleep challenges should begin with thorough assessment. This approach may include nomothetic approaches—such as the instruments described in **Table 1**—but should also include targeted questions, such as: Is anxiety a preexisting problem in other parts of the child's life? What aspects of bedtime or sleep does the child seem to be most concerned about? Does bedtime anxiety happen consistently across time (eg, different days of the week) and place (eg, sleeping over at a friend's house)?[a] If there are anxiety-related SRPs present, it is recommended to help the child to establish or strengthen healthy sleep hygiene habits (eg, a consistent and age-appropriate bedtime, a technologically free bedtime routine, and a dark and quiet sleep environment).[60] Following this several factors should be considered in the selection of the most effective and appropriate intervention, such as the developmental age and stage of the child, strategies that have been used to manage anxiety in other parts of the day, and the child and parent's ability to carry out an intervention.[5] Cognitive behavioral techniques are commonly recommended, and most have adequate research support, with comparatively less research on comprehensive cognitive behavioral therapy (CBT) packages to target SRPs and anxiety in youth. These techniques are summarized in **Table 2**.

Exposure and response prevention is often well-suited to disrupt anxious avoidance patterns during bedtime and sleep.[53] Based on the principles of both classical and operant conditioning, exposure and response prevention gradually exposes the child to increasingly anxiety-provoking stimuli or situations (eg, fear of the dark) without allowing them to engage in avoidance. Over time, fear often habituates and the child learns a sense of mastery. Systematic desensitization can also be used, in which the child is first taught relaxation strategies to use with exposure. Another variant of extinction learning can be used when working directly with parents. Such an approach is particularly useful for parents of children who have difficulty with independent sleep. In unmodified extinction, parents are instructed to put their child to sleep and not respond

**Table 2**
**Empirically supported psychotherapy intervention strategies**

| Intervention | Description | Applications |
|---|---|---|
| Exposure and response prevention | Behavioral strategy in which youth is gradually exposed to increasingly anxiety-provoking situations without engaging in avoidance.<br>In systematic desensitization, exposure is coupled with relaxation strategies. | Appropriate for children and adolescents.<br>Nighttime fears, often seen in GAD, SAD, and specific phobia.<br>Intrusive thoughts and compulsions at night, as seen in OCD. |
| Extinction | Behavioral strategy in which parents cease responding to bids for attention at night.<br>Can be unmodified or done gradually.<br>Parental fading involves the parent moving progressively further away from the child over several nights. | Appropriate for all ages; typically used with young children.<br>Difficulties with sleep onset and nighttime wakings.<br>High parental attention and accommodation at night. |
| Positive reinforcement | Behavioral strategy in which youth is reinforced for appropriate nighttime behaviors with stickers or other reward.<br>In bedtime passes, youth can trade in fixed number of passes per night for parental visits or assistance. | Appropriate for all ages; typically used with children.<br>Difficulties with bedtime routines, sleep onset, and nighttime wakings.<br>Low motivation to change behavior. |
| Cognitive self-instruction | Cognitive strategy in which youth uses positive self-talk to manage anxious thoughts at night. | Appropriate for children and adolescents.<br>Worries, often seen in GAD, SAD, and specific phobia. |
| Transitional object | Stuffed animal or other comfort object youth uses to self-soothe or youth provides care to at night. | Appropriate for young children.<br>Nighttime fears, often seen in GAD, SAD, and specific phobia. |

to crying or other bids for parental attention until morning. In graduated extinction, parents check on the child at intervals that are increasingly spaced out over time. Alternatively, parental fading can be used, in which the parent progressively moves further away from the child every few nights until they are no longer present in the room. Reviews of these various extinction approaches have generally demonstrated them to be efficacious in promoting shorter sleep onset and fewer night wakings, although it is noted that gradual approaches tend to be more acceptable to parents.[60,61]

Other CBT techniques that can be helpful include positive reinforcement and cognitive self-instruction. Positive reinforcement is designed to increase the frequency of desirable bedtime behaviors. In one application, the child is rewarded for taking steps toward a goal (such as completing steps of a bedtime routine), often with a sticker chart. Parents can also use bedtime passes—a system in which the child is given a limited number of passes that they can trade in each night for a parent visit. Research has demonstrated efficacy for the use of bedtime passes with young children (ages 3–6) in mitigating resistance to bedtime.[62,63] With cognitive self-instruction, youth are taught to develop positive self-talk around their ability to manage the fear-inducing situation (eg, "I can handle this") or to alter the valence of the feared stimulus (eg, "Being alone in the dark is calming and peaceful"). Such a strategy is often better suited to older children and adolescents who have more developed metacognitive skills; younger children can benefit from such cognitive tools when statements are more concrete.[5]

An adjunctive strategy for helping young children with fears of the dark can be providing them a transitional object. In one such application, children were provided with a stuffed animal called Huggy Puppy and either told that the puppy was frightened at night and needed the child's support or that the puppy was the child's companion to help the child at night when they were scared. Both versions have been shown to decrease nighttime fears.[64]

In devising a treatment plan to address SRPs among anxious youth, it is important to not only identify patterns of anxious avoidance but also possible secondary reinforcement[53] (for instance, prolonged access to electronic devices as a result of delaying bedtime). It is necessary to monitor for such secondary reinforcers as these can be treatment barriers. Limit setting around access to environmental reinforcers can be useful in this regard.

Evaluations of comprehensive CBT packages to target SRPs in anxious youth have been few but have demonstrated some potentially promising results.[65] For example, 1 study demonstrated that, when using a targeted sleep intervention as an adjunct to CBT, youth ages 9 to 14 years with anxiety demonstrated clinically significant decreases in sleep problems.[66] This intervention, called Sleeping TIGERS,[67] addressed thoughts, feelings, and behaviors that interfere with bedtime and sleep initiation while also enhancing personal motivation, helping youth to develop better sleep habits and sleep regularity, and promoting more effective limitations on media use at bedtime. Behavioral interventions for sleep issues in adolescents, including CBT for insomnia, have gained support as effective interventions in improving adolescent SRPs and have also demonstrated some effects on anxiety symptoms.[68,69]

A small body of research has also shown that CBT for youth anxiety, even when not directly targeting SRPs, also tends to improve SRPs. For example, the Child/Adolescent Anxiety Multimodal Study[70] examined the effects of a CBT intervention, Coping Cat,[71] sertraline (a selective serotonin reuptake inhibitor [SSRI]), combined therapy, and pill placebo on SRPs in youth with anxiety disorders. Both CBT and sertraline were shown to be effective in reducing SRPs in youth with anxiety.[72] Although all conditions showed improvements in SRPs, those conditions involving CBT showed greater improvements in dysregulated sleep. Other investigators have similarly found that parent-reported SRPs improved significantly after CBT for youth with anxiety and OCD, even in the absence of a targeted sleep intervention.[40,50] Further, children who are treatment responders to anxiety tend to demonstrate greater improvements in SRPs than nonresponders.[50] Proposed mechanisms for these improvements in SRPs via CBT have included decreased worry, improved mood, and decreased parental accommodation.[40,72]

Psychopharmacologic approaches are also often used to treat anxiety in youth. Medications such as SSRIs and selective serotonin norepinephrine reuptake inhibitors are among the most commonly prescribed.[73] Recent studies have shown that SSRIs (eg, fluvoxamine, sertraline) may improve not only anxiety but also lead to a decrease in insomnia and SRPs in this population as well.[2,72] Benzodiazepines have also shown some benefit in addressing SRPs. However, longer acting forms of these medications have been shown to cause daytime sleepiness. The risk for habituation or addiction with these medications also makes them higher risk for use in children, and they are typically recommended only for short-term use.[74] Finally, medications such as alpha-agonists, antihistamines, tricyclics, and melatonin have also been used to treat SRPs and insomnia in youth.[6] However, behavioral interventions are recommended as the first-line treatment, given their effectiveness and the possible side effects of these medications.[74]

## DISCUSSION

Empirical evidence suggests that sleep is a frequent and significant area of impairment across many of the anxiety conditions in childhood and adolescence. There is more research to support the notion that SRPs are a risk factor for the development of anxiety rather than the other way around.[37] In particular, there is more robust evidence to suggest SRPs are present for youth with GAD compared with other anxiety conditions. Yet, it is also possible that poor sleep is a transdiagnostic risk factor for psychiatric problems generally speaking, rather than sleep having specific relationships to individual anxiety disorders, as sleep disturbance broadly affects one's neurobiological arousal-regulating systems.[75] A range of SRPs have been documented using both subjective and objective assessment measures. However, self-reported sleep challenges have not always been corroborated by objective data. Further, empirical findings in this literature are somewhat constrained by assessment methods. As noted by a previous review, significant limitations include overreliance on parent-reported (vs child-reported data), the use of self-report measures that have not been empirically validated, and shared method variance across measures assessing sleep and anxiety.[6] Such limitations are important to keep in mind as well when interpreting the small body of intervention literature.

Differences emerge regarding sleep needs and patterns across normative development. Anxiety can interact with such patterns to create some general and some age-specific SRPs. Frequent problems for anxious younger children are often related to bedtime resistance and fears, whereas older children and adolescents tend to experience more difficulties with falling asleep owing to general worries and/or suffering the emotion regulation consequences associated with insufficient sleep.

Studies of specific cognitive and behavioral techniques have demonstrated empirical support for their ability to address some SRPs in anxious youth, such as behavioral difficulties at bedtime (eg, fear of the dark, overreliance on parents at bedtime) and nighttime wakings. CBT for insomnia can also importantly target more substantial sleep challenges for anxious youth. In addition, preliminary research suggests that comprehensive CBT approaches for anxiety have some beneficial secondary effects for SRPs, and psychopharmacology can also address SRPs as they relate to youth anxiety, although they are not typically recommended as first-line treatments.

There are a number of important future directions for clinical research to explore. Although it is apparent that SRPs are relevant to child anxiety, more research is needed using empirically validated, multimethod assessment approaches to clarify the nature of the relationship between particular SRPs and anxiety conditions. This literature would also be strengthened by taking care to look at samples more specifically by developmental stages. Given the critical changes in sleep development over time, looking at broad samples of age-varying youth might mask important differences. Additionally, the intervention literature is promising but still in a nascent stage. More rigorous interventions are needed to address the extent to which SRPs are mitigated by standard anxiety treatment approaches. If such research demonstrates significant residual sleep challenges, the development of psychotherapy interventions to specifically target SRPs as a standalone or adjunct treatment for youth anxiety may be warranted.

## CLINICS CARE POINTS

- CBT and psychopharmacology have demonstrated efficacy in the treatment of anxiety disorders, and a growing body of research demonstrates that both treatments may also improve SRPs in youth with anxiety even when sleep difficulties are not directly targeted.

- Interventions that include CBT have been generally shown to be more effective in targeting SRPs than those that do not include CBT.

- A limited body of research of specific cognitive and behavioral techniques to target sleep difficulties in anxious youth has demonstrated promising results.

- CBT for insomnia has demonstrated efficacy for the treatment of insomnia in adolescents, and treatment of insomnia has shown some positive effects on youth anxiety.

- Medications such as SSRIs have been shown to improve both youth anxiety as well as associated SRPs.

- Although other medications may also lead to improvements in youth anxiety and SRPs (such as benzodiazepines), behavioral interventions are recommended as the first-line treatment.

## REFERENCES

1. Beesdo K, Knappe S, Pine DS. Anxiety and anxiety disorders in children and adolescents: developmental issues and implications for DSM-V. Psychiatr Clin North Am 2009;32(3):483–524.
2. Alfano CA, Ginsburg GS, Kingery JN. Sleep-related problems among children and adolescents with anxiety disorders. J Am Acad Child Adolesc Psychiatry 2007;46(2):224–32.
3. Alfano CA, Pina AA, Zerr AA, et al. Pre-sleep arousal and sleep problems of anxiety-disordered youth. Child Psychiatry Hum Dev 2010;41(2):156–67.
4. Chase RM, Pincus DB. Sleep-related problems in children and adolescents with anxiety disorders. Behav Sleep Med 2011;9(4):224–36.
5. Meltzer LJ, McLaughlin Crabtree V. Pediatric sleep problems: a clinician's guide to behavioral interventions. Washington (DC): American Psychological Association; 2015.
6. Peterman JS, Carper MM, Kendall PC. Anxiety disorders and comorbid sleep problems in school-aged youth: review and future research directions. Child Psychiatry Hum Dev 2015;46(3):376–92.
7. American Psychiatric Association. Diagnostic and statistical manual of mental disorders. 5th edition. Washington (DC): American Psychiatric Association; 2013.
8. Alfano CA, Zakem AH, Costa NM, et al. Sleep problems and their relation to cognitive factors, anxiety, and depressive symptoms in children and adolescents. Depress Anxiety 2009;26(6):503–12.
9. Becker SP. External validity of children's self-reported sleep functioning: associations with academic, social, and behavioral adjustment. Sleep Med 2014; 15(9):1094–100.
10. Fletcher FE, Conduit R, Foster-Owens MD, et al. The association between anxiety symptoms and sleep in school-aged children: a combined insight from the children's sleep habits questionnaire and actigraphy. Behav Sleep Med 2018; 16(2):169–84.
11. Muris P, Merckelbach H, Ollendick TH, et al. Children's nighttime fears: parent–child ratings of frequency, content, origins, coping behaviors and severity. Behav Res Ther 2001;39(1):13–28.

12. Muris P, Merckelbach H, Mayer B, et al. How serious are common childhood fears? Behav Res Ther 2000;38(3):217–28.
13. El Rafihi-Ferreira R, Lewis KM, McFayden T, et al. Predictors of nighttime fears and sleep problems in young children. J Child Fam Stud 2019;28(4):941–9.
14. Reid GJ, Hong RY, Wade TJ. The relation between common sleep problems and emotional and behavioral problems among 2- and 3-year-olds in the context of known risk factors for psychopathology. J Sleep Res 2009;18(1):49–59.
15. Hudson JL, Gradisar M, Gamble A, et al. The sleep patterns and problems of clinically anxious children. Behav Res Ther 2009;47(4):339–44.
16. Fuligni AJ, Hardway C. Daily variation in adolescents' sleep, activities, and psychological well-being. J Adolesc 2006;16(3):353–78.
17. Ojio Y, Nishida A, Shimodera S, et al. Sleep duration associated with the lowest risk of depression/anxiety in adolescents. Sleep 2016;39(8):1555–62.
18. Zhang J, Paksarian D, Lamers F, et al. Sleep patterns and mental health correlates in US adolescents. J Pediatr 2017;182:137–43.
19. Rubens SL, Evans SC, Becker SP, et al. Self-reported time in bed and sleep quality in association with internalizing and externalizing symptoms in school-age youth. Child Psychiatry Hum Dev 2017;48(3):455–67.
20. Alfano CA, Patriquin MA, De Los Reyes A. Subjective-objective sleep comparisons and discrepancies among clinically-anxious and healthy children. J Abnorm Child Psychol 2015;43(7):1343–53.
21. Mullin BC, Pyle L, Haraden D, et al. A preliminary multimethod comparison of sleep among adolescents with and without generalized anxiety disorder. J Clin Child Adolesc Psychol 2017;46(2):198–210.
22. Steinsbekk S, Wichstrøm L. Stability of sleep disorders from preschool to first grade and their bidirectional relationship with psychiatric symptoms. J Dev Behav Pediatr 2015;36(4):243–51.
23. Armstrong JM, Ruttle PL, Klein MH, et al. Associations of child insomnia, sleep movement, and their persistence with mental health symptoms in childhood and adolescence. Sleep 2014;37(5):901–9.
24. Harvey AG, Stinson K, Whitaker KL, et al. The subjective meaning of sleep quality: a comparison of individuals with and without insomnia. Sleep 2008;31(3):383–93.
25. Forbes EE, Bertocci MA, Gregory AM, et al. Objective sleep in pediatric anxiety disorders and major depressive disorder. J Am Acad Child Adolesc Psychiatry 2008;47(2):148–55.
26. Kelly RJ, El-Sheikh M. Reciprocal relations between children's sleep and their adjustment over time. Dev Psychol 2014;50(4):1137–47.
27. Alfano CA, Beidel DC, Turner SM, et al. Preliminary evidence for sleep complaints among children referred for anxiety. Sleep Med 2006;7(6):467–73.
28. Muris P, Merckelbach H, Gadet B, et al. Fears, worries, and scary dreams in 4- to 12-year-old children: their content, developmental pattern, and origins. J Clin Child Psychol 2000;29(1):43–52.
29. Reynolds KC, Alfano CA. Things that go bump in the night: frequency and predictors of nightmares in anxious and nonanxious children. Behav Sleep Med 2016;14(4):442–56.
30. Steinsbekk S, Berg-Nielsen TS, Wichstrøm L. Sleep disorders in preschoolers: prevalence and comorbidity with psychiatric symptoms. J Dev Behav Pediatr 2013;34(9):633–41.
31. Gauchat A, Seguin J, Zadra A. Prevalence and correlates of disturbed dreaming in children. Pathol Biol (Paris) 2014;62(5):311–8.

32. Secrist ME, Dalenberg CJ, Gevirtz R. Contributing factors predicting nightmares in children: trauma, anxiety, dissociation, and emotion regulation. Psychol Trauma 2019;11(1):114–21.

33. Lebowitz ER, Shimshoni Y, Silverman WK. Family accommodation mediates nightmares and sleep-related problems in anxious children. J Anxiety Disord 2019;62:94–9.

34. Petit D, Touchette É, Tremblay RE, et al. Dyssomnias and parasomnias in early childhood. Pediatrics 2007;119(5):1016–25.

35. Gau S-F, Soong W-T. Psychiatric comorbidity of adolescents with sleep terrors or sleepwalking: a case-control study. Aust N Z J Psychiatry 1999;33(5):734–9.

36. Shanahan L, Copeland WE, Angold A, et al. Sleep problems predict and are predicted by generalized anxiety/depression and oppositional defiant disorder. J Am Acad Child Adolesc Psychiatry 2014;53(5):550–8.

37. Leahy E, Gradisar M. Dismantling the bidirectional relationship between paediatric sleep and anxiety. Clin Psychol 2012;16(1):44–56.

38. Lima RA, de Barros MVG, dos Santos MAM, et al. The synergic relationship between social anxiety, depressive symptoms, poor sleep quality and body fatness in adolescents. J Affect Disord 2020;260:200–5.

39. Nabinger de Diaz NA, Farrell LJ, Waters AM, et al. Sleep-related problems in pediatric obsessive-compulsive disorder and intensive exposure therapy. Behav Ther 2019;50(3):608–20.

40. Storch EA, Murphy TK, Lack CW, et al. Sleep-related problems in pediatric obsessive-compulsive disorder. J Anxiety Disord 2008;22(5):877–85.

41. Ivarsson T, Larsson B. Sleep problems as reported by parents in Swedish children and adolescents with obsessive-compulsive disorder (OCD), child psychiatric outpatients and school children. Nord J Psychiatry 2009;63(6):480–4.

42. Alfano CA, Kim KL. Objective sleep patterns and severity of symptoms in pediatric obsessive compulsive disorder: a pilot investigation. J Anxiety Disord 2011; 25(6):835–9.

43. Alfano CA. (Re)conceptualizing sleep among children with anxiety disorders: where to next? Clin Child Fam Psychol Rev 2018;21(4):482–99.

44. McMakin DL, Alfano CA. Sleep and anxiety in late childhood and early adolescence. Curr Opin Psychiatry 2015;28:483–9.

45. Gregory AM, Eley TC, O'Connor TG, et al. Etiologies of associations between childhood sleep and behavioral problems in a large twin sample. J Am Acad Child Adolesc Psychiatry 2004;43(6):744–51.

46. Whalen DJ, Gilbert KE, Barch DM, et al. Variation in common preschool sleep problems as an early predictor for depression and anxiety symptom severity across time. J Child Psychol Psychiatry 2017;58(2):151–9.

47. Sadeh A, Dahl RE, Shahar G, et al. Sleep and the transition to adolescence: a longitudinal study. Sleep 2009;32(12):1602–9.

48. Bai S, Ricketts EJ, Thamrin H, et al. Longitudinal study of sleep and internalizing problems in youth treated for pediatric anxiety disorders. J Abnorm Child Psychol 2020;48(1):67–77.

49. Cousins JC, Whalen DJ, Dahl RE, et al. The bidirectional association between daytime affect and nighttime sleep in youth with anxiety and depression. J Pediatr Psychol 2011;36(9):969–79.

50. Peterman JS, Carper MM, Elkins RM, et al. The effects of cognitive-behavioral therapy for youth anxiety on sleep problems. J Anxiety Disord 2016;37:78–88.

51. Mindell JA, Leichman ES, DuMond C, et al. Sleep and social-emotional development in infants and toddlers. J Clin Child Adolesc Psychol 2017;46(2):236–46.

52. Sharon T, Woolley JD. Do monsters dream? Young children's understanding of the fantasy/reality distinction. Br J Dev Psychol 2004;22(2):293–310.

53. Gordon J, King NJ, Gullone E, et al. Treatment of children's nighttime fears: the need for a modern randomised controlled trial. Clin Psychol Rev 2007;27(1): 98–113.

54. Crowley SJ, Acebo C, Carskadon MA. Sleep, circadian rhythms, and delayed phase in adolescence. Sleep Med 2007;8(6):602–12.

55. Hoyt LT, Maslowsky J, Olson JS, et al. Adolescent sleep barriers: profiles within a diverse sample of urban youth. J Youth Adolesc 2018;47(10):2169–80.

56. Wittmann M, Dinich J, Merrow M, et al. Social jetlag: misalignment of biological and social time. Chronobiol Int 2006;23(1–2):497–509.

57. Bartel KA, Gradisar M, Williamson P. Protective and risk factors for adolescent sleep: a meta-analytic review. Sleep Med Rev 2015;21:72–85.

58. Heath M, Johnston A, Dohnt H, et al. The role of pre-sleep cognitions in adolescent sleep-onset problems. Sleep Med 2018;46:117–21.

59. Stewart E, Gibb B, Strauss G, et al. Disruptions in the amount and timing of sleep and repetitive negative thinking in adolescents. Behav Sleep Med 2018;18(2): 217–25.

60. Moore M. Bedtime problems and night wakings: treatment of behavioral insomnia of childhood. J Clin Psychol 2010;66(11):1195–204.

61. Honaker SM, Meltzer LJ. Bedtime problems and night wakings in young children: an update of the evidence. Paediatr Respir Rev 2014;15(4):333–9.

62. Freeman KA. Treating bedtime resistance with the bedtime pass: a systematic replication and component analysis with 3-year-olds. J Appl Behav Anal 2006; 39(4):423–8.

63. Moore BA, Friman PC, Fruzzetti AE, et al. Brief report: evaluating the Bedtime Pass Program for child resistance to bedtime–A randomized, controlled trial. J Pediatr Psychol 2007;32(3):283–7.

64. Kushnir J, Sadeh A. Assessment of brief interventions for nighttime fears in preschool children. Eur J Pediatr 2012;171(1):67–75.

65. Clementi MA, Alfano CA. Targeted behavioral therapy for childhood generalized anxiety disorder: a time-series analysis of changes in anxiety and sleep. J Anxiety Disord 2014;28(2):215–22.

66. McMakin DL, Ricketts EJ, Forbes EE, et al. Anxiety treatment and targeted sleep enhancement to address sleep disturbance in pre/early adolescents with anxiety. J Clin Child Adolesc Psychol 2019;48(Suppl 1):S284–97.

67. Dahl R, Harvey A, Forbes E, et al. Sleeping TIGERS: a treatment for sleep problems in young people. Treatment manual. Pittsburgh (PA): University of Pittsburgh; 2009.

68. Blake MJ, Sheeber LB, Youssef GJ, et al. Systematic review and meta-analysis of adolescent cognitive–behavioral sleep interventions. Clin Child Fam Psychol Rev 2017;20(3):227–49.

69. Blake MJ, Trinder JA, Allen NB. Mechanisms underlying the association between insomnia, anxiety, and depression in adolescence: implications for behavioral sleep interventions. Clin Psychol Rev 2018;63:25–40.

70. Walkup JT, Albano AM, Piacentini J, et al. Cognitive behavioral therapy, sertraline, or a combination in childhood anxiety. N Engl J Med 2008;359(26):2753–66.

71. Kendall PC, Hedtke KA. Cognitive-behavioral therapy for anxious children: therapist manual. 3rd edition. Ardmore (PA): Workbook Publishing; 2006.

72. Caporino NE, Read KL, Shiffrin N, et al. Sleep-related problems and the effects of anxiety treatment in children and adolescents. J Clin Child Adolesc Psychol 2015; 46(5):675–85.

73. Wehry AM, Beesdo-Baum K, Hennelly MM, et al. Assessment and treatment of anxiety disorders in children and adolescents. Curr Psychiatry Rep 2015; 17(52):1–11.

74. Owens JA. Pharmacotherapy of pediatric insomnia. J Am Acad Child Adolesc Psychiatry 2009;48(2):99.

75. Baglioni C, Nanovska S, Regen W, et al. Sleep and mental disorders: a meta-analysis of polysomnographic research. Psychol Bull 2016;142(9):969–90.

76. Owens JA, Spirito A, McGuinn M. The Children's Sleep Habits Questionnaire (CSHQ): psychometric properties of a survey instrument for school-aged children. Sleep 2000;23(8):1043–52.

77. Bruni O, Ottaviano S, Guidetti V, et al. The Sleep Disturbance Scale for Children (SDSC): construction and validation of an instrument to evaluate sleep disturbances in childhood and adolescence. J Sleep Res 1996;5(4):251–61.

78. Buysse DJ, Ancoli-Israel S, Edinger JD, et al. Recommendations for a standard research assessment of insomnia. Sleep 2006;29(9):1155–73.

79. Sadeh A. Sleep assessment methods. Monogr Soc Res Child Dev 2015;80(1): 33–48.

# Afraid and Awake

## The Interaction Between Trauma and Sleep in Children and Adolescents

Veronica Fellman, DO[a],*, Patrick J. Heppell, Psy.D[a],
Suchet Rao, MD[b]

### KEYWORDS

- Sleep disorders • Children • Adolescents • Trauma • PTSD • Trauma treatment
- Sleep treatment

### KEY POINTS

- Traumatic experiences and sleep disturbances are both common in children and adolescents.
- Sleep-related issues and trauma responses share physiologic commonalities and thus interact with one another.
- A mental health evaluation should be trauma informed and should include a specific assessment of sleep complaints.
- Trauma-informed treatments, including both psychological and psychopharmacologic interventions, should directly address any identified sleep issues for best results.

### INTRODUCTION

"Maria, give me your phone right now! It's 1:43 AM and you have an algebra test in 6 hours!" screams Ms Vega, an exhausted but caring mother.

Ms Vega's 13-year-old daughter Maria hands the phone to her mother, who continues shouting: "I've warned you all night, I'm not paying your phone bills for the next 3 months!" Maria looks defeated but wired at the same time. She screams back, throws her heavy blanket over her head, and starts crying.

This kind of exchange has been happening nightly for the past 2 years. Family friends, school personnel, and even Maria's pediatrician have recommended for M.

This article originally appeared in *Child and Adolescent Psychiatric Clinics*, Volume 30 Issue 1, January 2021.
[a] Department of Child and Adolescent Psychiatry, NYU Grossman School of Medicine, Child Study Center, One Park Avenue, 7th Floor, New York City, NY 10016, USA; [b] Psychiatry and Behavioral Health, NYC Administration for Children's Services, 150 William Street, 11th Floor, New York City, NY 10038, USA
* Corresponding author.
*E-mail address:* Veronica.fellman@nyulangone.org

Psychiatr Clin N Am 47 (2024) 229–253
https://doi.org/10.1016/j.psc.2023.06.015

Vega to be stronger and more consistent. Warnings, removal of privileges, arguments, punishments, and behavioral charts have yielded the same results: a quiet and grumpy mother-daughter pair each morning.

When Ms Vega speaks to other adults, the same questions recur: Is Maria nocturnal? Defiant? Addicted to her phone? On drugs? Or just a typical 13-year-old in constant need of social interaction?

During a heated argument with her own mother, Ms Vega expresses her fear that "maybe she's bipolar like her dad ... I knew I shouldn't have stayed with that crazy man..."

Maria has never felt able to tell her mom, or anyone, about the things that keep her awake at night: the fear that her mother is in danger, or that her father will come back; her guilt that she is the reason he left; her worry about having to face more bullying from kids at school when they think she's being weird.

The fear that her daughter will end up like her ex-husband prompts Ms Vega to make an appointment for Maria to receive a mental health evaluation.

## BACKGROUND AND PREVALENCE

Sleep issues may be considered to be a part of the typical teenage experience, although less than 8% of teenagers sleep for the recommended number of hours each night.[1] Younger children also experience frequent sleep problems,[2] but what is normal, and what may be reflective of a mental health issue worthy of further evaluation?

Disturbance in sleep is common in many psychiatric disorders, including bipolar disorder, depressive disorders, and generalized anxiety disorder. Importantly for this article, sleep disturbances are also common in posttraumatic stress disorder (PTSD),[3] a combination that is under-recognized, and thus undertreated, in the pediatric population.

### What Is Trauma?

The National Child Traumatic Stress Network defines a traumatic event as "a frightening, dangerous, or violent event that poses a threat to a child's life or bodily integrity. Witnessing a traumatic event that threatens the life or physical security of a loved one can also be traumatic."[4] However, trauma is a reality for many young people in the United States. It comes in many forms (**Fig. 1**) and these forms often co-occur. According to the 2016 National Survey of Children's Health, 46% of the nation's youth aged 17 years and younger reported having experienced at least 1 trauma, whereas 22% had experienced more than 2 types of trauma.[5]

Maria has experienced various forms of trauma, but, as is often the case, only she has knowledge of this.

### Classic Posttraumatic Stress Disorder Versus Complex Trauma

Classic PTSD, as described in the Diagnostic Statistical Manual of Mental Disorders, Fifth Edition (DSM-5[3]) requires both an "exposure to actual or threatened death, serious injury, or sexual violence" and symptoms including "intrusion, persistent avoidance, negative alterations in cognitions and mood, and marked alterations in arousal and reactivity" that are experienced persistently for at least 1 month and cause an impairment in a person's functioning.

Since the groundbreaking Adverse Childhood Experiences (ACE) study,[6] further studies have shown that repeated trauma or multiple traumatic experiences can cause complex and wide-ranging damage across the lifespan.[7] Often referred to as complex

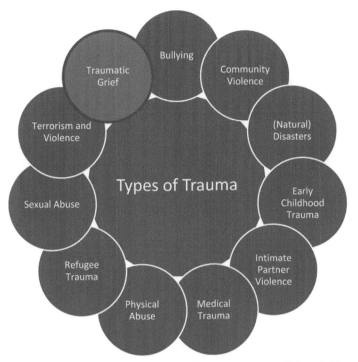

**Fig. 1.** Types of trauma. (*Data from* National Child Traumatic Stress Network. Trauma types. Available at: https://www.nctsn.org/what-is-child-trauma/trauma-types.)

trauma or developmental trauma disorder, traumatic experiences, especially when ongoing and chronic, affect the whole self and derail the developmental trajectories of children and adolescents in many ways (**Fig. 2**).

Despite efforts to make the DSM-5 criteria for PTSD more developmentally sensitive and to lower the threshold for diagnosing PTSD in children and adolescents,[8] and the International Classification of Diseases 11th Revision's inclusion of a separate and specific complex PTSD diagnosis,[9] complex trauma remains underidentified, misdiagnosed, and undertreated, especially in children and adolescents.[10]

### Diagnostic Pitfalls

Not all individuals with a trauma history meet criteria for PTSD, and those who do may also meet criteria for other disorders, most often anxiety and depressive disorders. Such comorbidity is common, and creates challenges with respect to accurate diagnosis and management. The varied presentation of complex trauma also leads to a risk of misdiagnosis with disorders including oppositional defiant disorder; attention-deficit/hyperactivity disorder (ADHD); and even conduct disorder, bipolar disorder, and schizophrenia.[10]

### The Biological Effects of Trauma

When faced with a threat, epinephrine, norepinephrine, and cortisol are released, triggering the body's natural and automatic fight-or-flight response. This response leads to increased blood flow to large muscles, intensification of the senses, and increased focused attention. Blood pressure and blood sugar concentrations increase to boost

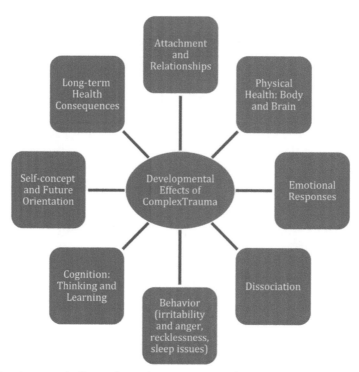

**Fig. 2.** Developmental effects of complex trauma on children and adolescents. (*Data from* National Child Traumatic Stress Network. Complex trauma effects. Available at: https://www.nctsn.org/what-is-child-trauma/trauma-types/complex-trauma/effects.)

the flow of energy to the muscles.[10] The same changes can also be activated when experiencing a trauma reminder or trigger (in Maria's case, this may include experiencing a flashback about scary disputes between her father and mother).

Ongoing trauma also leads to longer-term neurobiological effects on the brain, such as a greater role of the amygdala and the automatic fear reactions over the conscious thinking of the prefrontal cortex. Chronically increased cortisol levels leave adolescents constantly on edge and over-reactive, or, conversely, completely shut down, with inadequate reactions to real threats.[10] There are many factors influencing how any particular individual reacts to trauma (**Fig. 3**).

### Associations Between Sleep and Trauma/Posttraumatic Stress Disorder: a Reciprocal Relationship

Although the associations between sleep, mental disorder, and complex PTSD are still being studied, there is growing evidence supporting a reciprocal relationship between sleep disruption and mental disorder, including for adolescents with PTSD and anxiety, and adolescents who have a history of trauma.[25] Exposure to trauma may lead to sleep disturbances, whereas sleep disturbances may be a risk factor for the development of mental disorder,[11] especially depression and anxiety,[12] which then increases the likelihood of the person developing PTSD symptoms (**Fig. 4**).

### Exposure to Trauma and Its Impact on Sleep Disturbances

The physiology of sleep is complex and varies across the lifespan (discussed elsewhere in this issue). Although not all individuals who have experienced trauma develop

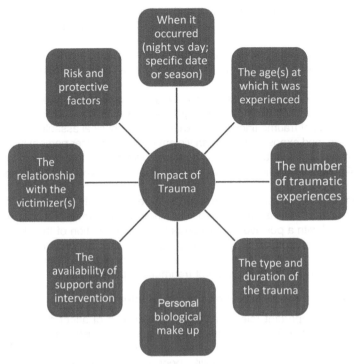

**Fig. 3.** Factors influencing reactions to trauma.

PTSD, most of those who are diagnosed with PTSD experience sleep disturbances.[13] These relationships are complex, not fully understood, and have been mostly studied in adults.

The findings regarding how trauma affects sleep physiology are also varied. For example, there is some agreement that adults with PTSD, especially older adults, tend to have more stage 1 sleep, less slow wave sleep, and increased rapid eye movement (REM) density.[14] Patients with PTSD show increased central arousal, which interferes with consolidation of REM sleep.[15,16]

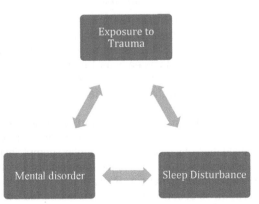

**Fig. 4.** The reciprocal relationship between trauma, sleep disturbance, and mental disorder.

It is well established that both acute and chronic childhood trauma are associated with sleep difficulties, not only soon after the event but continuing even decades later.[17–20]

Trauma is associated with sleep disturbances including nightmares, fragmented sleep, initial insomnia, fatigue, sensations (such as a feeling of falling) at night, light sleep, and night anxiety.[21–23]

What is less clear is whether a specific type of trauma results in a specific type of sleep disturbance. For example, although some studies have found that exposure to various types of trauma (including sexual trauma, physical assault, accidents, natural disasters, and exposure to sudden violent death of another person) increases the odds of insomnia 2-fold to 3-fold,[24] others have found that only childhood emotional neglect significantly predicted higher levels of insomnia for young adults[25] and college students.[26]

Childhood sexual abuse has been found to increase the rate of insomnia in adults. It is also associated with insomnia, sleep avoidance, and nightmares in children and adolescents,[27,28] with a positive correlation between the duration of the abuse and the severity of the symptoms.[29] However, it is also clear that, although nightmares are a frequent experience of children and adolescents and lead to poor sleep, they are not always associated with a history of traumatic experiences.[30]

### Sleep Disturbance and Its Impact on Trauma Symptoms

Sleep plays an important role in restoration, regulation of affect and behavior, and cognitive processing. There is some evidence that sleep disturbance interferes with normal emotional and cognitive processes and is thus potentially responsible for the attention issues, dysregulation, irritability, poor decision making, and poor anger management often associated with PTSD symptoms.[31] The impact of sleep disturbance on the development of mental disorder and trauma symptoms is thought to result not only from shared and overlapping regulatory systems but also from sleep disturbance itself being a risk factor for developing PTSD[32] and, interestingly, for being revictimized, as shown by Noll and colleagues[27] in a sample of young women with a history of childhood sexual abuse, even after controlling for PTSD and depression. Further evidence comes from adults' responses to trauma treatment: treatments that specifically target nightmares lead to greater PTSD symptom reduction, whereas treatments that fail to directly address sleep issues do not result in such improvement.[33]

### The Importance of Evaluating Both Trauma and Sleep

Sleep disturbances have been identified as a key risk factor for PTSD,[11] possibly because of shared neurologic pathways. Following a traumatic event, the impairment of normal sleep processes is one of the most frequent and distressing complaints.[34] Furthermore, from sleep complaints as early as 1 month after a trauma, it is possible to detect patients who will later develop chronic PTSD,[35] whereas the presence of nightmares may indicate how psychologically traumatic a stressful event or trauma could become.[36]

Given the widespread prevalence of trauma (particularly in children presenting for mental health evaluation or treatment) and the various ways in which trauma may affect sleep,[16] any evaluation of a child with a presenting complaint of a sleep problem should also include an evaluation of the child's trauma history and its possible impact. Similarly, any child who is found to have a history of trauma should be evaluated for a sleep disturbance. The value of such an approach is supported by the results of treatment studies, because trauma-informed treatments that do not address sleep complaints fail to significantly improve sleep disturbances, whereas treatments that specifically target nightmares lead to overall improvements in PTSD symptoms in adults.[37]

Thus, careful assessment of PTSD symptoms, trauma history, and sleep complaints is vital for a comprehensive evaluation, and, if both are present, both PTSD symptoms and sleep complaints should be directly targeted in treatment.

## HOW TO EVALUATE SLEEP DISTURBANCES IN THE CONTEXT OF TRAUMA (AND VICE VERSA)

A thorough mental health evaluation of a child presenting with trauma and a sleep disturbance should involve more than just a cursory examination asking whether the child has had any difficulty sleeping in the past 3 months. Such an evaluation may rely on the following, and the extent to which each is used depends on the circumstances under which the evaluation is occurring:

- Clinical interview of the child
- Obtaining collateral information from the primary, and other, caregivers (eg, a parent, a foster parent, a teacher)
- The use of semistructured/structured assessments such as the Pittsburgh Sleep Quality Index (PSQI)[38] or the Child PTSD Symptom Scale (CPSS)[39]
- Other tests (eg, polysomnography, sleep actigraphy)

### The Presenting Complaint

The nature of the presenting complaint for a child with a history of both trauma and sleep problems depends on various factors, including:

- The age of the child
- The person giving the presenting complaint
- The context in which the evaluation is occurring

### Age
Given that, as is developmentally appropriate, preschool and early school-aged children exposed to trauma are less likely to be able to articulate the presence of psychological distress or internalizing symptoms (eg, anxiety, depression), they are more likely to present with externalizing symptoms such as aggressive, impulsive, or otherwise inappropriate or unwanted behavior. Children of this age are also less likely to be able to provide a temporal relationship between the occurrence of trauma and the onset of a sleep problem. In such instances, the caregiver must be relied on to provide such contextual details.

### Person
Caregivers are more likely to report externalizing symptoms or behavioral problems but may be less aware of other sleep-related problems, particularly among adolescents.[40] **Table 1** outlines the likely source of different sleep-related complaints.

### Context
A sleep problem may be the first indicator of the hyperarousal associated with exposure to trauma,[35] or the sleep problem may occur simultaneously with or later than other signs and symptoms.[41,42] Regardless, a sleep problem is unlikely to result in a child being brought to a psychiatric emergency room or comprehensive psychiatric emergency program for evaluation unless there is an associated behavioral problem[43]

| Table 1 Presenting complaints for children with trauma and sleep difficulties | | |
|---|---|---|
| **Complaint Made Primarily by the Child** | **Complaint Made by Either the Child or the Caregiver** | **Complaint Made Primarily by the Caregiver** |
| Being unable to fall/stay asleep or return to sleep | The child is scared to go to bed or to sleep | The child is showing behavioral problems, especially at night |
| Hearing voices or seeing things (eg, shadows) at night[44] | The child is reporting nightmares | The child's school performance is poor, or teachers are complaining about the child's behavior |
| Daytime sleepiness | — | — |

or other psychiatric complaint. However, as frequently observed in clinical settings, a sleep issue may be the only presenting complaint given at the time of an initial evaluation in an outpatient clinic. As discussed earlier, any child presenting primarily with a sleep complaint should be evaluated for trauma.

As discussed earlier, the sleep-related symptoms of trauma may be divided into 3 broad categories. **Table 2** outlines some of the complaints that may accompany symptoms in each of these categories.

In order to ascertain whether a history of trauma is contributing to a child's sleep issue, it is necessary to determine a temporal relationship between the two. A clear timeline informed by child and collateral reporter, such as a parent/guardian, helps to establish whether symptoms developed following a trauma.

### Assessment of Trauma

Determining the nature of the trauma is important with respect to treatment of the trauma, although it may be of less relevance with respect to the treatment of the accompanying sleep issue. Although some studies[45] have found that children who had experienced physical abuse experienced more sleep disturbance than children who had been sexually abused, others have hypothesized that sexual abuse may be more likely to be implicated in the exacerbation of sleep-related trauma symptoms because such abuse may be more likely to occur either in a bedroom or at night.

| Table 2 Posttraumatic stress disorder criteria and sleep-related complaints | |
|---|---|
| **PTSD Criterion** | **How Might It Present?** |
| Criterion B: intrusion | • Increased reports of nightmares[a]<br>• Being unable to fall asleep or waking up at night<br>• The child asking to sleep with a caregiver<br>• The child complaining of hearing voices or seeing things |
| Criterion C: avoidance | • The child delaying the bedtime routine<br>• The child making excuses not to go to bed<br>• Increased use of substances at night |
| Criterion E: hyperarousal | • The child becoming more agitated, anxious, or argumentative at night<br>• Increased behavioral problems at night |

[a] The content of the nightmares is not necessarily related to the trauma.[42]

| Table 3 |  |
|---|---|
| **Externalizing and internalizing symptoms** |  |
| **Externalizing Symptoms** | **Internalizing Symptoms** |
| Behavioral problems | Psychological distress |
| Aggression | Anxiety |
| Oppositionality | Depression |
| Defiance | — |
| Substance use/misuse | — |

As discussed earlier, notwithstanding the amendments made to the criteria for PTSD with the arrival of DSM-5, the developmental effect of persistent and pervasive exposure to trauma remains incompletely captured by the DSM definition of PTSD,[46] and the impact of trauma on development may in part be linked, perhaps via the effect of trauma on the autonomic system as a whole, to alterations in sleep.[42,47,48]

Therefore, rather than presenting with classic PTSD, many children with a history of such trauma, regardless of the specific nature of the trauma, may present, for example, with symptoms consistent with disruptive mood dysregulation disorder, conduct disorder, an anxiety disorder, a mood disorder, or a substance use disorder in addition to their sleep disturbance. The child's presenting features may be broadly categorized as being either internalizing or externalizing symptoms (**Table 3**).

It should be noted that the same child may present at different times with features of either, or a combination of both, categories, and that either of the types of clinical features may contribute, directly or indirectly, to a sleep impairment, or, conversely, they may be exacerbated by impaired sleep.

Apparent behavioral problems may be secondary to the autonomic hyperarousal that is characteristically seen in people exposed to trauma. Depending on the specific nature of the problems that arise as a result of this hyperarousal, and the level of (or lack of) recognition of such symptoms as being attributable in large part to trauma, children presenting this way may or may not be treated with medication, which may have unintentional effects on sleep.

Beyond the contribution of hyperarousal to various sleep issues, the choice of medication may also have an impact: choosing a stimulant to treat what could be viewed as the hyperactivity of ADHD may result in further worsening of the child's hyperarousal, whereas opting for an atypical antipsychotic or mood-stabilizing medication to manage suspected bipolar disorder may worsen diurnal sedation and sleep phase shifts.

### Psychiatric Disorders to Rule Out

Given that mood, anxiety, trauma-related disorders, and stressor-related disorders, and of course primary sleep disorders, may all cause sleep disturbance, and that they all may co-occur, it is important that clinicians treating people with disordered sleep make attempts to determine what disorders are present and to what extent they are affecting the individuals' sleep.

### Bipolar and related disorders

As indicated earlier, significant behavioral problems are often attributed to early-onset bipolar disorder. When considering such a diagnosis, care must be taken to ascertain whether there exists a pattern of discrete episodes of mania or hypomania characteristic of bipolar disorder rather than the chronic emotional and behavioral dysregulation often associated with the combination of poor sleep and exposure to trauma. In addition, the sleep disturbance seen in bipolar disorder is the result of a reduced need and desire for sleep rather than an inability to sleep. In addition, given the low prevalence of mania in prepubertal children,[49,50] an abundance of caution should be exercised before making a bipolar diagnosis in young children.

### Schizophrenia spectrum and other psychotic disorders

Trauma can result in the emergence of psychosislike experiences (PLEs).[44] These PLEs should be differentiated from the psychotic symptoms seen in schizophrenia and related disorders. The absence of the so-called negative symptoms and cognitive decline that often accompany true psychotic disorders, in conjunction with the nature and timing of PLES, as well as the context within which PLEs occur, can be very informative in this regard. As with bipolar disorder, clinicians should remain mindful of the low prevalence of primary psychotic disorders in young children.[51] Sleep disturbances are a known factor that may exacerbate the expression of PLEs.[44]

As discussed earlier, problematic sleep may be both an effect of trauma and other disorders and also a contributing factor to the development of, or lack of ability to satisfactorily recover from, other disorders.

Maria meets with a reflective clinician:

"What keeps you up at night?"

"I talk to my friends on the phone, and some games I got into."

"Of course. Anything other than your phone? I mean, like, are you on your phone all day long?"

"No."

"So what's the purpose of the phone at night, or what keeps you up at night on your phone?"

"I just can't fall asleep ... I want to fall asleep, I'm tired, but I just can't."

"Is it your body keeping you awake, like feeling restless, full of energy ... or more your brain? Like you're thinking about things and you can't just turn it off?"

"Hmmmmm ... definitely my thoughts, and something else, but no, never mind ... it's my thoughts."

"It seems like there's something else you want to share with me ... just so you know, many kids and adults have a hard time sleeping, and there are many reason why that may be. I know it can be annoying, frustrating, confusing, and scary to not be able to fall asleep."

"Well ... sometimes ... I don't know how to say this, but it's like, I still hear my dad screaming at my mom, and like stuff being thrown around the living room ... you'll think I'm crazy, but he's been gone for like 6 years..."

She pauses.

"I miss him so much."

"It's like you are reliving some of those scary moments, and I'm guessing the phone helps you disconnect or distract yourself from all of it..."

"Something like that. And then, when my mom takes it away, she screams at me and it just makes it worse! So then I just throw myself under the covers, and try to cry so I don't hear it anymore."

"Just like..."

"Just like I used to do when it was actually happening ... wait, are you going to put me in the mental ward 'cause I'm like schizophrenic or something?

"I don't think so ... you are describing a pretty normal response to something scary. Let me ask you, why do you think you don't need the phone during the day, at school or even at home?

"I don't know. At school I have my friends, and anyway, it never happens during the day."

"It?"

"Me hearing things."

"And what about the fighting back then?"

"Mom and dad would only fight at night when my dad would come back late from work...."

"It must have been scary ... it must still be scary."

"Can we talk about something else ... I'm not crazy right?"

# TREATMENT
## Importance of Treating Sleep in Posttraumatic Stress Disorder

If sleep is one of the pathways by which the long-term effects of trauma are perpetuated, then sleep may also represent a potential behavioral target for intervention to reduce the negative, long-term health effects of childhood trauma.[37] Data repeatedly indicate that sleep-related symptoms of PTSD tend to persist despite otherwise successful treatments of daytime symptoms[52–54] (although many studies do not include sleep assessment). Following successful treatment of veterans' PTSD, clinically significant sleep disturbance remained 5 to 10 years later.[55] Similarly, clinically significant insomnia remained in adolescent girls following a successful use of a developmentally adapted exposure protocol.[55]

In addition to being refractory to treatment, sleep disturbance also disrupts the ability to heal from trauma and benefit from psychotherapy for PTSD. Sleep is integral to the mechanisms by which psychotherapy modalities create change. These mechanisms include cognitive processing, affective learning, consolidation of emotional memories, and fear extinction, all of which are disrupted by sleep dysregulation.[56] REM sleep is important for processing of traumatic memories and decoupling these memories from their emotional power.[57] It seems to be essential for fear extinction, the process by which a conditioned trigger for fear is relearned as safe. There is evidence suggesting that treating sleep symptoms may improve regulation of neuroendocrine and inflammatory pathways, possibly improving readiness for treatment.[58]

Treatment of PTSD may be more successful if it incorporates treatment of associated sleep disorders.[59] Treatments that target sleep-related symptoms can reduce daytime symptoms[60,61] and enhance readiness for psychotherapy by increasing confidence and compliance,[62] as well as biological capacity, as described earlier.

For all these reasons, specific treatment of sleep symptoms can be an important component of trauma treatment. However, as with so many areas of child psychiatry, there is a limited evidence base and so clinicians must extrapolate from adult data. This situation is complicated by age-dependent pharmacodynamics, different pharmacokinetics, and disease variations seen across the lifespan.[63] The specific phenomenology of PTSD in children further complicates a false equivalency. However, given the dearth of evidence, this article uses adult research to explore treatment options.

## Psychoeducation

Teaching children and families about symptoms, treatment, and therapeutic goals is the essential first step in treatment and must remain a component of care in an ongoing way. Clinicians can provide a specific rationale for each intervention and expectations for the timing of symptom relief.[64] For example, it may be helpful to

**Table 4**
**Psychological interventions for posttraumatic stress disorder that improve sleep**

| Treatment | Description | Citation | Population | Results |
|---|---|---|---|---|
| Prolonged exposure | Manualized treatment that includes imaginal and in vivo exposures to traumatic reminders | Brownlow et al,[55] 2016 | 61 adolescent girls | Improved sleep disturbance, but clinically significant insomnia symptoms remained |
| | | Gutner et al,[56] 2013 | 171 women | Improved insomnia and nightmare severity |
| Cognitive processing therapy[a] | Cognitive restructuring of maladaptive beliefs about trauma | Galovski et al,[71] 2009 | 108 women | Improved overall sleep and had large effects on insomnia and nightmare severity, but did not result in normal sleep |
| Eye movement desensitization and reprocessing | Based on the adaptive information processing model and the hypothesis that traumatic memories are inadequately stored | Raboni et al,[72] 2014 | 24 adults | More consolidated sleep, reduced awakenings |
| | | Meentken et al,[73] (2020) | 74 children with medically related subthreshold PTSD symptoms | Improved both subjective and parent reports of sleep |

[a] Developmentally adapted cognitive processing therapy has shown good efficacy for adolescents with PTSD but sleep-related specific measurements were not reported.[69,70]

describe that exposures will be necessarily uncomfortable but, over time, will decrease nightmares.

### Behavioral Approaches

Sleep hygiene is a necessary component of many interventions and should be introduced early. Simple interventions such as exercise and listening to relaxing music before bed have shown benefits.[65–67]

### Psychological Approaches

Psychological interventions are the first-line treatment of sleep disorders associated with PTSD. Choosing a modality of psychotherapy depends on treatment targets (ie, nightmares vs insomnia). **Table 4** includes a summary of interventions for PTSD that do not directly target sleep-related symptoms but show improvements in those symptoms. **Table 5** includes specific interventions for PTSD-related insomnia. **Table 6** includes specific interventions for PTSD-related nightmares. It is helpful to develop a clear treatment plan for specific symptoms in order to track progress, which can best be done with the use of rating scales (eg, The Pittsburgh Sleep Quality Index[38]) or a sleep diary.[68]

**Table 5**
**Psychological interventions for posttraumatic stress disorder–related insomnia**

| Treatment | Description | Citation | Population | Results |
|---|---|---|---|---|
| Cognitive behavior treatment of insomnia | Protocol typically includes (1) sleep restriction, (2) stimulus control, (3) sleep hygiene, (4) cognitive restructuring, (5) relaxation techniques | Talbot et al,[61] 2014 | 45 adults | Improved sleep and overall functioning |
| | | Kanady et al,[74] 2018, further analysis of Talbot et al's[61] data | 45 adults | Decreased fear of sleep |
| Narrative exposure therapy | Evidence-based, manualized treatment designed specifically for survivors of multiple traumatic exposures; it focuses on each exposure in chronologic order, taking a lifeline approach[75] | Park et al,[76] 2020 | 20 North Korean adolescent refugees | Substantially decreased insomnia and improved sleep quality after 5–10 sessions (lasting 6 mo after treatment) |

## Psychopharmacology

Psychotherapy remains the treatment of choice for PTSD and related sleep symptoms in children. The addition of medication can be considered when sleep symptoms are debilitating or refractory to treatment.[52,59,82] Some of the most commonly used medications are briefly discussed later, followed by a summary (**Table 7**) of significant research on patients with PTSD that can be used to guide decision making.

Although selective serotonin reuptake inhibitors (SSRIs) are widely acknowledged as a first-line treatment of PTSD (sertraline and paroxetine have US Food and Drug Administration approval for adults), they do not have consistent data supporting their efficacy in sleep symptoms in adults or children.[52] Activation and disinhibition in children are widely recognized side effects that could worsen sleep problems.[83]

Prazosin has long been a mainstay for the treatment of PTSD-related nightmares in both adults and increasingly in children.[84] It is a α1-adrenergic receptor antagonist that is able to cross the blood-brain barrier and therefore decrease sympathetic blood flow.[85] A 2017 multisite, randomized controlled trial compared prazosin with placebo in 304 veterans.[86] Results revealed no significant improvement in sleep or nightmares and prazosin has since been downgraded in the American Academy of Sleep (AAS) recommendations for treatment of nightmares. However, there are many other studies showing prazosin's efficacy,[87] and the AAS recognizes that prazosin remains a primary treatment.[87,88]

A 2017 retrospective chart review analyzed the use of prazosin in 34 children with PTSD.[89] It showed a clinically significant decrease in nightmares and sleep problems, with tolerability and efficacy in a larger dose range than has been typically been

**Table 6**
**Psychological interventions for posttraumatic stress disorder–related nightmares**

| Treatment | Description | Citation | Population | Results |
|---|---|---|---|---|
| Imagery rehearsal | Reimagining a benign ending to a NM and then rehearsing the new scripted ending during waking hours | Casement and Swanson,[77] 2012, a meta-analysis | Adults | Reduced NM frequency, improved sleep, and improved global PTSD symptoms |
| | | Krakow et al[78] 2001 | 168 women | Reduced NMs and improved sleep |
| | | Krakow et al,[79] 2001 | 19 adjudicated adolescent girls with high prevalence of sexual abuse | Significantly decreased NM frequency (3 mo after a 1-d workshop) |
| | | Nappi et al,[34] 2012, a review of current literature | Adults | Decreased NM frequency and severity; sleep problems, PTSD symptoms, and depression |
| Exposure, relaxation, and rescripting therapy | Rewriting and rehearsing a NM, often in a group setting; includes psychoeducation, relaxation techniques | Davis and Wright,[80] 2007 | 32 adults | Decreased NM frequency and severity; improved sleep quality and quantity |
| | | Fernandez et al,[81] 2013, case series | 2 children with trauma-related NM | Decreased NMs and improved sleep |

*Abbreviation:* NM, nightmare.

**Table 7**
Psychopharmacologic interventions for posttraumatic stress disorder

| Drug | Citation | Population | Results |
|---|---|---|---|
| Prazosin | Ferrafiat et al,[84] 2020, case series | 18 adolescent inpatients | Significant, rapid improvements in all PTSD symptom clusters, including sleep-related symptoms |
| | Raskind et al,[86] 2018, RPC | 304 veterans | No benefit compared with placebo in sleep or NMs |
| | Keeshin et al,[89] 2017, chart review | 34 children | Significant decrease in sleep problems and NMs |
| Clonidine | De Bellis et al,[90] 2001, case report | 9-y-old child | Improved insomnia and nightmares |
| | Harmon and Riggs [91] 1996, open label | 7 preschoolers | 5 of 7 had reduced insomnia and nightmares |
| Guanfacine | Horrigan[92] 1996, case report | 7-y-old child | Improved NMs |
| | Connor et al,[93] 2013, open-label pilot of guanfacine ER | 19 youth, some with ADHD | Improved PTSD but not NMs |
| Propranolol | Famularo et al,[94] 1988, case series | 11 children | Improved insomnia |
| Sertraline | Davidson et al,[95] 2001, DBRPC | 208 adults | Insomnia was significant side effect |
| | Brady et al,[96,97] 2000, DBRPC | 187 adults | Insomnia was significant side effect |
| Venlafaxine ER | Stein et al,[96] 2013, pooled analysis of 2 RCTs | 685 adults | Did not improve NMs |
| Fluvoxamine | Morgenthaler et al,[87] 2018, position paper | Adults | Improved NMs |
| | Good and Petersen[98] 2001, case report | 8-y-old child | Taken with mirtazapine, improved sleep |
| Trazodone | Warner et al,[99] 2001 | 74 adult inpatients | Reduced insomnia and NMs |
| Imipramine | Robert et al,[100] 1999, prospective randomized | 25 children with acute stress disorder | Improved flashbacks and insomnia |
| Eszopiclone | Dowd et al,[101] 2020, DBRPC | 25 adults | No significant improvement in insomnia |
| | Pollack et al,[102] 2011, DBRPC | 24 adults | Improved sleep symptoms and daytime function |

*(continued on next page)*

**Table 7**
*(continued)*

| Drug | Citation | Population | Results |
|---|---|---|---|
| Benzodiazepines | Guina et al,[103] 2015, meta-analysis | Review of adult literature | Risks outweigh usefulness |
| Clonazepam | Cates et al,[104] 2004 | 6 adults, single-blind PBO control | Minimal effect on early insomnia; no improvement in NMs |
| Olanzapine | Stein et al,[105] 2002, DBPC / Jakovljević et al,[106] 2003, case series | 19 adults, (resistant to SSRIs) / 5 adults | Adjunctive olanzapine improved sleep / Adjunctive olanzapine rapidly improved NMs and insomnia |
| Risperidone | Krystal et al,[107] 2016, RPC | 267 male veterans | Adjunctive risperidone produced small but significant improvement in sleep and NMs |
| Aripiprazole | Lambert,[108] 2006, case series | 5 male veterans | Improved NMs |
| Quetiapine | Villarreal et al,[109] 2016, RPC | 80 adults | Transient, mild improvement in insomnia that was lost by week 5 |
|  | Byers et al,[110] 2010, historical prospective cohort, quetiapine vs prazosin | 324 veterans | Recommended prazosin rather than quetiapine for sleep symptoms because of longer-term effectiveness, better tolerability |
| Carbamazepine | Loof et al,[111] 1995, open label | 28 youth | 78% had remission of all PTSD symptoms, including NMs and hypnogogic hallucinations |
| Gabapentin | Hamner et al,[112] 2001, chart review | 30 adults | Adjunctive gabapentin improved insomnia and NMs in 77% |
| Topiramate | Alderman et al[113] 2009, 8-wk open label | 43 veterans | Significant decrease in number of patients who experienced NMs or anxiety that interfered with sleep |
|  | Berlant et al,[114] 2002, chart review | 35 adults | Significantly decreased NMs and flashbacks |
| Nabilone | Jetly et al,[115] 2015, RDBP | 10 adults | Significantly improved NMs |
|  | Fraser,[116] 2009, open label | 47 adults with treatment-resistant NMs | 72% subjects, total remission of NMs |

*Abbreviations:* ER, extended release; RCT, randomized controlled trial; SSRIs, selective serotonin reuptake inhibitors; DBRPC, Double Bind Randomized Placebo Controlled; PBO, Placebo; RPC, Randomized Placebo Controlled.

described. Thirty-five percent of children required doses of more than 5 mg, and 17% of the 34 children received doses greater than or equal to 10 mg. The investigators hypothesized that children were able to tolerate the higher doses in part because of the slow titration with frequent reassessment. Interestingly, 2 children discontinued treatment because of increased anxiety after taking prazosin, describing that they felt more vulnerable because of their decreased hypervigilance. On discontinuation, no patients reported rebound hypertension (unlike what is often seen with $\alpha$2-agonists).

A recently published prospective case series of 18 adolescent inpatients with PTSD showed rapid and significant improvements in all symptom clusters of PTSD, including sleep-related symptoms.[84] Effective dosing seemed to be at or more than 2 mg/d.

### Integration

Addressing sleep disruption in the context of PTSD requires trauma-focused treatment. The gold standard treatment of PTSD is psychotherapeutic interventions.[25] Most successful trauma treatments use variations of the following core components: (1) ensuring that a child is safe; (2) providing psychoeducation about trauma and treatment; (3) skills building; (4) addressing avoidance of trauma, often using exposures; and (5) integrating family work to both educate and improve relationships.[82] Elements of treatment of sleep disruption may be integrated into these various components. For example, ensuring a safe environment for sleep may include removal of traumatic reminders. Psychoeducation should include the significant bidirectional impact PTSD has on sleep with explanation of the links between DSM-5 criteria and symptoms: hyperarousal (insomnia), intrusion (nightmares), and avoidance (avoidance of sleep). Skills building can include basic sleep hygiene practice. Exposures can address nightmare content and fear of the dark/bedtime.

After completing a comprehensive evaluation, the therapist explains to Maria and her mother that Maria has PTSD including hyperarousal (insomnia), intrusive memories triggered by reminders (mother screaming, night time), and avoidance of memories (using her phone as distraction). The therapist normalizes her reaction and explains goals of treatment, including symptom targets (reduction of sleep latency and neutralization of triggers with reduction of avoidance). For Maria, treatment will consist of prolonged exposure therapy plus cognitive behavior treatment of insomnia. The therapist also describes a realistic timeline of symptom reduction. The therapist's conclusion, clarity, and hopefulness renew Maria's and mother's hope that things can improve.

### SUMMARY

Traumatic experiences and resulting PTSD are under-recognized in children and adolescents but may underlie or exacerbate sleep complaints. Any evaluation of sleep symptoms should include developmentally appropriate screening for trauma, keeping in mind that PTSD often presents differently in children than in adults. Sleep disturbances associated with trauma are shaped by both physiologic responses and psychological ones. Sleep-related symptoms may be refractory to otherwise successful treatment of PTSD. These residual symptoms interfere with functioning but also may disrupt the ability to benefit from psychotherapy, because restorative sleep is necessary for fear extinction and neutralizing of traumatic memories. Psychotherapeutic interventions remain the necessary first-line treatment of trauma-related sleep disturbance with their larger evidence base, although there are some data to support medication use in children. Regardless of the intervention used, treatment of sleep symptoms should be integrated into treatment of PTSD.

## CLINICS CARE POINTS

- In an assessment of sleep complaints, consider the possible role of trauma and perform a screen.
- In an assessment of PTSD, sleep should be evaluated specifically with questions about quantity of sleep, sleep latency, awakenings, bedtime routine, and subjective quality.
- Early identification and treatment of disrupted sleep improves daytime functioning, academic performance, and behavioral and emotional regulation.
- Use rating scales and a sleep diary to assess and track changes.
  - Pittsburgh Sleep Quality Index[38]
  - University of California, Los Angeles, PTSD Reaction Index[117]
  - Children's sleep diary[68]
- Consider supplementation of evidence-based PTSD treatment with specific treatment targeted at sleep symptoms.
  - There may be benefit to starting sleep treatment before beginning trauma treatment.
- Research suggests normalization of sleep may have benefit in reducing daytime PTSD symptoms.
- Further research is needed to assess sleep disruption in children with PTSD and appropriate treatments, including the option of combining treatments.

## DISCLOSURE

The authors have nothing to disclose.

## REFERENCES

1. Eaton DK, McKnight-Eily LR, Lowry R, et al. Prevalence of insufficient, borderline, and optimal hours of sleep among high school students - United States, 2007. J Adolesc Health 2010;46(4):399–401.
2. Meltzer LJ, Mindell JA. Sleep and sleep disorders in children and adolescents. Psychiatr Clin North Am 2006;29(4):1059–76 [abstract: x].
3. American Psychiatric Association. American psychiatric association. DSM-5 task force. In: Diagnostic and statistical manual of mental disorders: DSM-5. 5th edition. Washington, D.C.: American Psychiatric Association. xliv; 2013. p. 947.
4. The national child traumatic stress Network (n.d.). Available at: https://www.nctsn.org/what-is-child-trauma/trauma-types/complex-trauma/effects. Accessed October 6, 2020.
5. Sacks V, Murphey D. 2018. Available at: https://www.childtrends.org/publications/prevalence-adverse-childhood-experiences-nationally-state-race-ethnicity/. Accessed October 6, 2020.
6. Felitti VJ, Anda RF, Nordenberg D, et al. Relationship of childhood abuse and household dysfunction to many of the leading causes of death in adults. The Adverse Childhood Experiences (ACE) Study. Am J Prev Med 1998;14(4):245–58.
7. Gerson R, Rappaport N. Traumatic stress and posttraumatic stress disorder in youth: recent research findings on clinical impact, assessment, and treatment. J Adolesc Health 2013;52(2):137–43.
8. Substance, A. and A. Mental Health Services. CBHSQ methodology report. In: DSM-5 changes: implications for child serious emotional disturbance. Rockville (MD): Substance Abuse and Mental Health Services Administration (US); 2016.

9. Cloitre M, Garvert DW, Brewin CR, et al. Evidence for proposed ICD-11 PTSD and complex PTSD: a latent profile analysis. Eur J Psychotraumatol 2013;4.

10. Gerson R, Heppell P. Beyond PTSD: helping and healing teens exposed to trauma. Washington, DC: American Psychiatric Pub; 2018.

11. Kovachy B, O'Hara R, Hawkins N, et al. Sleep disturbance in pediatric PTSD: current findings and future directions. J Clin Sleep Med 2013;9(5):501–10.

12. Orchard F, Gregory AM, Gradisar M, et al. Self-reported sleep patterns and quality amongst adolescents: cross-sectional and prospective associations with anxiety and depression. J Child Psychol Psychiatry 2020. https://doi.org/10.1111/jcpp.13288.

13. Seelig AD, Jacobson IG, Smith B, et al. Sleep patterns before, during, and after deployment to Iraq and Afghanistan. Sleep 2010;33(12):1615–22.

14. Kobayashi I, Boarts JM, Delahanty DL. Polysomnographically measured sleep abnormalities in PTSD: a meta-analytic review. Psychophysiology 2007;44(4):660–9.

15. Chapman DP, Wheaton AG, Anda RF, et al. Adverse childhood experiences and sleep disturbances in adults. Sleep Med 2011;12(8):773–9.

16. Kajeepeta S, Gelaye B, Jackson CL, et al. Adverse childhood experiences are associated with adult sleep disorders: a systematic review. Sleep Med 2015;16(3):320–30.

17. Baiden P, Fallon B, den Dunnen W, et al. The enduring effects of early-childhood adversities and troubled sleep among Canadian adults: a population-based study. Sleep Med 2015;16(6):760–7.

18. Brindle RC, Cribbet MR, Samuelsson LB, et al. The relationship between childhood trauma and poor sleep health in adulthood. Psychosom Med 2018;80(2):200–7.

19. Singh GK, Kenney MK. Rising prevalence and neighborhood, social, and behavioral determinants of sleep problems in US children and adolescents, 2003-2012. Sleep Disord 2013;2013:394320.

20. Lavie P. Sleep disturbances in the wake of traumatic events. N Engl J Med 2001;345(25):1825–32.

21. Germain A, Buysse DJ, Nofzinger E. Sleep-specific mechanisms underlying posttraumatic stress disorder: integrative review and neurobiological hypotheses. Sleep Med Rev 2008;12(3):185–95.

22. Spilsbury JC, Babineau DC, Frame J, et al. Association between children's exposure to a violent event and objectively and subjectively measured sleep characteristics: a pilot longitudinal study. J Sleep Res 2014;23(5):585–94.

23. Ho FY, Chan CS, Tang KN. Cognitive-behavioral therapy for sleep disturbances in treating posttraumatic stress disorder symptoms: a meta-analysis of randomized controlled trials. Clin Psychol Rev 2016;43:90–102.

24. Hall Brown TS, Akeeb A, Mellman TA. The role of trauma type in the risk for insomnia. J Clin Sleep Med 2015;11(7):735–9.

25. Cohen JA, Bukstein O, Walter H, et al. Practice parameter for the assessment and treatment of children and adolescents with posttraumatic stress disorder. J Am Acad Child Adolesc Psychiatry 2010;49(4):414–30.

26. John-Henderson NA, Williams SE, Brindle RC, et al. Changes in sleep quality and levels of psychological distress during the adaptation to university: the role of childhood adversity. Br J Psychol 2018;109(4):694–707.

27. Noll JG, Trickett PK, Susman EJ, et al. Sleep disturbances and childhood sexual abuse. J Pediatr Psychol 2006;31(5):469–80.

28. Goldston DB, Turnquist DC, Knutson JF. Presenting problems of sexually abused girls receiving psychiatric services. J Abnorm Psychol 1989;98(3): 314–7.

29. Rimsza ME, Berg RA, Locke C. Sexual abuse: somatic and emotional reactions. Child Abuse Negl 1988;12(2):201–8.

30. Manni R, Ratti MT, Marchioni E, et al. Poor sleep in adolescents: a study of 869 17-year-old Italian secondary school students. J Sleep Res 1997;6(1):44–9.

31. Dahl RE, Lewin DS. Pathways to adolescent health sleep regulation and behavior. J Adolesc Health 2002;31(6 Suppl):175–84.

32. Dahl RE. Sleeplessness and aggression in youth. J Adolesc Health 2006;38(6): 641–2.

33. Spoormaker VI, Montgomery P. Disturbed sleep in post-traumatic stress disorder: secondary symptom or core feature? Sleep Med Rev 2008;12(3):169–84.

34. Nappi CM, Drummond SP, Hall JM. Treating nightmares and insomnia in posttraumatic stress disorder: a review of current evidence. Neuropharmacology 2012;62(2):576–85.

35. Koren D, Arnon I, Lavie P, et al. Sleep complaints as early predictors of posttraumatic stress disorder: a 1-year prospective study of injured survivors of motor vehicle accidents. Am J Psychiatry 2002;159(5):855–7.

36. Thompson A, Lereya ST, Lewis G, et al. Childhood sleep disturbance and risk of psychotic experiences at 18: UK birth cohort. Br J Psychiatry 2015;207(1):23–9.

37. Charuvastra A, Cloitre M. Safe enough to sleep: sleep disruptions associated with trauma, posttraumatic stress, and anxiety in children and adolescents. Child Adolesc Psychiatr Clin N Am 2009;18(4):877–91.

38. Buysse DJ, Reynolds CF, Monk TH, et al. The Pittsburgh sleep quality index: a new instrument for psychiatric practice and research. Psychiatry Res 1989; 28(2):193–213.

39. Foa EB, Johnson KM, Feeny NC, et al. The child PTSD Symptom Scale: a preliminary examination of its psychometric properties. J Clin Child Psychol 2001; 30(3):376–84.

40. Alfano CA, Beidel DC, Turner SM, et al. Preliminary evidence for sleep complaints among children referred for anxiety. Sleep Med 2006;7(6):467–73.

41. Nunes ML, Bruni O. Insomnia in childhood and adolescence: clinical aspects, diagnosis, and therapeutic approach. J Pediatr (Rio J) 2015;91(6 Suppl 1): S26–35.

42. Ramtekkar U, Ivanenko A. Sleep in children with psychiatric disorders. Semin Pediatr Neurol 2015;22(2):148–55.

43. Sheridan DC, Spiro DM, Fu R, et al. Mental health utilization in a pediatric emergency department. Pediatr Emerg Care 2015;31(8):555–9.

44. Andorko ND, Millman ZB, Klingaman E, et al. Association between sleep, childhood trauma and psychosis-like experiences. Schizophr Res 2018;199:333–40.

45. Glod CA, Teicher MH, Hartman CR, et al. Increased nocturnal activity and impaired sleep maintenance in abused children. J Am Acad Child Adolesc Psychiatry 1997;36(9):1236–43.

46. Karatzias T, Cloitre M, Maercker A, et al. PTSD and complex PTSD: ICD-11 updates on concept and measurement in the UK, USA, Germany and Lithuania. Eur J Psychotraumatol 2018;8(sup7):1418103.

47. Beilharz JE, Paterson M, Fatt S, et al. The impact of childhood trauma on psychosocial functioning and physical health in a non-clinical community sample of young adults. Aust N Z J Psychiatry 2020;54(2):185–94.

48. Gregory AM, O'Connor TG. Sleep problems in childhood: a longitudinal study of developmental change and association with behavioral problems. J Am Acad Child Adolesc Psychiatry 2002;41(8):964–71.
49. Duffy A, Carlson G, Dubicka B, et al. Pre-pubertal bipolar disorder: origins and current status of the controversy. Int J Bipolar Disord 2020;8(1):18.
50. Harrington R, Myatt T. Is preadolescent mania the same condition as adult mania? A British perspective. Biol Psychiatry 2003;53(11):961–9.
51. Gordon CT, Frazier JA, McKenna K, et al. Childhood-onset schizophrenia: an NIMH study in progress. Schizophr Bull 1994;20(4):697–712.
52. Brownlow JA, Harb GC, Ross RJ. Treatment of sleep disturbances in post-traumatic stress disorder: a review of the literature. Curr Psychiatry Rep 2015; 17(6):41.
53. Zayfert C, DeViva JC. Residual insomnia following cognitive behavioral therapy for PTSD. J Trauma Stress 2004;17(1):69–73.
54. Walters EM, Jenkins MM, Nappi CM, et al. The impact of prolonged exposure on sleep and enhancing treatment outcomes with evidence-based sleep interventions: a pilot study. Psychol Trauma 2020;12(2):175–85.
55. Brownlow JA, McLean CP, Gehrman PR, et al. Influence of sleep disturbance on global functioning after posttraumatic stress disorder treatment. J Trauma Stress 2016;29(6):515–21.
56. Gutner CA, Casement MD, Stavitsky Gilbert K, et al. Change in sleep symptoms across cognitive processing therapy and prolonged exposure: a longitudinal perspective. Behav Res Ther 2013;51(12):817–22.
57. Sanford LD, Suchecki D, Meerlo P. In: Meerlo P, Benca RM, Abel T, editors. Stress, arousal, and sleep, in sleep, neuronal plasticity and brain function. Berlin, Heidelberg (Baden-Württemberg): Springer Berlin Heidelberg; 2015. p. 379–410.
58. Pigeon WR, Heffner KL, Crean H, et al. Responding to the need for sleep among survivors of interpersonal violence: a randomized controlled trial of a cognitive-behavioral insomnia intervention followed by PTSD treatment. Contemp Clin Trials 2015;45(Pt B):252–60.
59. Waltman SH, Shearer D, Moore BA. Management of post-traumatic nightmares: a review of pharmacologic and nonpharmacologic treatments since 2013. Curr Psychiatry Rep 2018;20(12):108.
60. Nappi CM, Drummond SP, Thorp SR, et al. Effectiveness of imagery rehearsal therapy for the treatment of combat-related nightmares in veterans. Behav Ther 2010;41(2):237–44.
61. Talbot LS, Maguen S, Metzler TJ, et al. Cognitive behavioral therapy for insomnia in posttraumatic stress disorder: a randomized controlled trial. Sleep 2014; 37(2):327–41.
62. Baddeley JL, Gros DF. Cognitive behavioral therapy for insomnia as a preparatory treatment for exposure therapy for posttraumatic stress disorder. Am J Psychother 2013;67(2):203–14.
63. Stephenson T. How children's responses to drugs differ from adults. Br J Clin Pharmacol 2005;59(6):670–3.
64. Donnelly CL. Pharmacologic treatment approaches for children and adolescents with posttraumatic stress disorder. Child Adolesc Psychiatr Clin N Am 2003;12(2):251–69.
65. Jespersen KV, Vuust P. The effect of relaxation music listening on sleep quality in traumatized refugees: a pilot study. J Music Ther 2012;49(2):205–29.

66. Bosch J, Weaver TL, Neylan TC, et al. Impact of engagement in exercise on sleep quality among veterans with posttraumatic stress disorder symptoms. Mil Med 2017;182(9):e1745–50.

67. Rosenbaum S, Sherrington C, Tiedemann A. Exercise augmentation compared with usual care for post-traumatic stress disorder: a randomized controlled trial. Acta Psychiatr Scand 2015;131(5):350–9.

68. Children's sleep diary, adapted by CHOC children's from the national sleep foundation. 2016. Available at: https://www.choc.org/wp/wp-content/uploads/2016/04/Children-Sleep-Diary-Vers_2.pdf. Accessed October 6, 2020.

69. Rosner R, Rimane E, Frick U, et al. Effect of developmentally adapted cognitive processing therapy for youth with symptoms of posttraumatic stress disorder after childhood sexual and physical abuse: a randomized clinical trial. JAMA Psychiatry 2019;76(5):484–91.

70. Matulis S, Resick PA, Rosner R, et al. Developmentally adapted cognitive processing therapy for adolescents suffering from posttraumatic stress disorder after childhood sexual or physical abuse: a pilot study. Clin Child Fam Psychol Rev 2014;17(2):173–90.

71. Galovski TE, Monson C, Bruce SE, et al. Does cognitive-behavioral therapy for PTSD improve perceived health and sleep impairment? J Trauma Stress 2009; 22(3):197–204.

72. Raboni MR, Alonso FF, Tufik S, et al. Improvement of mood and sleep alterations in posttraumatic stress disorder patients by eye movement desensitization and reprocessing. Front Behav Neurosci 2014;8:209.

73. Meentken MG, van der Mheen M, van Beynum IM, et al. EMDR for children with medically related subthreshold PTSD: short-term effects on PTSD, blood-injection-injury phobia, depression and sleep. Eur J Psychotraumatol 2020;11(1):1705598.

74. Kanady JC, Talbot LS, Maguen S, et al. Cognitive behavioral therapy for insomnia reduces fear of sleep in individuals with posttraumatic stress disorder. J Clin Sleep Med 2018;14(7):1193–203.

75. Fazel M, Stratford HJ, Rowsell E, et al. Five applications of narrative exposure therapy for children and adolescents presenting with post-traumatic stress disorders. Front Psychiatry 2020;11:19.

76. Park JK, Park J, Elbert T, et al. Effects of narrative exposure therapy on posttraumatic stress disorder, depression, and insomnia in traumatized north Korean refugee youth. J Trauma Stress 2020;33(3):353–9.

77. Casement MD, Swanson LM. A meta-analysis of imagery rehearsal for post-trauma nightmares: effects on nightmare frequency, sleep quality, and posttraumatic stress. Clin Psychol Rev 2012;32(6):566–74.

78. Krakow B, Hollifield M, Johnston L, et al. Imagery rehearsal therapy for chronic nightmares in sexual assault survivors with posttraumatic stress disorder: a randomized controlled trial. JAMA 2001;286(5):537–45.

79. Krakow B, Sandoval D, Schrader R, et al. Treatment of chronic nightmares in adjudicated adolescent girls in a residential facility. J Adolesc Health 2001; 29(2):94–100.

80. Davis JL, Wright DC. Randomized clinical trial for treatment of chronic nightmares in trauma-exposed adults. J Trauma Stress 2007;20(2):123–33.

81. Fernandez S, DeMarni Cromer L, Borntrager C, et al. A case series: Cognitive-behavioral treatment (exposure, relaxation, and rescripting therapy) of trauma-related nightmares experienced by children. Clin Case Stud 2013;12(1):39–59.

82. Keeshin BR, Strawn JR. Psychological and pharmacologic treatment of youth with posttraumatic stress disorder: an evidence-based review. Child Adolesc Psychiatr Clin N Am 2014;23(2):399–411x.

83. Luft MJ, Lamy M, DelBello MP, et al. Antidepressant-induced activation in children and adolescents: risk, recognition and management. Curr Probl Pediatr Adolesc Health Care 2018;48(2):50–62.

84. Ferrafiat V, Soleimani M, Chaumette B, et al. Use of prazosin for pediatric posttraumatic stress disorder with nightmares and/or sleep disorder: case series of 18 patients prospectively assessed. Front Psychiatry 2020;11:724.

85. Akinsanya A, Marwaha R, Tampi RR. Prazosin in children and adolescents with posttraumatic stress disorder who have nightmares: a systematic review. J Clin Psychopharmacol 2017;37(1):84–8.

86. Raskind MA, Peskind ER, Chow B, et al. Trial of prazosin for post-traumatic stress disorder in military veterans. N Engl J Med 2018;378(6):507–17.

87. Morgenthaler TI, Auerbach S, Casey KR, et al. Position paper for the treatment of nightmare disorder in adults: an american academy of sleep medicine position paper. J Clin Sleep Med 2018;14(6):1041–55.

88. Khachatryan D, Groll D, Booij L, et al. Prazosin for treating sleep disturbances in adults with posttraumatic stress disorder: a systematic review and meta-analysis of randomized controlled trials. Gen Hosp Psychiatry 2016;39:46–52.

89. Keeshin BR, Ding Q, Presson AP, et al. Use of prazosin for pediatric PTSD-associated nightmares and sleep disturbances: a retrospective chart review. Neurol Ther 2017;6(2):247–57.

90. De Bellis MD, Keshavan MS, Harenski KA. Anterior cingulate N-acetylaspartate/creatine ratios during clonidine treatment in a maltreated child with posttraumatic stress disorder. J Child Adolesc Psychopharmacol 2001;11(3):311–6.

91. Harmon RJ, Riggs PD. Clonidine for posttraumatic stress disorder in preschool children. J Am Acad Child Adolesc Psychiatry 1996;35(9):1247–9.

92. Horrigan JP. Guanfacine for PTSD nightmares. J Am Acad Child Adolesc Psychiatry 1996;35(8):975–6.

93. Connor DF, Grasso DJ, Slivinsky MD, et al. An open-label study of guanfacine extended release for traumatic stress related symptoms in children and adolescents. J Child Adolesc Psychopharmacol 2013;23(4):244–51.

94. Famularo R, Kinscherff R, Fenton T. Propranolol treatment for childhood posttraumatic stress disorder, acute type. A pilot study. Am J Dis Child 1988;142(11):1244–7.

95. Davidson JR, Rothbaum BO, van der Kolk BA, et al. Multicenter, double-blind comparison of sertraline and placebo in the treatment of posttraumatic stress disorder. Arch Gen Psychiatry 2001;58(5):485–92.

96. Stein DJ, Rothbaum BO, Baldwin DS, et al. A factor analysis of posttraumatic stress disorder symptoms using data pooled from two venlafaxine extended-release clinical trials. Brain Behav 2013;3(6):738–46.

97. Brady K, Pearlstein T, Asnis GM, et al. Efficacy and safety of sertraline treatment of posttraumatic stress disorder: a randomized controlled trial. JAMA 2000;283(14):1837–44.

98. Good C, Petersen C. SSRI and mirtazapine in PTSD. J Am Acad Child Adolesc Psychiatry 2001;40(3):263–4.

99. Warner MD, Dorn MR, Peabody CA. Survey on the usefulness of trazodone in patients with PTSD with insomnia or nightmares. Pharmacopsychiatry 2001;34(4):128–31.

100. Robert R, Blakeney PE, Villarreal C, et al. Imipramine treatment in pediatric burn patients with symptoms of acute stress disorder: a pilot study. J Am Acad Child Adolesc Psychiatry 1999;38(7):873–82.

101. Dowd SM, Zalta AK, Burgess HJ, et al. Double-blind randomized controlled study of the efficacy, safety and tolerability of eszopiclone vs placebo for the treatment of patients with post-traumatic stress disorder and insomnia. World J Psychiatry 2020;10(3):21–8.

102. Pollack MH, Hoge EA, Worthington JJ, et al. Eszopiclone for the treatment of posttraumatic stress disorder and associated insomnia: a randomized, double-blind, placebo-controlled trial. J Clin Psychiatry 2011;72(7):892–7.

103. Guina J, Rossetter SR, DeRHODES BJ, et al. Benzodiazepines for PTSD: a systematic review and meta-analysis. J Psychiatr Pract 2015;21(4):281–303.

104. Cates ME, Bishop MH, Davis LL, et al. Clonazepam for treatment of sleep disturbances associated with combat-related posttraumatic stress disorder. Ann Pharmacother 2004;38(9):1395–9.

105. Stein MB, Kline NA, Matloff JL. Adjunctive olanzapine for SSRI-resistant combat-related PTSD: a double-blind, placebo-controlled study. Am J Psychiatry 2002; 159(10):1777–9.

106. Jakovljevic M, Sagud M, Mihaljevic-Peles A. Olanzapine in the treatment-resistant, combat-related PTSD–a series of case reports. Acta Psychiatr Scand 2003;107(5):394–6 [discussion: 396].

107. Krystal JH, Pietrzak RH, Rosenheck RA, et al. Sleep disturbance in chronic military-related PTSD: clinical impact and response to adjunctive risperidone in the Veterans Affairs cooperative study #504. J Clin Psychiatry 2016;77(4): 483–91.

108. Lambert MT. Aripiprazole in the management of post-traumatic stress disorder symptoms in returning Global War on Terrorism veterans. Int Clin Psychopharmacol 2006;21(3):185–7.

109. Villarreal G, Hamner MB, Cañive JM, et al. Efficacy of quetiapine monotherapy in posttraumatic stress disorder: a randomized, placebo-controlled trial. Am J Psychiatry 2016;173(12):1205–12.

110. Byers MG, Allison KM, Wendel CS, et al. Prazosin versus quetiapine for night-time posttraumatic stress disorder symptoms in veterans: an assessment of long-term comparative effectiveness and safety. J Clin Psychopharmacol 2010;30(3):225–9.

111. Looff D, Grimley P, Kuller F, et al. Carbamazepine for PTSD. J Am Acad Child Adolesc Psychiatry 1995;34(6):703–4.

112. Hamner MB, Brodrick PS, Labbate LA. Gabapentin in PTSD: a retrospective, clinical series of adjunctive therapy. Ann Clin Psychiatry 2001;13(3): 141–6.

113. Alderman CP, McCarthy LC, Condon JT, et al. Topiramate in combat-related posttraumatic stress disorder. Ann Pharmacother 2009;43(4):635–41.

114. Berlant J, van Kammen DP. Open-label topiramate as primary or adjunctive therapy in chronic civilian posttraumatic stress disorder: a preliminary report. J Clin Psychiatry 2002;63(1):15–20.

115. Jetly R, Heber A, Fraser G, et al. The efficacy of nabilone, a synthetic cannabinoid, in the treatment of PTSD-associated nightmares: a preliminary randomized, double-blind, placebo-controlled cross-over design study. Psychoneuroendocrinology 2015;51:585–8.

116. Fraser GA. The use of a synthetic cannabinoid in the management of treatment-resistant nightmares in posttraumatic stress disorder (PTSD). CNS Neurosci Ther 2009;15(1):84–8.

117. Rodriguez N SA, Pynoos RS. UCLA post traumatic stress disorder reaction index for DSM-IV, child, adolescent, and parent versions. Los Angeles (CA): UCLA Trauma Psychiatry Service; 1998.

# Sleep and Mood Disorders Among Youth

Lauren D. Asarnow, PhD, Riya Mirchandaney, BA

## KEYWORDS

- Depression • Sleep • Insomnia • Cognitive behavioral therapy for insomnia
- Delayed sleep phase • Evening preference

## KEY POINTS

- Evidence indicates that sleep problems often predict and predate the development of mood disorders.
- Rates of sleep disorders among youth with mood disorders are high and comorbidity between mood episodes and sleep problems are associated with more severe mood episodes.
- Sleep problems are associated with poor depression treatment response and may be associated with recurrence of mood episodes.
- Cognitive behavioral therapy for insomnia is an effective psychosocial intervention for improving insomnia symptoms among youth.
- Sleep improvement seems to be an important mediator of depression treatment among youth.

Research suggests that sleep plays an important role in the development, progression, and maintenance of mood disorder symptoms among children and adolescents.[1–4] Although most of the extant research focuses on the relationship between insomnia and mood disorders, other sleep disorders such as delayed sleep phase, inadequate total sleep duration, and bedtime resistance in younger children may play important roles in mood episodes.[1,4,5] Although there are no medications approved by the US Food and Drug Administration specifically for sleep disorders in children and adolescents, fortunately there are effective behavioral sleep interventions. Research indicates that these behavioral interventions do effectively improve sleep in children and adolescents with depression and indicate that sleep improvement is an important mediator of depression treatment outcome.[6–8] There is far less literature on bipolar disorders among youth and sleep, and more research is needed

This article originally appeared in *Child and Adolescent Psychiatric Clinics*, Volume 30 Issue 1, January 2021.
The authors have nothing to disclose.
University of California, San Francisco, Department of Psychiatry and Behavioral Sciences, 401 Parnassus Avenue, RM LP-A307, San Francisco, CA 94143, USA
*E-mail address:* Lauren.Asarnow@ucsf.edu

**psych.theclinics.com**

to examine the potential role of a sleep intervention on the course of mood episodes among youth.

## DEFINING SLEEP PROBLEMS AMONG CHILDREN AND ADOLESCENTS

Although there are many sleep disorders that have been associated with depression, this review highlights the 3 most common sleep disorders studied in the context of mood disorders among youth (1) insomnia, (2) delayed sleep phase, and (3) hypersomnia. Other sleep disorders and behaviors such as nightmares and obstructive sleep apnea are also important factors to consider; however, they are not the focus of the present review.[9,10]

### Insomnia

Most research on sleep disorders among youth has focused on insomnia. Insomnia is defined as difficulty initiating, maintaining, or returning to sleep after an early morning awakening at least 3 nights per week for 3 months or more.[11] The *Diagnostic and Statistical Manual of Mental Disorders*, 5th edition, also specifies that the difficulty sleeping must occur despite adequate opportunity for sleep.

Psychophysiologic (sometimes termed "conditioned") insomnia is among the most common forms of insomnia in adults and may occur in older children and adolescents. Psychophysiologic insomnia is characterized by heightened physiologic and emotional arousal related to sleep and the sleep environment. Children with psychophysiologic insomnia often report anxiety about sleep, including maladaptive cognitions about the consequences of their sleep problems that often exacerbate their difficulties falling asleep.

In children, another distinct form of insomnia is behaviorally based insomnia. It typically presents as bedtime resistance, characterized by prolonged sleep onset and/or night wakings. Many children present with both bedtime resistance and prolonged nighttime awakenings, which often require parental intervention and therefore disrupt parents' sleep as well. This behaviorally based insomnia is often related to either inconsistent or inadequate parental limit setting or maladaptive sleep-onset associations. The limit setting type of behavioral insomnia is characterized by bedtime resistance with verbal protests, and repeated requests or demands at bedtime ("curtain calls"). The delayed sleep onset resulting from bedtime resistance may result in inadequate sleep and subsequent moodiness and irritability the following day. The type of behavioral insomnia that is generally the result of certain sleep-onset associations is characterized by prolonged night waking and often results in insufficient sleep. In this disorder, the child has learned to fall asleep with specific sleep associations that typically require parental intervention, such as being held, rocked, or fed. During the night, when the child awakens, they are not able to return to sleep (or self-soothe) unless those same sleep associations are available. The child then seeks the parents' attention to provide the necessary associations.

It is developmentally appropriate for some degree of transient bedtime resistance or insomnia to occur in children. To be considered a sleep disorder, the symptoms must occur frequently ($\geq$3 times per week) and persistently (for $\geq$3 months) and result in significant impairment of functioning in the child, parent(s), or family.

Insomnia is more common in children than in adolescents. Behavioral insomnia is most common in young children aged 0 to 5 years, but it can persist into the school-age years.[12,13] Indeed, bedtime resistance has been reported in 10% to 15% of toddlers, and estimates indicate that 15% to 30% of preschool-aged children have insomnia.[14] Among school aged-children (4–10 years of age), 25% to 40% report a sleep problem; 15% of these children have behavioral insomnia and approximately 11% have psychophysiologic insomnia.[15] Approximately 11% of adolescents (13–16 years of age) report significant insomnia symptoms.[16]

Importantly, evidence indicates that insomnia tends to be chronic. Indeed, 88% of adolescents with a history of insomnia report current insomnia.[16] Therefore, insomnia in children is an important problem to address.

### Delayed Sleep Phase

Another important factor, particularly during adolescence, are sleep disorders affecting the circadian system; specifically, the focus of this review is on delayed sleep phase. Adolescence is associated with a biological shift in the circadian system at puberty in the direction of a delayed sleep phase, characterized by a preference for later sleep onset and offset, and sometimes referred to as an evening circadian preference or evening chronotype.[17] This biological shift in the circadian system at puberty in the direction of a delayed sleep phase is often compounded by social changes during adolescence, such as less parental control, increased access to stimulating social activities (music, the Internet, text messaging, etc), increased academic demands at school, early school start times, increased social pressures, and increased use of alcohol and drugs.[18–20] These social and hormonal influences can be synergistic in their effects, resulting in delayed bedtimes, less time available for sleep, and greater difficulty falling and staying asleep. Not surprisingly, adolescents report that they find it difficult to wake up for school and stay awake at school; they then attempt to catch up on sleep on the weekends, resulting in variability in timing of sleep and contributing to poor sleep quality. As a result, adolescents with delayed sleep phase also frequently experience insomnia, short sleep duration, poor sleep quality, and daytime sleepiness.

In community samples, rates of evening circadian preference or delayed sleep phase range between 30% and 40% of adolescents.[1,21] Although this delay in circadian preference can be problematic for many youth, for youth that are able to adjust their sleep and wake times to accommodate this biologically driven delay, there may be few adverse consequences. Indeed, the American Academy of Sleep Medicine[22] and the Centers for Disease Control and Prevention[23] recommend that middle and high schools implement start times no earlier than 8:30 AM to promote adolescents' sleep needs, alertness, learning, safety, mental health, and well-being.

### Hypersomnia

Although not as clearly defined or thoroughly researched as insomnia and delayed sleep phase, hypersomnia (or hypersomnolence) is a crucial sleep disorder to consider among youth. Based on diagnostic criteria in the *Diagnostic and Statistical Manual of Mental Disorders*, 5th edition, the International Classification of Sleep Disorders-2, and the *International Classification of Diseases*, 10th edition, hypersomnia can be characterized by a combination of prolonged nighttime sleep episodes, increased nighttime wakefulness, frequent daytime napping, and, most notably, excessive daytime sleepiness.[24] However, excessive daytime sleepiness is neither synonymous with nor unique to hypersomnia—for example, in the International Classification of Sleep Disorders-2, excessive daytime sleepiness is also listed as an essential feature of both narcolepsy and behaviorally induced insufficient syndrome, and is associated with a variety of syndromes (eg, Kleine–Levin syndrome) and other sleep disorders, including insomnia and delayed sleep phase.[25] Because excessive daytime sleepiness is implicated in so many other diagnoses, idiopathic hypersomnia—that is, hypersomnia not explained by sleep deprivation, substance use, or other medical or psychiatric conditions—is significantly less common than excessive day-time sleepiness itself, which, as a symptom, is reported at fairly high rates among both adults and children.[26] Idiopathic hypersomnia is chronic, and patients tend to experience onset of symptoms during adolescence or early adulthood.[27] In addition to excessive daytime sleepiness combined with normal or prolonged (>10 hours) major sleep periods, patients with idiopathic hypersomnia often report a symptom known as sleep drunkenness, or waking up with confusion, automatic behavior, and repeated returns to sleep.[27]

Epidemiologic studies of hypersomnia have been inconsistent, focusing on the presence of one of 2 primary symptoms: excessive quantity of sleep or, more commonly, excessive daytime sleepiness.[25] Excessive daytime sleepiness among children and adolescents seems to be both prevalent and influenced by age: in pediatric clinics, excessive daytime sleepiness was twice as common among middle school-aged children than preschool-aged children,[28] and prevalence rates among preadolescents average to 4%, compared with 20% among high school seniors.[29] A confluence of factors—including physiologic changes that occur with maturation, sociocultural factors, and certain pathologies—predisposes teenagers in particular to excessive daytime sleepiness.[29]

## RATES OF SLEEP DISORDERS AMONG YOUTH WITH MOOD DISORDERS

As noted elsewhere in this article, the prevalence of insomnia, delayed sleep phase, and hypersomnia are quite common among community samples of children and adolescents; however, among samples of youth with a mood disorder, the prevalence rates are even higher. In a study of 553 youth (ages 7.3–14.9 years) with major depression,[30] 72.7% also reported a sleep disturbance (mostly insomnia). In adolescents with major depression, the rates of insomnia vary between 33% and 51%.[30] Although there are fewer studies that estimate rates of evening circadian preference among depressed youth, there are numerous studies that indicate a strong association between depression and evening circadian preference,[31–33] with some studies of depressed youth indicating evening preference in as much as 81% of some depressed samples.[31] Based on prevalence rates alone, it is clear that the relationship between sleep disorders and depression among youth is important.

Importantly, in a review by Gregory and Sadeh[34] the authors note that the concurrent relationship between sleep problems and depression may change over time. Indeed, 1 study[16] found that the association between sleep problems and depression was greater in children aged 11 years (odds ratio, 9.7) than aged 6 years (odds ratio, 4.7). Additionally, Gregory and Sadeh[34] reference a report[35] showing an increase in the magnitude of the association between sleep problems and depression from childhood (age 4 years; correlation, 0.39) to adolescence (age 13–15 years; correlation, 0.52). Gregory and Sadeh posit that a possible explanation for this trend is that sleep problems may be more common in children than adolescents and therefore perhaps more part of a typical development trajectory and less significant or indicative of a problem.

Bipolar disorder, with a weighted average prevalence rate across subtypes of 3.9% among children and adolescents, is also inextricably linked with sleep disorders.[36] Sleep disturbances associated with bipolar disorder may differ across manic, depressive, and euthymic states. Interestingly, the diagnostic criteria suggest that individuals in manic states may experience a decreased need for sleep, and community studies show the prevalence of decreased sleep need to be between 21% and 87.5% among youth affected by bipolar disorder.[37] In a sample of 8- to 11-year-olds with early onset bipolar spectrum disorders, 82% report having depression-related sleep problems, with initial insomnia being the most pervasive.[38] Hypersomnia is also particularly salient in youth with bipolar disorder—a study by Parker and colleagues[39] found hypersomnia to be present in 75% of patients with bipolar disorder younger than 25 years, but with increasing age, early morning awakening emerged as the dominant pattern instead.

Additionally, major depression, as well as subsyndromal depression, during adolescence and prepuberty seems to precede the development of bipolar disorder in emerging adulthood—this association has been replicated in a variety of prospective and retrospective studies.[40–42]

## SLEEP PROBLEMS MAY PREDICT AND PREDATE THE DEVELOPMENT OF MOOD DISORDERS

The relationship between sleep problems and the development of depression can be linked back to the perinatal period. Research suggests that maternal perinatal sleep quality has the potential to influence vulnerabilities in children's affective development. A large birth cohort study[43] found a prospective effect of prenatal insomnia symptoms on the social–emotional development of the child at 2 years of age, even after adjusting for confounding factors. However, the authors found the effect of perinatal insomnia on social–emotional child development to be mediated by postnatal factors—specifically, insomnia and depression symptoms—suggesting a potential chain of mechanisms characterizing this longitudinal process.[43] Indeed, in a review of the relationship between sleep quality and depression during the perinatal period, Okun[44] concluded that prenatal sleep disturbance is predictive of increased risk for development of postpartum depression.

Sleep characteristics in early infancy and toddlerhood seem to predict internalizing symptoms among toddlers and children. In a longitudinal study of 32,662 children, Sivertsen and colleagues[3] found short sleep duration and nocturnal awakenings at 18 months of age to be significantly predictive, in a dose–response manner, of internalizing problems at 5 years. Similarly, a recent study by Morales-Muñoz and colleagues[45] also found short sleep duration and nocturnal awakenings in infancy to be prospectively related to internalizing symptoms in toddlers. Another large population-based prospective study[46] found dyssomnia (frequent nocturnal awakenings), parasomnia (the presence of nightmares), and short sleep duration in infancy and toddlerhood to be associated with an increased risk for depressive symptoms at 3 years of age. Results from several studies indicate a significant path from sleep problems among preschool aged children to internalizing problems at school age.[47–49]

Among school-age children and adolescents, research indicates that insomnia likely precedes and predicts depressive episodes. A study of 289 twin pairs[50] found that sleep problems at age 8 predicted depression at age 10. Importantly, the authors also found that genetic influences played a significant role in the prospective relationship between insomnia and depression in this sample.[50] In another sample of youth age 13 to 16 years with comorbid insomnia and depression,[2] insomnia preceded depression in 69% of the sample; the authors also found a significant association between prior insomnia and onset of depression even after adjusting for gender, race/ethnicity, and any prior anxiety disorder.[2] Data from the Great Smoky Mountains Study[51] suggests a bidirectional relationship between sleep and depression, such that sleep problems during childhood predicted increases in the prevalence of later depression and anxiety symptoms in adolescents, and depression in childhood predicted later increases in sleep problems. Using a nationally representative sample of adolescents, our research group[1] examined specific sleep parameters that predict future depressive episodes. We found that late bedtime in middle school predicted more depression symptoms in young adulthood.[1] This study and others[32,33] suggest that evening circadian preference (indexed by late bedtime) may also be an important predictor of depression.

In a review, Alvaro, Roberts, and Harris[52] concluded, with caution, that the association between childhood sleep problems and depression is likely unidirectional. Indeed, several long-term longitudinal studies indicate that school-age childhood insomnia can predict adolescent and adult depression. As part of the British Cohort Study 1970, a prospective birth cohort with 30 years of follow-up (1975–2005), 7437 parents reported on the sleep difficulties of their 5-year-olds.[53] These children were followed up over 30 years, and when the participants were aged 34 years they were asked if they had been treated for depression in the past year.[53] After adjusting for a number of potential cofounds (including maternal depression and sleep), severe sleep problems at 5 years was a significant predictor of depression at age 34.[53] In another sample of 490 children from a large longitudinal study,[35] analyses indicate that sleep problems at age 4 predicted behavioral and emotional problems in mid adolescence. However, some researchers have failed to find evidence for this long-term relationship between sleep and depression. For example, Armstrong and colleagues[54] failed to find a prospective relationship between insomnia persistence and depression over 15 years.

Relatedly, there is increasing evidence that insomnia is also a prospective risk factor for self-harm, suicidal ideation, and suicidal behavior. In a longitudinal sample of adolescents, self-reported difficulties initiating or maintaining sleep at ages 12 to 14 significantly predicted suicidal thoughts and self-harm behaviors at ages 15 to 17.[55] In another sample of 101 youth selected for the presence of repeated self-harm behavior and high suicidality, self-reported sleep quality was significantly associated with elevated levels of overall self-harm, suicide attempts, nonsuicidal self-injurious behavior, and suicidal ideation at the same assessment, and predicted future self-harm within 30 days.[31]

Taken together, sleep problems as early as the perinatal period may be an opportunity for early identification of those at risk for depression. Sleep problems may also be a potential prevention intervention target for youth at risk for depression.

Sleep disorders may also indicate a risk for the later development of bipolar disorders. Evidence from adult experimental sleep research studies indicate that induced sleep deprivation is associated with the onset of mania or hypomania. In a study by Wehr and colleagues,[56] 9 rapidly cycling adult patients with bipolar disorder who were in a depressed phase were sleep deprived for 40 hours (ie, 1 night's sleep deprivation), triggering mania or hypomania in 7 of the 9 individuals. In another study, Colombo and colleagues (1999)[57] recruited 206 depressed bipolar patients and randomized them to receive 1 night of total sleep deprivation followed by either a recovery night or a recovery night in combination with several medications (lithium salts, fluoxetine, amineptine, and pindolol). The results indicated that, after only 1 night of sleep deprivation, 9% of patients switched into mania or hypomania.[57] These results point to the possibility that chronic sleep deprivation could greatly influence relapse to mania.

Similarly, evidence suggests that the development of bipolar disorder is often preceded by sleep disturbance in childhood and adolescence. In a sample of offspring (ages 10–16 years) with at least 1 parent with bipolar disorder, youth with poor sleep had nearly twice the odds of developing bipolar disorder relative to good or variable sleepers.[58] Another study using a distinct sample of offspring with at least 1 parent with bipolar disorder found that over an average of 3.8 years, disturbed sleep patterns accounted for nearly one-third (33.1%) of the explained variance in psychiatric symptom change; specifically, changes in mania, depression, anxiety, and mood lability were associated with shorter sleep duration, later sleep timing preference, poorer sleep continuity, and worsening daytime sleepiness.[59] In a community sample of 3021 young adults and adolescents, symptoms of trouble falling asleep and early morning awakening at baseline were predictive of subsequent onset of bipolar disorder.[60] Additionally, according to a meta-analysis of sleep disturbance predicting the onset of bipolar disorder, sleep disturbances during childhood and adolescence frequently precede bipolar episodes—specifically, insomnia seems to precede the onset of manic episodes (with a frequency range of 48.8% to 54.8%), and both insomnia (14.0% to 66.7%), and hypersomnia (14.0% to 33.3%) seem to precede the onset of depressive episodes.[61]

Given the evidence for a prodromal role of sleep disturbance in depression and mood episodes in bipolar disorder, sleep disturbance presents itself as a rich opportunity for the early detection of and intervention for youth at risk for mood disorders. However, for youth who already have mood disorders, the data on the prospective relationship between mood disorders and the development of sleep disorders are reviewed elsewhere in this article.

## THE RELATIONSHIP BETWEEN MOOD DISORDERS AND THE DEVELOPMENT OF SLEEP DISORDERS

Although the evidence reviewed elsewhere in this article points to a unidirectional relationship between sleep problems and mood disorders, there is also evidence to suggest the reverse relationship—that is, mood disorders as risk factors for later sleep problems—as well as a bidirectional relationship between the two.

There is a body of perinatal depression research that supports the idea that maternal perinatal depression may predict sleep problems among children, although it is unclear to what extent this association is mediated by concurrent maternal depression. In the Avon Longitudinal Study of Parents and Children (ALSPAC) cohort, O'Connor and colleagues[62] found that prenatal mood disturbance predicted offspring sleep problems at 18 and 30 months, independent of postnatal mood covariates. Similarly, results from the Finnish PREDO cohort showed that toddler-aged children of women with clinically significant depressive symptomology during pregnancy had, on average, shorter sleep duration, longer sleep latency, and more night awakenings (although this was fully mediated by concurrent maternal depressive symptomology) and were more likely to have a sleep disorder.[63] Interestingly, concurrent maternal depression added to the effect of prenatal depression on sleep disorders, such that children were most likely to have sleep disorders if their mothers had clinically significant depressive symptoms both during pregnancy and at the time of assessment.[63] Also using the ALSPAC cohort, Taylor and colleagues[64] found evidence that maternal postnatal depression was associated with an increased risk of sleep problems in adolescent offspring, suggesting that this association has the potential to persist beyond early childhood.

Most studies tend to support a unidirectional relationship where sleep problems precede and predict depression symptoms among children; however, a few studies have found a bidirectional relationship between sleep problems and depression. A longitudinal study[65] conducted among 2475 Norwegian children gathered from a primary care setting found a bidirectional relationship such that depression at age 4 was associated with insomnia at age 6 and insomnia at age 4 increased the risk for developing symptoms of depression at age 6. As mentioned elsewhere in this article, in data from the Great Smokey Mountain Study conducted among 1420 children followed longitudinally from ages 9 to 16 years, Shanahan and colleagues[51] found that sleep problems both predict and are predicted by depression.

Although most of the longitudinal data seem to support the idea that sleep problems commonly predict and predate depression, there are also data to support a more complex and bidirectional model where depression can also predict later development of sleep problems. These studies support the idea that perinatal depression is likely a predictor of sleep problems among offspring and that depressed youth may also be at risk for developing future sleep problems, thus creating a vicious cycle between sleep problems and depression.

A review of the literature found no such studies indicating the mania may precede sleep problems. However, as noted elsewhere in this article, depression symptoms during adolescence and the prepubertal period appear to precede the development of bipolar disorder in emerging adulthood.[40–42]

## COMORBIDITY BETWEEN MOOD DISORDERS AND SLEEP PROBLEMS IS ASSOCIATED WITH GREATER SYMPTOM SEVERITY

Sleep problems are associated with greater depression symptom severity. In a sample of more than 500 patients between the ages of 7.0 and 14.9 years,[30] sleep disturbance (observed in >70% of the sample) was associated with greater depression severity and a greater likelihood of presenting depressed mood, irritability, distinct sadness, psychomotor agitation, fatigue, anhedonia, inappropriate guilt, weight loss, and diurnal variation. Emslie and colleagues[66] found that, among children and adolescents with depressive disorders, insomnia symptoms, which were present in more than one-half the sample, were associated with a greater severity of specific depressive symptoms, including fatigue, suicidal ideation, physical complaints, and concentration. Similarly, among young adults with depressive symptoms, those reporting sleep disturbance had more anxiety symptoms than those without sleep disturbance.[67]

In children and adolescents, there is a growing body of research documenting the connection between sleep and suicidal ideation and self-harm. One community-based study of more than 600 school-aged children[68] found that significantly more children with self-harm behaviors reported subjective insomnia symptoms, even after adjusting for symptoms of depression. A cross-sectional, national and representative sample consisting of more than 75,000 students (grades 7–12) in Korea[69] found that sleep disturbance was significantly associated with suicidal ideation in adolescents. In a study conducted by Goldstein, Bridge, and Brent,[70] sleep disturbances were assessed in 140 adolescent who died by suicide and in 131 controls with a psychological autopsy protocol. The authors found that, when rates of sleep disturbances were compared between groups, suicide completers had higher rates of overall sleep disturbance within both the last week and the current affective episode.[70] In another study of Korean adolescents,[71] weekend catch-up sleep duration (an indicator of insufficient weekday sleep and a common behavior among evening preference teens) was associated with suicide attempts and self-injury.

Youth that present with both sleep problems and depression represent a particularly high-risk group. These youth tend to have more severe depression and higher rates of self-harm and suicidality. Sleep problems may be a marker of disease severity in these patients.

To date, there are little to no published data on the relationship between sleep and disease severity among youth with bipolar disorder. One study conducted by Lunsford-Avery and colleagues[72] among youth with bipolar disorder who were entering a treatment trial found that sleep disturbance was associated with greater depression severity but not mania; Another study using a functional MRI paradigm found that long and short sleep disturbance among youth with bipolar disorder was associated with less cognitive control under stress, an important factor for regulating impulsivity, which is characteristic of the disorder[73] and a correlate of disease severity.

Among adults with bipolar disorder, there are much more data to support the hypothesis that sleep problems correlate with disease severity. For example, in a sample of more than 400 adults with bipolar disorder in a euthymic phase, a shorter sleep duration was associated with increased mania severity, and greater sleep variability was associated with increased mania and depression severity.[74] A study of adolescents with bipolar disorder compared with control adolescents, found that increased awakenings and wakefulness on weekends predicted depression symptoms among adolescents with bipolar disorder.[75] In the STEP-BD trial, conducted among more than 2000 adults with bipolar disorder, a short sleep duration was associated with a more severe symptom presentation, whereas both short and long sleep durations were associated with poorer function and quality of life compared with a normal sleep duration.[76]

## SLEEP PROBLEMS MAY BE ASSOCIATED WITH POOR MOOD DISORDER TREATMENT RESPONSE

Problematically, sleep problems may also be associated with poor response to both psychosocial and psychopharmacological antidepressant treatments. One study conducted among 166 depressed adolescents treated with either a 12-week course of sertraline, cognitive-behavioral therapy, or a combination, found that, across treatment groups, pretreatment and persistent sleep disturbance was associated with lower response and remission rates.[77] In another study of 309 children and adolescents randomized to fluoxetine or placebo, the authors found similar antidepressant response in those with or without insomnia symptoms; however, there was a significant difference by age group.[66] Among adolescents, those with insomnia symptoms were less likely to respond to fluoxetine than those without, whereas in children, the reverse was true (ie, those with insomnia symptoms were more likely to respond to fluoxetine than those without insomnia).[66] Although it is not clear why age moderated the association between disturbed sleep and response to fluoxetine, the authors suggest that this might be related to developmental differences in sleep architecture between depressed children and adolescents.[66] This finding may also be related to the point made by Gregory and Sadeh[34] that sleep problems are more common among children than adolescents and may therefore be less associated with risk. In a study of psychotherapy conducted by McGlinchey and colleagues (2017),[78] the authors found that among depressed adolescents undergoing interpersonal psychotherapy for adolescents or treatment as usual, sleep disturbance predicted more depression and interpersonal stress across treatments and led to a slower improvement in depression and interpersonal functioning. Interestingly, in a retrospective study of adults being treated for comorbid depression and insomnia, the authors found that childhood onset insomnia predicted worse treatment outcomes, underlying the importance of treating insomnia for a successful course of depression treatment at all developmental stages.[79]

Taken together, the data point to sleep problems among adolescents as a risk factor for poor depression treatment response. These data highlight the clinical importance of evaluating sleep problems among child and adolescent health care providers, especially among youth with comorbid depression.

Among adults and adolescents with bipolar disorder the data are more mixed. Youth with bipolar disorder who received either family-focused treatment or a control therapy did not demonstrate improved sleep symptoms compared with the control treatment; however, their mood symptoms were significantly improved.[72] Moreover, in a study of adults with bipolar disorder who participated in the STEP-BD trial, sleep duration was not a moderator of psychotherapy outcomes. However, this study did not look at other important sleep outcomes such as sleep irregularity or insomnia symptoms.[80]

## SLEEP PROBLEMS MAY BE ASSOCIATED WITH RECURRENCE OF MOOD EPISODES

Recovery from depression occurs in more than 90% of depressed children and adolescents within 1 to 2 years.[81,82] However, once recovered, depressed children and adolescents experience high rates of recurrence of their depression. When reevaluated 6 to 7 years later, depression remained a problem in 25% to 50% of youth, and a new episode of depression was reported in 54% to 72% of depressed children and adolescents followed for 3 to 8 years.[83-88]

In adults and adolescents, insomnia is the most common residual symptom in remitted depression.[89-91] Moreover, adult data point to insomnia as an important predictor of recurrent depressive episodes.[92-94] In adolescents and children, there is less evidence for insomnia as a predictor of recurrence; however, 1 study providing evidence that sleep disruption may be a predictor of depression recurrence is highlighted here. Emslie and colleagues[95] (2001) conducted a naturalistic 1 year follow-up of 113 depressed children and adolescents. Using sleep polysomnography, the authors found that decreased sleep efficiency and delayed sleep onset (both indices of insomnia symptoms) at baseline predicted depression recurrence at the 1-year follow-up.[95] More research is needed in children and adolescents to further investigate sleep problems as a risk factor for depression recurrence.

Results from samples of adults and youth with bipolar disorder similarly find that sleep problems are associated with mood episode reoccurrence. Results from one study of youth with bipolar disorder indicated that sleep impairment and severity of manic and depressive symptoms were significantly intercorrelated over a 2-year period after treatment for mood symptoms.[72] As noted elsewhere in this article, in adults with bipolar disorder enrolled in the STEP-BD trial for whom follow-up data were available, a shorter sleep duration was associated with increased mania severity, and greater sleep variability was associated with increased mania and depression severity over a 12-month period.[76]

## TREATMENT OF COMORBID MOOD DISORDERS AND SLEEP PROBLEMS

Given the severity and clinical implications of samples of depressed youth with comorbid sleep problems, the natural conclusion is to address both conditions with evidence-based psychotherapy and psychopharmacology. In the Treatment of Resistant Depression in Adolescents Study (TORDIA),[96] 334 treatment-resistant adolescents with depression received 1 of the 4 treatment strategies in a 2 × 2 balanced factorial design: (a) switch to another selective serotonin reuptake inhibitor, (b) switch to venlafaxine, (c) switch to another selective serotonin reuptake inhibitor plus cognitive-behavioral therapy (CBT); or (d) switch to venlafaxine plus cognitive behavioral therapy (CBT). Those adolescents who received pharmacologic treatment for sleep difficulties showed a poorer response rate than did those who did not receive medication for sleep, indicating that nonpharmacologic therapies may be a preferable first line of treatment for adolescents with treatment resistant depression receiving antidepressant pharmacotherapy.[96]

CBT for insomnia (CBT-I) is the first-line recommended treatment for insomnia in adults. Numerous studies have demonstrated its effectiveness in treating insomnia with and without medical and psychiatric comorbidities. Several systematic reviews and meta-analyses[7,8,97] focused on the effectiveness of CBT-I in children and adolescents have found that CBT-I can effectively improve sleep in school-age children and adolescents and that improvements are maintained over time.

In the preparation of this review, only 1 trial that tested concomitant treatment of depression and insomnia among adolescents was identified. The study compared the combination of CBT for depression plus CBT-I to CBT for depression plus sleep hygiene control therapy for insomnia among adolescents with comorbid insomnia and depression; the authors found no difference in rates of recovery from depression between the 2 conditions.[6] However, when limiting the analysis to those who remitted from depression, the researchers found a trend for faster remission among those in the CBT-I group,[6] indicating that sleep improvement does play an important role in depression remission. Interestingly, this mirrors the findings in adult trials of depression treatment augmentation with CBT-I.[98–100] More research is needed in this important domain to identify potential moderators of depression treatment outcome among youth with comorbid depression and sleep problems.

Although sleep pharmacotherapy may be contraindicated in some samples of youth with comorbid depression and sleep problems, CBT-I is an effective psychosocial intervention for improving insomnia symptoms among youth. However, although sleep improvement seems to be an important mediator of depression treatment among youth with depression and sleep problems, augmenting antidepressant treatment (psychosocial or pharmacologic) with CBT-I may not necessarily improve depression outcomes. Of note, individuals with delayed sleep phase (who also very commonly have insomnia) have been left out of many of these trials[6,98,99] owing to concerns that CBT-I does not adequately address circadian concerns. As noted elsewhere in this article, delayed sleep phase is a very common concern among adolescents and particularly among depressed adolescents.[1,17,32] A report published by our group provides some evidence from the adult literature that those with a delayed sleep preference and depression may be at risk for poor depression treatment response unless their sleep problems are addressed.[101]

There are no studies conducted to date that directly address treatment of sleep disturbance among youth with bipolar disorder and there is only one trial of CBT-I among adults with bipolar disorder. This study, conducted by Allison Harvey and colleagues,[102] found that relative to a psychoeducation condition, CBT-I for bipolar disorder (CBTI-BP) decreased insomnia severity and led to higher rates of insomnia remission after treatment and marginally higher rates at 6 months of follow-up, indicating that CBTI-BP is safe and effective for patients with bipolar disorder. Moreover, during the 6-month follow-up, the CBTI-BP group had fewer days in a bipolar episode (3.3 days vs 25.5 days), experienced a significantly lower hypomania/mania relapse rate (4.6% vs 31.6%), and a marginally lower overall mood episode relapse rate (13.6% vs 42.1%) compared with the control group.[102] In summary, this study indicates that CBTI-BP is effective for insomnia among patients with bipolar disorder and may also reduce the frequency and intensity of mood episodes among patients with bipolar disorder. The authors recommend that practitioners should encourage regularity in sleep and wake times as a first step in treatment, and carefully monitor changes in mood and daytime sleepiness throughout the intervention.[103] However, it should be noted that this is the only study to date to specifically test CBT-I in patients with bipolar disorder and the results should be replicated.

## SUMMARY

Sleep problems play an important role in the development, progression, and maintenance of unipolar and bipolar depression symptoms among children and adolescents. Identification of sleep problems as early as maternal perinatal insomnia may predict and predate depression among youth. Depression prevention through the early identification and treatment of sleep problems is an important future direction for research. Data suggest that children and adolescents who go on to develop comorbid mood symptoms and sleep problems represent a particularly high-risk group. Children and adolescents with comorbid mood symptoms and sleep problems tend to have more severe depressive symptoms, higher rates of self-harm and suicidality, and their depression symptoms tend to be less responsive to treatment. Even when depression and bipolar disorder treatments successfully improve mood symptoms, sleep problems tend to be among the most common residual symptoms and, if untreated, may be associated with recurrent depression and/or mania. Treatment research supports the idea that sleep problems can be improved through CBT-I among youth with and without depression. Although limited, the treatment research also indicates that, although CBT-I may not significantly augment depression treatment outcomes, sleep improvement is an important mediator of depression treatment outcomes. Although there are no CBT-I data among youth with bipolar disorder, adult data suggest that CBTI-BP may improve both insomnia and mood symptoms among adults with bipolar disorder. Moreover, more research is needed on sleep problems that have been underevaluated and undertreated, such as delayed sleep phase.

## CLINICS CARE POINTS

- Sleep problems such as delayed sleep phase, hypersomnia, and insomnia should be evaluated in clinical care for both the treatment and prevention of mood symptoms among youth.
- Youth who present with comorbid mood and sleep problems are a particularly high-risk group.
- CBT-I is an effective treatment for sleep problems among youth with and without depression.
- If left untreated, sleep problems are among the most common residual symptoms after mood episode remission and are likely a risk factor for mood episode recurrence.

## ACKNOWLEDGMENT

This project was supported by 1K23MH116520-01A1 from the National Institute of Mental Health, a fellowship for Access to Care from the Klingenstein Third Generation Foundation, and a NARSAD Young Investigator Award from the Brain and Behavior Research Foundation awarded to LDA.

## REFERENCES

1. Asarnow LD, McGlinchey E, Harvey AG. The effects of bedtime and sleep duration on academic and emotional outcomes in a nationally representative sample of adolescents. J Adolesc Health 2014;54(3):350–6.

2. Johnson EO, Roth T, Breslau N. The association of insomnia with anxiety disorders and depression: exploration of the direction of risk. J Psychiatr Res 2006; 40(8):700–8.

3. Sivertsen B, Harvey AG, Reichborn-Kjennerud T, et al. Later emotional and behavioral problems associated with sleep problems in toddlers: a longitudinal study. JAMA Pediatr 2015;169(6):575–82.

4. McGlinchey EL, Harvey AG. Risk behaviors and negative health outcomes for adolescents with late bedtimes. J Youth Adolesc 2015;44(2):478–88.

5. Harvey AG, Hein K, Dolsen MR, et al. Modifying the impact of eveningness chronotype ("night-owls") in youth: a randomized controlled trial. J Am Acad Child Adolesc Psychiatry 2018;57(10):742–54.

6. Clarke G, McGlinchey EL, Hein K, et al. Cognitive-behavioral treatment of insomnia and depression in adolescents: a pilot randomized trial. Behav Res Ther 2015;69:111–8.

7. Åslund L, Arnberg F, Kanstrup M, et al. Cognitive and behavioral interventions to improve sleep in school-age children and adolescents: a systematic review and meta-analysis. J Clin Sleep Med 2018;14(11):1937–47.

8. Blake MJ, Sheeber LB, Youssef GJ, et al. Systematic review and meta-analysis of adolescent cognitive–behavioral sleep interventions. Clin Child Fam Psychol Rev 2017;20(3):227–49.

9. Schredl M, Fricke-Oerkermann L, Mitschke A, et al. Longitudinal study of nightmares in children: stability and effect of emotional symptoms. Child Psychiatry Hum Dev 2009;40(3):439–49.

10. Yilmaz E, Sedky K, Bennett DS. The relationship between depressive symptoms and obstructive sleep apnea in pediatric populations: a meta-analysis. J Clin Sleep Med 2013;9(11):1213–20.

11. Association AP. Diagnostic and statistical manual of mental disorders (DSM-5®). American Psychiatric Pub; 2013.

12. Combs D, Goodwin JL, Quan SF, et al. Insomnia, health-related quality of life and health outcomes in children: a seven year longitudinal cohort. Sci Rep 2016;6:27921.

13. Medicine AAoS. International classification of sleep disorders. 3rd edition. American Academy Of Sleep Medicine; 2014.

14. Kerr S, Jowett S. Sleep problems in pre-school children: a review of the literature. Child Care Health Dev 1994;20(6):379–91.

15. Owens JA, Spirito A, McGuinn M, et al. Sleep habits and sleep disturbance in elementary school-aged children. J Dev Behav Pediatr 2000;21(1):27–36.

16. Johnson EO, Chilcoat HD, Breslau N. Trouble sleeping and anxiety/depression in childhood. Psychiatry Res 2000;94(2):93–102.

17. Carskadon MA, Vieira C, Acebo C. Association between puberty and delayed phase preference. Sleep 1993;16(3):258–62.

18. Orzech KM, Grandner MA, Roane BM, et al. Digital media use in the 2 h before bedtime is associated with sleep variables in university students. Comput Hum Behav 2016;55(A):43–50.

19. Carskadon MA. Patterns of sleep and sleepiness in adolescents. Pediatrician 1990;17(1):5–12.

20. Wolfson AR, Carskadon MA. Sleep schedules and daytime functioning in adolescents. Child Dev 1998;69(4):875–87.

21. Gradisar M, Wolfson AR, Harvey AG, et al. The sleep and technology use of Americans: findings from the National Sleep Foundation's 2011 Sleep in America poll. J Clin Sleep Med 2013;9(12):1291–9.

22. Watson NF, Martin JL, Wise MS, et al. Delaying middle school and high school start times promotes student health and performance: an American Academy of Sleep Medicine position statement. J Clin Sleep Med 2017;13(4):623–5.

23. Prevention CfDCa. Schools start too early. Available at: https://www.cdc.gov/sleep/features/schools-start-too-early.html.

24. Kaplan KA, Harvey AG. Hypersomnia across mood disorders: a review and synthesis. Sleep Med Rev 2009;13(4):275–85.

25. Ohayon MM. From wakefulness to excessive sleepiness: what we know and still need to know. Sleep Med Rev 2008;12(2):129–41.

26. Saini P, Rye DB. Hypersomnia: evaluation, treatment, and social and economic aspects. Sleep Med Clin 2017;12(1):47–60.

27. Kothare SV, Kaleyias J. Narcolepsy and other hypersomnias in children. Curr Opin Pediatr 2008;20(6):666–75.

28. Archbold KH, Pituch KJ, Panahi P, et al. Symptoms of sleep disturbances among children at two general pediatric clinics. The J Pediatr 2002;140(1):97–102.

29. Kotagal S. Hypersomnia in children. Sleep Med Clin 2012;7(2):379–89.

30. Liu X, Buysse DJ, Gentzler AL, et al. Insomnia and hypersomnia associated with depressive phenomenology and comorbidity in childhood depression. Sleep 2007;30(1):83–90.

31. Asarnow JB, S Babeva, K Adrian, et al. Sleep in youths with repeated self-harm and high suicidality: does sleep predict self-harm risk?, in press.

32. Selvi Y, Aydin A, Boysan M, et al. Associations between chronotype, sleep quality, suicidality, and depressive symptoms in patients with major depression and healthy controls. Chronobiol Int 2010;27(9–10):1813–28.

33. Chan JW, Lam SP, Li SX, et al. Eveningness and insomnia: independent risk factors of nonremission in major depressive disorder. Sleep 2014;37(5):911–7.

34. Gregory AM, Sadeh A. Sleep, emotional and behavioral difficulties in children and adolescents. Sleep Med Rev 2012;16(2):129–36.

35. Gregory AM, O'connor TG. Sleep problems in childhood: a longitudinal study of developmental change and association with behavioral problems. J Am Acad Child Adolesc Psychiatry 2002;41(8):964–71.

36. Van AM, Moreira ALR, Youngstrom E. Updated meta-analysis of epidemiologic studies of pediatric bipolar disorder. J Clin Psychiatry 2019;80(3):18r12180.

37. Harvey AG, Talbot LS, Gershon A. Sleep disturbance in bipolar disorder across the lifespan. Clin Psychol (New York) 2009;16(2):256–77.

38. Lofthouse N, Fristad M, Splaingard M, et al. Parent and child reports of sleep problems associated with early-onset bipolar spectrum disorders. J Fam Psychol 2007;21(1):114.

39. Parker G, Malhi G, Hadzi-Pavlovic D, et al. Sleeping in? The impact of age and depressive sub-type on hypersomnia. J Affect Disord 2006;90(1):73–6.

40. Geller B, Zimerman B, Williams M, et al. Bipolar disorder at prospective follow-up of adults who had prepubertal major depressive disorder. Am J Psychiatry 2001;158(1):125–7.

41. Strober M, Carlson G. Bipolar illness in adolescents with major depression: clinical, genetic, and psychopharmacologic predictors in a three-to four-year prospective follow-up investigation. Arch Gen Psychiatry 1982;39(5):549–55.

42. Skjelstad DV, Malt UF, Holte A. Symptoms and signs of the initial prodrome of bipolar disorder: a systematic review. J Affect Disord 2010;126(1–2):1–13.

43. Adler I, Weidner K, Eberhard-Gran M, et al. The impact of maternal symptoms of perinatal insomnia on social-emotional child development: a population-based, 2-year follow-up study. Behav Sleep Med 2020;1–15.
44. Okun ML. Disturbed sleep and postpartum depression. Curr Psychiatry Rep 2016;18(7):66.
45. Morales-Muñoz I, Lemola S, Saarenpää-Heikkilä O, et al. Parent-reported early sleep problems and internalising, externalising and dysregulation symptoms in toddlers. BMJ Paediatr Open 2020;4(1):e000622.
46. Jansen PW, Saridjan NS, Hofman A, et al. Does disturbed sleeping precede symptoms of anxiety or depression in toddlers? The generation R study. Psychosom Med 2011;73(3):242–9.
47. Troxel WM, Trentacosta CJ, Forbes EE, et al. Negative emotionality moderates associations among attachment, toddler sleep, and later problem behaviors. J Fam Psychol 2013;27(1):127.
48. Whalen DJ, Gilbert KE, Barch DM, et al. Variation in common preschool sleep problems as an early predictor for depression and anxiety symptom severity across time. J Child Psychol Psychiatry 2017;58(2):151–9.
49. Hatzinger M, Brand S, Perren S, et al. In pre-school children, sleep objectively assessed via sleep-EEGs remains stable over 12 months and is related to psychological functioning, but not to cortisol secretion. J Psychiatr Res 2013;47(11):1809–14.
50. Gregory AM, Rijsdijk FV, Lau JY, et al. The direction of longitudinal associations between sleep problems and depression symptoms: a study of twins aged 8 and 10 years. Sleep 2009;32(2):189–99.
51. Shanahan L, Copeland WE, Angold A, et al. Sleep problems predict and are predicted by generalized anxiety/depression and oppositional defiant disorder. J Am Acad Child Adolesc Psychiatry 2014;53(5):550–8.
52. Alvaro PK, Roberts RM, Harris JK. A systematic review assessing bidirectionality between sleep disturbances, anxiety, and depression. Sleep 2013;36(7):1059–68.
53. Greene G, Gregory AM, Fone D, et al. Childhood sleeping difficulties and depression in adulthood: the 1970 British Cohort Study. J Sleep Res 2015;24(1):19–23.
54. Armstrong JM, Ruttle PL, Klein MH, et al. Associations of child insomnia, sleep movement, and their persistence with mental health symptoms in childhood and adolescence. Sleep 2014;37(5):901–9.
55. Wong MM, Brower KJ, Zucker RA. Sleep problems, suicidal ideation, and self-harm behaviors in adolescence. J Psychiatr Res 2011;45(4):505–11.
56. Wehr TA, Goodwin FK, Wirz-Justice A, et al. 48-hour sleep-wake cycles in manic-depressive illness: naturalistic observations and sleep deprivation experiments. Arch Gen Psychiatry 1982;39(5):559–65.
57. Colombo C, Benedetti F, Barbini B, et al. Rate of switch from depression into mania after therapeutic sleep deprivation in bipolar depression. Psychiatry Res 1999;86(3):267–70.
58. Levenson JC, Soehner A, Rooks B, et al. Longitudinal sleep phenotypes among offspring of bipolar parents and community controls. J Affect Disord 2017;215:30–6.
59. Soehner AM, Bertocci MA, Levenson JC, et al. Longitudinal associations between sleep patterns and psychiatric symptom severity in high-risk and community comparison youth. J Am Acad Child Adolesc Psychiatry 2019;58(6):608–17.

60. Ritter PS, Höfler M, Wittchen H-U, et al. Disturbed sleep as risk factor for the subsequent onset of bipolar disorder–data from a 10-year prospective-longitudinal study among adolescents and young adults. J Psychiatr Res 2015;68:76–82.

61. Pancheri C, Verdolini N, Pacchiarotti I, et al. A systematic review on sleep alterations anticipating the onset of bipolar disorder. Eur Psychiatry 2019;58:45–53.

62. O'Connor TG, Caprariello P, Blackmore ER, et al. Prenatal mood disturbance predicts sleep problems in infancy and toddlerhood. Early Hum Dev 2007; 83(7):451–8.

63. Toffol E, Lahti-Pulkkinen M, Lahti J, et al. Maternal depressive symptoms during and after pregnancy are associated with poorer sleep quantity and quality and sleep disorders in 3.5-year-old offspring. Sleep Med 2019;56:201–10.

64. Taylor AK, Netsi E, O'Mahen H, et al. The association between maternal postnatal depressive symptoms and offspring sleep problems in adolescence. Psychol Med 2017;47(3):451–9.

65. Steinsbekk S, Wichstrøm L. Stability of sleep disorders from preschool to first grade and their bidirectional relationship with psychiatric symptoms. J Dev Behav Pediatr 2015;36(4):243–51.

66. Emslie GJ, Kennard BD, Mayes TL, et al. Insomnia moderates outcome of serotonin-selective reuptake inhibitor treatment in depressed youth. J Child Adolesc Psychopharmacol 2012;22(1):21–8.

67. Nyer M, Farabaugh A, Fehling K, et al. Relationship between sleep disturbance and depression, anxiety, and functioning in college students. Depress Anxiety 2013;30(9):873–80.

68. Singareddy R, Krishnamurthy VB, Vgontzas AN, et al. Subjective and objective sleep and self-harm behaviors in young children: a general population study. Psychiatry Res 2013;209(3):549–53.

69. Park JH, Yoo JH, Kim SH. Associations between non-restorative sleep, short sleep duration and suicidality: findings from a representative sample of Korean adolescents. Psychiatry Clin Neurosci 2013;67(1):28–34.

70. Goldstein TR, Bridge JA, Brent DA. Sleep disturbance preceding completed suicide in adolescents. J Consult Clin Psychol 2008;76(1):84.

71. Kang SG, Lee YJ, Kim SJ, et al. Weekend catch-up sleep is independently associated with suicide attempts and self-injury in Korean adolescents. Compr Psychiatry 2014;55(2):319–25.

72. Lunsford-Avery JR, Judd CM, Axelson DA, et al. Sleep impairment, mood symptoms, and psychosocial functioning in adolescent bipolar disorder. Psychiatry Res 2012;200(2–3):265–71.

73. Soehner AM, Goldstein TR, Gratzmiller SM, et al. Cognitive control under stressful conditions in transitional age youth with bipolar disorder: diagnostic and sleep-related differences in fronto-limbic activation patterns. Bipolar Disord 2018;20(3):238–47.

74. Gruber J, Miklowitz DJ, Harvey AG, et al. Sleep matters: sleep functioning and course of illness in bipolar disorder. J Affect Disord 2011;134(1–3):416–20.

75. Gershon A, Singh MK. Sleep in adolescents with bipolar I disorder: stability and relation to symptom change. J Clin Child Adolesc Psychol 2017;46(2):247–57.

76. Gruber J, Harvey AG, Wang PW, et al. Sleep functioning in relation to mood, function, and quality of life at entry to the Systematic Treatment Enhancement Program for Bipolar Disorder (STEP-BD). J Affect Disord 2009;114(1–3):41–9.

77. Manglick M, Rajaratnam SM, Taffe J, et al. Persistent sleep disturbance is associated with treatment response in adolescents with depression. Aust N Z J Psychiatry 2013;47(6):556–63.

78. McGlinchey EL, Reyes-Portillo JA, Turner JB, et al. Innovations in practice: the relationship between sleep disturbances, depression, and interpersonal functioning in treatment for adolescent depression. Child Adolesc Ment Health 2017;22(2):96–9.

79. Edinger JD, Manber R, Buysse DJ, et al. Are patients with childhood onset of insomnia and depression more difficult to treat than are those with adult onsets of these disorders? A report from the TRIAD study. J Clin Sleep Med 2017;13(2):205–13.

80. Sylvia L, Salcedo S, Peters A, et al. Do sleep disturbances predict or moderate the response to psychotherapy in bipolar disorder? J Nerv Ment Dis 2017;205(3):196.

81. McCauley E, Myers K, Mitchell J, Calderon R, et al. Depression in young people: initial presentation and clinical course. J Am Acad Child Adolesc Psychiatry 1993;32(4):714–22.

82. Kovacs M, Feinberg TL, Crouse-Novak MA, et al. Depressive disorders in childhood: I. A longitudinal prospective study of characteristics and recovery. Arch Gen Psychiatry 1984;41(3):229–37.

83. Strober M, Lampert C, Schmidt S, et al. The course of major depressive disorder in adolescents: I. Recovery and risk of manic switching in a follow-up of psychotic and nonpsychotic subtypes. J Am Acad Child Adolesc Psychiatry 1993;32(1):34–42.

84. Emslie GJ, Rush AJ, Weinberg WA, et al. Recurrence of major depressive disorder in hospitalized children and adolescents. J Am Acad Child Adolesc Psychiatry 1997;36(6):785–92.

85. Keller MB, Beardslee W, Lavori PW, et al. Course of major depression in non-referred adolescents: a retrospective study. J Affective Disord 1988;15(3):235–43.

86. Asarnow JR, Bates S. Depression in child psychiatric inpatients: cognitive and attributional patterns. J Abnormal Child Psychol 1988;16(6):601–15.

87. Eastgate J, Gilmour L. Long-term outcome of depressed children: a follow-up study. Dev Med Child Neurol 1984;26(1):68–72.

88. Goodyer I, Germany E, Gowrusankur J, et al. Social influences on the course of anxious and depressive disorders in school-age children. Br J Psychiatry 1991;158:676–84.

89. Kennard B, Silva S, Vitiello B, et al. Remission and residual symptoms after short-term treatment in the treatment of adolescents with depression study (TADS). J Am Acad Child Adolesc Psychiatry 2006;45(12):1404–11.

90. Nierenberg A, Husain M, Trivedi M, et al. Residual symptoms after remission of major depressive disorder with citalopram and risk of relapse: a STAR* D report. Psychol Med 2010;40(1):41.

91. Tao R, Emslie GJ, Mayes TL, et al. Symptom improvement and residual symptoms during acute antidepressant treatment in pediatric major depressive disorder. J Child Adolesc Psychopharmacol 2010;20(5):423–30.

92. Perils ML, Giles DE, Buysse DJ, et al. Self-reported sleep disturbance as a prodromal symptom in recurrent depression. J Affect Disord 1997;42(2-3):209–12.

93. Dombrovski AY, Cyranowski JM, Mulsant BH, et al. Which symptoms predict recurrence of depression in women treated with maintenance interpersonal psychotherapy? Depress Anxiety 2008;25(12):1060–6.

94. Franzen PL, Buysse DJ. Sleep disturbances and depression: risk relationships for subsequent depression and therapeutic implications. Dialogues Clin Neurosci 2008;10(4):473–81.

95. Emslie GJ, Armitage R, Weinberg WA, et al. Sleep polysomnography as a predictor of recurrence in children and adolescents with major depressive disorder. Int J Neuropsychopharmacol 2001;4(2):159–68.

96. Brent D, Emslie G, Clarke G, et al. Switching to another SSRI or to venlafaxine with or without cognitive behavioral therapy for adolescents with SSRI-resistant depression: the TORDIA randomized controlled trial. JAMA 2008; 299(8):901–13.

97. Meltzer LJ, Mindell JA. Systematic review and meta-analysis of behavioral interventions for pediatric insomnia. J Pediatr Psychol 2014;39(8):932–48.

98. Manber R, Buysse DJ, Edinger J, et al. Efficacy of cognitive-behavioral therapy for insomnia combined with antidepressant pharmacotherapy in patients with comorbid depression and insomnia: a randomized controlled trial. J Clin Psychiatry 2016;77(10):e1316–23.

99. Carney CE, Edinger JD, Kuchibhatla M, et al. Cognitive behavioral insomnia therapy for those with insomnia and depression: a randomized controlled clinical trial. Sleep 2017;40(4):zsx019.

100. McCall WV, Benca RM, Rosenquist PB, et al. Reducing suicidal ideation through insomnia treatment (REST-IT): a randomized clinical trial. Am J Psychiatry 2019; 176(11):957–65.

101. Asarnow LD, Bei B, Krystal A, et al. Circadian preference as a moderator of depression outcome following cognitive behavioral therapy for insomnia plus antidepressant medications: a report from the TRIAD study. J Clin Sleep Med 2019;15(4):573–80.

102. Harvey AG, Soehner AM, Kaplan KA, et al. Treating insomnia improves mood state, sleep, and functioning in bipolar disorder: a pilot randomized controlled trial. J Consul Clin Psychol 2015;83(3):564–77.

103. Kaplan KA, Harvey AG. Behavioral treatment of insomnia in bipolar disorder. Am J Psychiatry 2013;170(7):716–20.

# When Night Falls Fast

## Sleep and Suicidal Behavior Among Adolescents and Young Adults

Sara N. Fernandes, MA[a], Emily Zuckerman, BA[b],
Regina Miranda, PhD[c], Argelinda Baroni, MD[d],*

**KEYWORDS**

- Suicide • Sleep • Nightmares • Insomnia • Adolescent • Young adult

**KEY POINTS**

- Sleep disturbances, including insomnia and nightmares, are associated with suicidal behaviors in youth and predictive of future suicidal ideation.
- Data regarding hypersomnia, sleep apnea, and suicide risk in youth are mixed.
- Interconnected biological and psychological mechanisms may underlie the relationship between sleep and suicidal behaviors: executive functioning, hyperarousal, thwarted belongingness, and perceived burdensomeness, among others.

## INTRODUCTION

Suicide is a leading cause of death worldwide; in the United States it is the tenth leading cause of death across the lifespan and the second leading cause of death among youth. Adolescents are at increased risk for both suicidal ideation and behaviors.[1,2] Notably, most youth who move from ideation to suicide planning do so within 1 year of the onset of their ideation.[3] Despite decades of research on risk factors for youth suicidal behavior, clinicians are not able to accurately predict or effectively prevent these catastrophic events.[4] Historically, many risk factor studies have focused on psychiatric diagnoses, distal and time-invariant risk factors such as history of child

This article originally appeared in *Child and Adolescent Psychiatric Clinics*, Volume 30 Issue 1, January 2021.

Funding: This work was partially funded with grant MH120846.

[a] New York State Psychiatric Institute, Columbia University Irving Medical Center, 1051 Riverside Drive, Room 1600C, New York, NY 10032, USA; [b] Department of Child and Adolescent Psychiatry, NYU Langone Health, One Park Avenue, 7th Floor, New York, NY 10016, USA; [c] Department of Psychology, Hunter College and The Graduate Center, City University of New York, 695 Park Avenue, Room 611HN, New York, NY 10065, USA; [d] Department of Child and Adolescent Psychiatry, NYU Grossman School of Medicine, One Park Avenue, 7th Floor, New York, NY 10016, USA

* Corresponding author.

*E-mail address:* Argelinda.Baroni@nyulangone.org

Psychiatr Clin N Am 47 (2024) 273–286

https://doi.org/10.1016/j.psc.2023.06.017

0193-953X/24/© 2023 Elsevier Inc. All rights reserved.

abuse, and demographic variables, which have not been useful in short-term detection and prediction of suicide risk.[4]

Accordingly, it is critical to identify transdiagnostic and proximal suicide risk factors that can be objectively assessed and are amenable to interventions. Sleep problems, especially insomnia and nightmares, represent a promising area in suicide research and prevention.[4] This article discusses (1) what is known regarding the relationships between sleep symptoms and suicide, (2) potential mechanisms underlying these associations, and (3) assessments and treatments currently used in clinical practice.

## SLEEP DISTURBANCES AND SUICIDAL IDEATION AND BEHAVIORS

Insomnia, short sleep duration, and nightmares have repeatedly been found to be associated with increased suicide risk (ie, ideation and/or behaviors, such as planning and attempts) in children, adolescents, and young adults, even if several limitations have been noted.[5–11] Main limitations include paucity of prospective studies and lack of use of reliable sleep measures; most studies have extracted a few sleep questions rather than using validated questionnaires focusing on sleep.[4,11]

### Insomnia and Short Sleep Duration

Insomnia, common across all ages, includes difficulties going to sleep or staying asleep, accompanied by daytime dysfunction.[12] Large cross-sectional adolescent surveys show that experiencing insomnia or insufficient sleep duration is associated with increased rates of suicidal ideation after adjusting for covariates such as age, sex, socioeconomic status, depressive symptoms, and mood disorders.[4,6,13,14] A recent meta-analysis of cross-sectional data from 37,536 adolescents estimated that sleep disturbances substantially and significantly increase risk of suicidal ideation (odds ratio [OR], 2.35), plans (OR, 1.58) and attempts (OR, 1.92), with girls at higher risk of sleep-related suicide attempts than boys.[11]

Data from the Youth Risk Behavior Survey found that short sleep duration was associated with suicidal ideation and behaviors in a dose-dependent manner among 67,615 adolescents surveyed, independently of causes (eg, insomnia vs volitional sleep restriction). Adolescents who slept less than 6 hours (vs 8 hours) had more than 3 times higher odds of considering suicide, planning to attempt suicide, or attempting suicide, and more than 4 times higher odds of reporting an attempt that resulted in treatment.[15] Similarly, a recent review noted that an additional hour of sleep was associated with significantly decreased suicidal ideation among adolescents.[16] A study of adolescent monozygotic twins found short sleep durations to be related to both suicidal ideation and behaviors, adjusting for genetics and shared environments.[17] Similar results were found in studies linking insomnia with suicidal behaviors, including planning and attempts.[6,7,18,19] A study of adolescent suicide completers versus community controls found that the presence of insomnia, both within the week before death and within the current affective episode, significantly distinguished completers from controls, even after adjusting for affective disorders and depressive symptom severity.[18]

Moving beyond cross-sectional and self-report methods, prospective studies have also supported insomnia and short sleep duration as independent risk factors for future suicidal ideation and attempts.[11,20] A systematic review found that, in 7 of 10 studies, sleep problems significantly predicted suicidal ideation and behaviors among adolescents. However, a meta-analysis on the role of sleep in suicidal behaviors was inconclusive.[11] However, in one of the few studies that assessed sleep and suicide prospectively and proximally (after 1-week and 3-week periods) using both subjective and objective (ie, actigraphic) methods, insomnia significantly predicted future ideation among young adults.[20] Altogether, the literature supports insomnia as an independent risk factor for present and future suicidal ideation and behaviors. Accordingly, assessing insomnia subjectively and/or objectively may help clinicians determine an adolescent's current and future risk of suicidal ideation and behaviors. The literature supporting this conclusion spans a wide range of adolescent populations (eg, community based, nationally representative, and clinically severe), further supporting its potential use in a variety of clinical and community settings.[4]

### Extended Sleep Time

Hypersomnia has also been associated with heightened suicide risk in adolescents.[16] However, the literature on hypersomnia is mixed, possibly because of inconsistent definitions across studies. One study found that extended sleep time (>10 hours) was associated with increased suicidal ideation and behaviors (ie, ideation, planning, and/or attempts; OR, 4.7) in adolescents,[21] whereas another noted that daytime sleepiness was associated with suicidal behaviors.[22] In a study comparing adolescent suicide completers and community controls, sleeping longer than usual yielded a significant group difference.[18] Incidentally, Diagnostic and Statistical Manual of Mental Disorders, Fifth Edition (DSM-5), defines hypersomnia as excessive daytime sleepiness and extended sleep periods as the main criteria.[12] At the same time, some studies have found no significant relation between longer sleep periods and suicidal behavior, and some have reported the opposite effect: that hypersomnia was protective.[6,23,24] Guo and colleagues[6] found that sleeping more than 9 hours (vs 7–9 hours) was associated with significantly higher odds of suicide attempts (OR, 2.5) in adolescents, but it was not associated with ideation. Of note, 9 hours is the normal sleep time for adolescents. In contrast, another study found that insomnia was related to suicidal ideation and attempts, but hypersomnia was not.[23] Moreover, Kim and colleagues[7] found that adolescents who self-reported typically spending 10 or more hours in bed had lower odds (OR, 0.61) of endorsing suicidal ideation and plans, compared with youth sleeping around 7 h/d. A few large, cross-sectional studies support a U-shaped relationship between suicidal behavior and sleep, with both short sleep periods and extended ones (>9 or 10 hours) being associated with more suicidal events (ideation and/or attempts).[16] Overall, more research is needed to understand the relationship between hypersomnia and suicidal behaviors and differentiate between total sleep time, total time in bed, and daytime sleepiness.

### Sleep Regularity

Although less commonly studied than insomnia and sleep duration, sleep regularity and circadian rhythms have been found to be associated with increased suicide risk among adolescents and young adults.[20,25] Both self-report and actigraphy measures revealed that having highly variable sleep patterns was not only related to current suicidal ideation but also predictive of ideation 7 and 21 days later, adjusting for depressive symptoms and baseline ideation in young adults.[20] Intriguingly, sleep variability outperformed depressive symptoms in predicting future ideation. Similarly, sleep rhythm reversals (ie, sleeping during the day and being active at night) have been found to be associated with suicide attempts among adolescent outpatients.[23]

### Obstructive Sleep Apnea

Pediatric obstructive sleep apnea is a common condition, with an estimated prevalence of 1% to 6% in the general population and 19% to 61% in obese children and adolescents.[26] It is included in the DSM-5 and should be suspected in youth with frequent loud snoring, witnessed apneas (pauses in nocturnal breathing), restless sleep, and mouth breathing.[12,27] Sleep apnea severely disrupts sleep continuity, and individuals with sleep apneas are functionally sleep deprived. Despite the high prevalence of obstructive sleep apnea, research regarding its relationship with suicide risk is scarce. Although a few large-scale and small-scale investigations among adults found significant associations between sleep apnea and suicide risk,[28–30] studies of children and adolescents have been mixed.[28] A recent survey of 746 children and adolescents that used daytime sleepiness as a proxy for sleep apnea found that obstructive sleep apnea was significantly associated with suicidal ideation even when adjusting for depressive symptoms and perceived stress.[24] This study suggests that sleep apnea is a significant independent risk factor for ideation in youth, with the limitation that the diagnosis did not include history of snoring or objective measures for sleep apnea. Similarly, a large (N = 7072), rigorous prospective study of adolescents found that excessive daytime sleepiness at baseline increased risk of ideation (OR, 1.6) and suicidal plans (OR, 2.6) 1 year later, whereas self-reported loud snoring did not.[31] Thus, the impact of sleep apnea and snoring on youth suicide risk is currently inconclusive, with initial evidence suggesting that excessive daytime sleepiness confers additional risk beyond other risk factors, such as depressive symptoms, anxiety, and perceived stress.

### Nightmares

Nightmares are "extended, extremely dysphoric, and well-remembered dreams."[12] Clinicians often consider nightmares a feature of posttraumatic stress disorder (PTSD), but nightmares are often idiopathic, and frequent distressing nightmares are main features of nightmare disorder in the DSM-5 Sleep-Wake Disorder section.[12] Nightmares are usually described by frequency, level of distress caused, and chronicity.[32,33] Research examining nightmares in children and adolescents is limited,[34] but existing work suggests that nightmares are common, especially in younger youth. Approximately 22% to 28% of children aged 5 through 11 years experience nightmares, with a prevalence up to 41% for children in psychiatric care,[35,36] whereas 8% of older adolescents (15–18 years old) experience frequent nightmares.[35]

Nightmares have emerged as an important risk factor for suicidal behavior in adults.[10] Recent studies also support associations between nightmares and suicidal ideation and behaviors in adolescents and young adults, even when adjusting for mental disorder,[10,20,37,38] with a few exceptions.[10,11] A study of 503 college students found an association between nightmares and suicide attempts, even after adjusting for PTSD severity, highlighting that the morbidity of nightmares goes beyond PTSD.[39] A study of 50 inpatient adolescents showed an association between nightmares and suicidal ideation, independent of other sleep measures.[37] Two longitudinal studies suggested that nightmares precede both suicidal ideation and behaviors.[20,38] One study found that higher scores on a nightmare rating scale at baseline predicted increased ideation at 7-day and 21-day follow-ups in young adults,[20] and another study found that frequent nightmares increased the odds of suicidal behavior almost 2-fold (OR, 1.96) after 1 year among adolescents, even after adjusting for demographic factors and mental disorder.[38] Thus, available evidence suggests that nightmares are associated with increased risk of both suicidal ideation and attempts among adolescents and young adults.

## POTENTIAL MECHANISMS IN THE RELATION BETWEEN SLEEP DISTURBANCES AND SUICIDE RISK

Several studies have examined biological and psychological factors that may account for the impact of sleep disturbances on suicide risk. Biological factors include executive functioning, frontal lobe processes, and hyperarousal, whereas psychological factors range from thwarted belonging, perceived burdensomeness, and acquired capability to specific cognitions and appraisals such as defeat, entrapment, rumination, hopelessness, and negative self-appraisals (**Fig. 1**).[40]

### Executive Functioning

Sleep loss negatively affects executive functioning,[4] and executive function deficits have been associated with suicidal behavior. Accordingly, researchers suggest that insomnia and sleep disruptions may increase susceptibility to suicidal behavior via executive dysfunction.[4,11,41,42] Deficits in problem solving, decision making, attention, and impulse control have been found among suicide attempters and individuals with insomnia.[4,43–45] Likewise, insufficient sleep has been linked to impaired emotion regulation and heightened emotional reactivity, aspects of executive functioning linked to suicide risk.[4] Sleep restriction worsens mood and decreases adolescents' abilities to modulate negative emotions; these features have been found to be more severely impaired among adolescent suicide attempters compared with ideators,[46] as well as among adolescents with multiple attempts compared with 1-time attempters.[47] In adults, emotion regulation has been suggested to mediate the relationship between nightmares and suicidal behavior.[48]

### Hyperarousal

Hyperarousal has also been linked to suicide risk. Studies have connected increased agitation, hyperarousal, and night awakenings with susceptibility to suicidal behaviors.[40,49–52] In addition, hyperarousal states can amplify suicidal ideation and risk in adults with high levels of capability for suicide, operationalized as lowered fear of death and increased tolerance for physical pain, per Joiner's (https://www.ncbi.nlm.nih.gov/pmc/articles/PMC5730496/) interpersonal theory of suicide.[40] Similarly, nightmares might interact with acquired capability to predict suicidal behavior via hyperarousal.[53] Altogether, pairing increased arousal with other deficits in executive

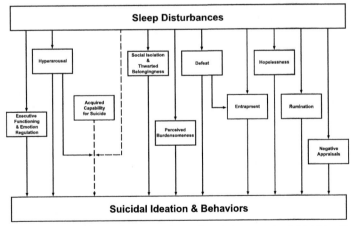

**Fig. 1.** Solid lines show pathways between sleep disturbances and suicidal ideation and behaviors via underlying biological and psychological mechanisms, as described in the text. Dotted lines show related pathways with mixed support from the literature, as described in the text. (*Adapted from* Littlewood D, Kyle SD, Pratt D, et al. Examining the role of psychological factors in relationship between sleep problems and suicide. Clin Psychol Rev 2017;54:10; with permission.)

functioning (ie, increased impulsivity, decreased problem solving, and so forth) that accompany sleep disturbances may increase susceptibility to suicidal ideation and behaviors in adolescents.[4]

## Thwarted Belonging, Perceived Burdensomeness, and Acquired Capability

The literature on psychological mechanisms underlying the impact of sleep disturbances on youth suicide risk is growing.[40] The interpersonal theory of suicide introduced 3 constructs that may determine suicide risk: thwarted belonging, perceived burdensomeness, and the aforementioned acquired capability for suicide.[40] Thwarted belonging represents feelings of loneliness, isolation, and lack of belonging, as well as limited social relationships. Perceived burdensomeness reflects individuals seeing themselves and their existence as a burden to family, friends, or society. The theory suggests that thwarted belonging and perceived burdensomeness lead to suicidal ideation, and people attempt suicide when they have also acquired the capability for suicide. The literature supports the idea that those with sleep disturbances and insomnia experience increased feelings of loneliness, isolation, and thwarted belonging.[9,54,55] Others are often asleep and unavailable at night, leaving those who are awake to feel more alone and without support. Insomnia has also been linked with increased perceived burdensomeness.[9,55] Thwarted belonging was found to mediate the association between insomnia and suicidal ideation in cross-sectional and longitudinal research with young adults.[56,57] Similarly, perceived burdensomeness mediated the relationship between insomnia and suicide risk in a cross-sectional study of adolescent inpatients.[55] However, studies investigating the links between sleep disturbances and acquired capability are scarce, particularly in adolescents, and the literature is mixed. For example, 2 studies found that insomnia was not associated with acquired capability in samples of young adults and adolescents, whereas it was positively associated with thwarted belongingness and perceived burdensomeness.[9,55] In contrast, a study involving mainly young adults found that insomnia and nightmares interacted with levels of acquired capability to predict concurrent suicidal ideation or attempts.[53] Altogether, data supporting a link between sleep disturbances and increased thwarted belonging and perceived burdensomeness are growing, as is support for associations between these psychological factors and increases in suicidal ideation and behaviors. However, the link between sleep disturbances and acquired capability is less clear.

## Defeat and Entrapment

Defeat (ie, the self-perception of low social rank) and entrapment (ie, the desire to escape without the means of doing so) are also linked to suicidal behavior.[40,58] In the context of sleep disturbances, some investigators see sleep as an escape from the physical or emotional pain individuals experience during the day.[59] However, insomnia and similar sleep disturbances that prevent sleep serve as barriers that prevent escape. Thus, a feeling of entrapment develops or is emphasized, which, in turn, may lead to heightened risk of suicidal behavior. For some, suicide-related behaviors may represent an alternative escape. Nightmares might trigger the perception of defeat, which may enhance the sense of entrapment, resulting in suicidal behavior. Perceptions of defeat and entrapment have also been found to mediate the concurrent relationship between insomnia or nightmares and suicidal ideation among adolescents.[8]

## Rumination, Hopelessness, and Negative Self-Appraisals

Other cognitions commonly explored in relation to suicide risk include rumination (ie, repetitive thinking about negative emotional states, their related causes, and their potential consequences), feelings of hopelessness, and negative appraisals.[40] As

**Table 1**
**Screeners and assessments**

| | Format | Description |
|---|---|---|
| **Suicide Risk** | | |
| Ask Suicide Screening Questions Tool | 4-question screener for youth 10–24 y of age | Suicide risk screener designed for emergency departments, inpatient units, and outpatient care settings. Available in multiple languages at http://www.nimh.nih.gov/asq |
| Columbia Suicide Severity Rating Scale | 17-item scale for children, adolescents, and adults | Suicide risk scale assessing past and present suicidal ideation and behaviors. Training and PDF versions for all ages and settings available at https://cssrs.columbia.edu/the-columbia-scale-c-ssrs/cssrs-for-communities-and-healthcare |
| Self-Injurious Thoughts and Behaviors Interview | 5 screening items and up to (long form) 169 or (short form) 72 variable-format items for youth and young adults | Suicide risk structured interview assessing suicidal ideation, planning, gestures, attempts, and nonsuicidal self-injury. Available at https://nocklab.fas.harvard.edu/tasks |
| **Sleep Disturbances** | | |
| BEARS | 5-item screener for youth 2–12 y of age; based on parent and/or child reports | Clinical interview and/or self-report form assessing bedtime issues, excessive daytime sleepiness, awakenings and abnormal sleep behaviors, regularity and duration of sleep, and snoring. Available in original article[65] |
| Child Sleep Habits Questionnaire | 45-item measure for youth 4–10 y of age; based on parent report | Parent-report measure designed to assess sleep disturbances, including bedtime issues, sleep-disordered breathing, daytime sleepiness, and parasomnias. Available in original article[80] |
| The Sleep Disturbance Scale for Children | 26-item rating scale for youth 6–15 y of age; based on parent report | Likert-style rating scale designed to capture sleep disturbances in youth. Available in original article[81] |

(*continued on next page*)

**Table 1**
*(continued)*

| | Format | Description |
|---|---|---|
| Children's Chronotype Questionnaire | 27-item measure for youth 4–11 y of age; based on parent report | Parent-report measure assessing chronotype in youth. Available in original article[82] |
| Sleep diaries | Self-report tracking tool for all ages | Self-report tool for tracking sleep regularity and duration. Recommended for long-term care. Template available at http://yoursleep.aasmnet.org/pdf/sleepdiary.pdf |
| **Nightmares** | | |
| Nightmare Distress Questionnaire | 13-item measure for young adults and adults; has been used with adolescents | Self-report measure using Likert scales to assess distress and impact of nightmares. Available in original article[83] |
| Disturbing Dream and Nightmare Severity Index | 5-item measure designed for adults; has been used with adolescents | Self-report measure assessing frequency, severity, and impact of nightmares. Available through the author[84] |

previously highlighted, many sleep disturbances often involve lack of sleep and increased time awake at night. During these late hours, individuals are often without support or social interaction, while others are asleep and unavailable. These times can leave individuals susceptible to feelings of hopelessness and rumination. A study of 27,929 adolescents found that every hour of less sleep was associated with significantly heightened odds of experiencing sadness and hopelessness.[60] Hopelessness may also partially mediate the relationship between insomnia or nightmares and suicidal ideation.[40] Similarly, diminished sleep durations and sleep quality have been linked with increased rumination and related repetitive negative cognitions,[61–63] and rumination has been found to mediate the link between sleep disturbances and suicidal behavior.[63] Relatedly, both negative cognitive self-appraisals and dysfunctional attitudes toward sleep have been found to relate to suicidal ideation.[37,64] Negative sleep appraisals were even found to mediate associations between sleep disturbances and ideation in individuals with depressive disorders.[64] Altogether, lack of sleep seems to have a cascade effect on perceptions and cognitions that may increase susceptibility to suicidal ideation or behaviors.

## APPLICATION TO CLINICAL CARE

Considering the literature's support that sleep disturbances are a modifiable risk factor for suicide in youth, it is imperative that effective and appropriate assessments for these phenomena be made available to clinicians and others. Screeners and assessments come in a variety of forms to adapt to various clinical and community settings: clinical interviews, self-report forms, and parent reports, among others. Resources for clinicians are summarized in **Table 1**. For sleep, the authors recommend a stepwise approach, starting with the BEARS (bedtime issues, excessive daytime sleepiness, awakenings and abnormal sleep behaviors, regularity and duration of sleep, and snoring) and proceeding with a more granular assessment if positive findings emerge from questionnaires or clinical interviews. Notably, using the BEARS in a primary pediatric setting increased detection of sleep disturbances 4-fold, compared with usual care.[65]

Although still untested, addressing sleep disturbances might ameliorate suicidal ideation and behaviors among children and adolescents. A few targeted studies of adults have found improvements in suicidal ideation by cognitive behavior therapy for insomnia (CBT-I) or hypnotics (1 trial used zolpidem and 1 mirtazapine).[4,66–69] No trials have been designed to measure change in suicidal behavior with specific interventions for insomnia or nightmares in youth, but a few trials have found improvements in mental health in youth receiving CBT-I.[70,71] Preliminary research on nightmares also suggests that imagery rehearsal therapy and exposure, relaxation, and rescripting therapy may be effective in reducing suicidal ideation in adults with nightmares.[72–74] Although there is some evidence that prazosin might reduce nightmares, 2 recent rigorous studies found that prazosin improved neither nightmares nor suicidal ideation in adult patients with PTSD.[75,76] However, there are no studies addressing suicidal ideation and nightmare treatment in youth, but imagery rehearsal therapy has been effectively adapted for adolescents.[77,78]

## SUMMARY

Sleep problems, especially insomnia, short sleep duration, and chronic nightmares, are potential risk factors for suicidal ideation and behaviors in adolescents and young adults, and they often precede the onset of suicidal ideation or behaviors. Disturbed sleep is present across diagnoses and is modifiable.[4] As such, it represents a promising area in suicide prevention. Appropriate screening for sleep problems should be done systematically for all youth endorsing suicidal ideation or behaviors or with risk factors such as mood or trauma-related symptoms.[4] More work is needed to clarify the role of extended sleep periods, excessive daytime sleepiness, and the possible contribution of other sleep disorders to suicide risk. Nightmares are rarely explored or addressed beyond PTSD, but they seem to be an independent risk factor for suicide. Importantly, the association between sleep symptoms and suicidal ideation and behavior endures in most studies, even when demographic factors or mood symptoms are taken into account. Of note, the links between sleep disturbances and suicidal ideation and behaviors in younger children and preadolescents are rarely studied, and more research is needed in this area. Previous work suggests that sleep problems precede depression in children, and it is possible that disturbed sleep precedes suicidal ideation in younger children as well.[79] Further research is needed to understand the relationship between sleep disturbances and suicidal ideation and behaviors in children and adolescents, because improving sleep may represent one of the most tractable opportunities to address the problem of adolescent suicide.

## CLINICS CARE POINTS

- Sleep disturbances are transdiagnostic, modifiable, and treatable.
- Screening for sleep disturbances in suicidal adolescents and vice versa is strongly encouraged, because sleep disturbances are associated with suicidal ideation and behaviors.
- Nightmares are often neglected symptoms associated with suicidal behaviors.

- Clinicians should consider a stepwise approach for assessing sleep, screening all youth with BEARS and then using questionnaires and clinical interviews if needed.
- Cognitive behavior therapies are effective in treating insomnia and nightmares.

## DISCLOSURE

The authors have nothing to disclose.

## REFERENCES

1. Balazs J, Miklosi M, Kereszteny A, et al. Adolescent subthreshold-depression and anxiety: psychopathology, functional impairment and increased suicide risk. J Child Psychol Psychiatry 2013;54(6):670–7.
2. Nock MK, Borges G, Bromet EJ, et al. Cross-national prevalence and risk factors for suicidal ideation, plans and attempts. Br J Psychiatry 2008;192(2):98–105.
3. Nock MK, Green JG, Hwang I, et al. Prevalence, correlates, and treatment of life-time suicidal behavior among adolescents: results from the National Comorbidity Survey Replication Adolescent Supplement. JAMA Psychiatry 2013;70(3): 300–10.
4. Kearns JC, Coppersmith DDL, Santee AC, et al. Sleep problems and suicide risk in youth: a systematic review, developmental framework, and implications for hospital treatment. Gen Hosp Psychiatry 2020;63:141–51.
5. Baiden P, Tadeo SK, Tonui BC, et al. Association between insufficient sleep and suicidal ideation among adolescents. Psychiatry Res 2019;287:112579.
6. Guo L, Xu Y, Deng J, et al. Association between sleep duration, suicidal ideation, and suicidal attempts among Chinese adolescents: the moderating role of depressive symptoms. J Affect Disord 2017;208:355–62.
7. Kim JH, Park EC, Lee SG, et al. Associations between time in bed and suicidal thoughts, plans and attempts in Korean adolescents. BMJ Open 2015;5(9): e008766.
8. Russell K, Rasmussen S, Hunter SC. Insomnia and nightmares as markers of risk for suicidal ideation in young people: investigating the role of defeat and entrapment. J Clin Sleep Med 2018;14(5):775–84.
9. Nadorff MR, Anestis MD, Nazem S, et al. Sleep disorders and the interpersonal-psychological theory of suicide: independent pathways to suicidality? J Affect Disord 2014;152:505–12.
10. Bernert RA, Nadorff MR. Sleep disturbances and suicide risk. Sleep Med Clin 2015;10(1):35–9.
11. Liu JW, Tu YK, Lai YF, et al. Associations between sleep disturbances and suicidal ideation, plans, and attempts in adolescents: a systematic review and meta-analysis. Sleep 2019;42(6):zsz054.
12. American Psychiatric Association. Diagnostic and statistical manual of mental disorders (DSM-5®). Washington, DC: American Psychiatric Pub; 2013.
13. Kim Y, Kim K, Kwon HJ, et al. Associations between adolescents' sleep duration, sleep satisfaction, and suicidal ideation. Salud Mental 2016;39(4):213–9.
14. Park JH, Yoo JH, Kim SH. Associations between non-restorative sleep, short sleep duration and suicidality: findings from a representative sample of Korean adolescents. Psychiatry Clin Neurosci 2013;67(1):28–34.
15. Weaver MD, Barger LK, Malone SK, et al. Dose-dependent associations between sleep duration and unsafe behaviors among us high school students. JAMA Pediatr 2018;172(12):1187–9.

16. Chiu HY, Lee HC, Chen PY, et al. Associations between sleep duration and suicidality in adolescents: a systematic review and dose-response meta-analysis. Sleep Med Rev 2018;42:119–26.
17. Matamura M, Tochigi M, Usami S, et al. Associations between sleep habits and mental health status and suicidality in a longitudinal survey of monozygotic twin adolescents. J Sleep Res 2014;23(3):290–4.
18. Goldstein TR, Bridge JA, Brent DA. Sleep disturbance preceding completed suicide in adolescents. J Consult Clin Psychol 2008;76(1):84.
19. Kim SY, Sim S, Choi HG. High stress, lack of sleep, low school performance, and suicide attempts are associated with high energy drink intake in adolescents. PLoS One 2017;12(11):e0187759.
20. Bernert RA, Hom MA, Iwata NG, et al. Objectively assessed sleep variability as an acute warning sign of suicidal ideation in a longitudinal evaluation of young adults at high suicide risk. J Clin Psychiatry 2017;78(6):e678–87.
21. Fitzgerald CT, Messias E, Buysse DJ. Teen sleep and suicidality: results from the youth risk behavior surveys of 2007 and 2009. J Clin Sleep Med 2011;7(4):351–6.
22. Lopes MC, Boronat AC, Wang YP, et al. Sleep complaints as risk factor for suicidal behavior in severely depressed children and adolescents. CNS Neurosci Ther 2016;22(11):915–20.
23. McGlinchey EL, Courtney-Seidler EA, German M, et al. The role of sleep disturbance in suicidal and nonsuicidal self-injurious behavior among adolescents. Suicide Life Threat Behav 2017;47(1):103–11.
24. Tseng WC, Liang YC, Su MH, et al. Sleep apnea may be associated with suicidal ideation in adolescents. Eur Child Adolesc Psychiatry 2019;28(5):635–43.
25. Lee YJ, Cho SJ, Cho IH, et al. Insufficient sleep and suicidality in adolescents. Sleep 2012;35(4):455–60.
26. Andersen IG, Holm JC, Homøe P. Obstructive sleep apnea in obese children and adolescents, treatment methods and outcome of treatment - a systematic review. Int J Pediatr Otorhinolaryngol 2016;87:190–7.
27. Kaditis AG, Alonso Alvarez ML, Boudewyns A, et al. Obstructive sleep disordered breathing in 2- to 18-year-old children: diagnosis and management. Eur Respir J 2016;47(1):69–94.
28. Bishop TM, Ashrafioun L, Pigeon WR. The association between sleep apnea and suicidal thought and behavior: an analysis of national survey data. J Clin Psychiatry 2018;79(1):17m11480.
29. Choi SJ, Joo EY, Lee YJ, et al. Suicidal ideation and insomnia symptoms in subjects with obstructive sleep apnea syndrome. Sleep Med 2015;16(9):1146–50.
30. Kaufmann CN, Susukida R, Depp CA. Sleep apnea, psychopathology, and mental health care. Sleep Health 2017;3(4):244–9.
31. Liu X, Liu Z-Z, Wang Z-Y, et al. Daytime sleepiness predicts future suicidal behavior: a longitudinal study of adolescents. Sleep 2019;42(2):1–10.
32. Nielsen T, Zadra A. Idiopathic nightmares and dream disturbances associated with sleep–wake transitions. In: Kryger MH, Roth T, Dement WC, editors. Principles and practice of sleep medicine. 5th edition. Saunders; 2011. p. 1106–15.
33. Sandman N, Valli K, Kronholm E, et al. Nightmares: prevalence among the Finnish general adult population and war veterans during 1972-2007. Sleep 2013;36(7):1041–50.
34. Munezawa T, Kaneita Y, Osaki Y, et al. Nightmare and sleep paralysis among Japanese adolescents: a nationwide representative survey. Sleep Med 2011;12(1):56–64.

35. Simonds JF, Parraga H. Prevalence of sleep disorders and sleep behaviors in children and adolescents. J Am Acad Child Adolesc Psychiatry 1982;21(4): 383–8.
36. Salzarulo P, Chevalier A. Sleep problems in children and their relationship with early disturbances of the waking-sleeping rhythms. Sleep 1983;6(1):47–51.
37. Kaplan SG, Ali SK, Simpson B, et al. Associations between sleep disturbance and suicidal ideation in adolescents admitted to an inpatient psychiatric unit. Int J Adolesc Med Health 2014;26(3):411–6.
38. Liu X, Liu ZZ, Chen RH, et al. Nightmares are associated with future suicide attempt and non-suicidal self-injury in adolescents. J Clin Psychiatry 2019; 80(4):18m12181.
39. Nadorff MR, Nazem S, Fiske A. Insomnia symptoms, nightmares, and suicidal ideation in a college student sample. Sleep 2011;34(1):93–8.
40. Littlewood D, Kyle SD, Pratt D, et al. Examining the role of psychological factors in the relationship between sleep problems and suicide. Clin Psychol Rev 2017; 54:1–16.
41. Fortier-Brochu É, Beaulieu-Bonneau S, Ivers H, et al. Insomnia and daytime cognitive performance: a meta-analysis. Sleep Med Rev 2012;16(1):83–94.
42. Lo JC, Ong JL, Leong RL, et al. Cognitive performance, sleepiness, and mood in partially sleep deprived adolescents: the need for sleep study. Sleep 2016;39(3): 687–98.
43. Miranda R, Gallagher M, Bauchner B, et al. Cognitive inflexibility as a prospective predictor of suicidal ideation among young adults with a suicide attempt history. Depress Anxiety 2012;29(3):180–6.
44. Bridge JA, McBee-Strayer SM, Cannon EA, et al. Impaired decision making in adolescent suicide attempters. J Am Acad Child Adolesc Psychiatry 2012; 51(4):394–403.
45. Keilp JG, Gorlyn M, Russell M, et al. Neuropsychological function and suicidal behavior: attention control, memory and executive dysfunction in suicide attempt. Psychol Med 2013;43(3):539–51.
46. Zlotnick C, Donaldson D, Spirito A, et al. Affect regulation and suicide attempts in adolescent inpatients. J Am Acad Child Adolesc Psychiatry 1997;36(6):793–8.
47. Esposito C, Spirito A, Boergers J, et al. Affective, behavioral, and cognitive functioning in adolescents with multiple suicide attempts. Suicide Life Threat Behav 2003;33(4):389–99.
48. Ward-Ciesielski EF, Winer ES, Drapeau CW, et al. Examining components of emotion regulation in relation to sleep problems and suicide risk. J Affect Disord 2018;241:41–8.
49. Han KS, Kim L, Shim I. Stress and sleep disorder. Exp Neurobiol 2012;21(4): 141–50.
50. Dolsen MR, Cheng P, Arnedt JT, et al. Neurophysiological correlates of suicidal ideation in major depressive disorder: hyperarousal during sleep. J Affect Disord 2017;212:160–6.
51. Perlis ML, Grandner MA, Brown GK, et al. Nocturnal wakefulness as a previously unrecognized risk factor for suicide. J Clin Psychiatry 2016;77(6):e726–33.
52. Mars B, Heron J, Klonsky ED, et al. Predictors of future suicide attempt among adolescents with suicidal thoughts or non-suicidal self-harm: a population-based birth cohort study. Lancet Psychiatry 2019;6(4):327–37.
53. Hochard KD, Heym N, Townsend E. Investigating the interaction between sleep symptoms of arousal and acquired capability in predicting suicidality. Suicide Life Threat Behav 2017;47(3):370–81.

54. Kurina LM, Knutson KL, Hawkley LC, et al. Loneliness is associated with sleep fragmentation in a communal society. Sleep 2011;34(11):1519–26.
55. Zullo L, Horton S, Eaddy M, et al. Adolescent insomnia, suicide risk, and the interpersonal theory of suicide. Psychiatry Res 2017;257:242–8.
56. Chu C, Hom MA, Rogers ML, et al. Is insomnia lonely? exploring thwarted belongingness as an explanatory link between insomnia and suicidal ideation in a sample of South Korean university students. J Clin Sleep Med 2016;12(5):647–52.
57. Chu C, Hom MA, Rogers ML, et al. Insomnia and suicide-related behaviors: a multi-study investigation of thwarted belongingness as a distinct explanatory factor. J Affect Disord 2017;208:153–62.
58. O'Connor RC, Smyth R, Ferguson E, et al. Psychological processes and repeat suicidal behavior: a four-year prospective study. J Consult Clin Psychol 2013; 81(6):1137–43.
59. Littlewood DL, Gooding P, Kyle SD, et al. Understanding the role of sleep in suicide risk: qualitative interview study. BMJ Open 2016;6(8):e012113.
60. Winsler A, Deutsch A, Vorona RD, et al. Sleepless in Fairfax: the difference one more hour of sleep can make for teen hopelessness, suicidal ideation, and substance use. J Youth Adolesc 2015;44(2):362–78.
61. Pillai V, Steenburg LA, Ciesla JA, et al. A seven day actigraphy-based study of rumination and sleep disturbance among young adults with depressive symptoms. J Psychosom Res 2014;77(1):70–5.
62. Takano K, Iijima Y, Tanno Y. Repetitive thought and self-reported sleep disturbance. Behav Ther 2012;43(4):779–89.
63. Weis D, Rothenberg L, Moshe L, et al. The effect of sleep problems on suicidal risk among young adults in the presence of depressive symptoms and cognitive processes. Arch Suicide Res 2015;19(3):321–34.
64. McCall WV, Batson N, Webster M, et al. Nightmares and dysfunctional beliefs about sleep mediate the effect of insomnia symptoms on suicidal ideation. J Clin Sleep Med 2013;9(02):135–40.
65. Owens JA, Dalzell V. Use of the 'BEARS' sleep screening tool in a pediatric residents' continuity clinic: a pilot study. Sleep Med 2005;6(1):63–9.
66. Trockel M, Karlin BE, Taylor CB, et al. Effects of cognitive behavioral therapy for insomnia on suicidal ideation in veterans. Sleep 2015;38(2):259–65.
67. McCall WV, Benca RM, Rosenquist PB, et al. Reducing suicidal ideation through insomnia treatment (REST-IT): a randomized clinical trial. Am J Psychiatry 2019; 176(11):957–65.
68. Gandotra K, Chen P, Jaskiw GE, et al. Effective treatment of insomnia with mirtazapine attenuates concomitant suicidal ideation. J Clin Sleep Med 2018;14(5): 901–2.
69. Manber R, Bernert RA, Suh S, et al. CBT for insomnia in patients with high and low depressive symptom severity: adherence and clinical outcomes. J Clin Sleep Med 2011;7(6):645–52.
70. Trockel M, Manber R, Chang V, et al. An e-mail delivered CBT for sleep-health program for college students: effects on sleep quality and depression symptoms. J Clin Sleep Med 2011;7(3):276–81.
71. Blake MJ, Sheeber LB, Youssef GJ, et al. Systematic review and meta-analysis of adolescent cognitive–behavioral sleep interventions. Clin Child Fam Psychol Rev 2017;20(3):227–49.
72. Germain A, Nielsen T. Impact of imagery rehearsal treatment on distressing dreams, psychological distress, and sleep parameters in nightmare patients. Behav Sleep Med 2003;1(3):140–54.

73. Ellis TE, Rufino KA, Nadorff MR. Treatment of nightmares in psychiatric inpatients with imagery rehearsal therapy: an open trial and case series. Behav Sleep Med 2017;17(2):112–23.

74. Cogan CM, Lee JY, Cranston CC, et al. The impact of exposure, relaxation, and rescripting therapy for post-trauma nightmares on suicidal ideation. J Clin Psychol 2019;75(12):2095–105.

75. McCall WV, Pillai A, Case D, et al. A pilot, randomized clinical trial of bedtime doses of prazosin versus placebo in suicidal posttraumatic stress disorder patients with nightmares. J Clin Psychopharmacol 2018;38(6):618–21.

76. Raskind MA, Peskind ER, Chow B, et al. Trial of prazosin for post-traumatic stress disorder in military veterans. N Engl J Med 2018;378(6):507–17.

77. Krakow B, Sandoval D, Schrader R, et al. Treatment of chronic nightmares in adjudicated adolescent girls in a residential facility. J Adolesc Health 2001; 29(2):94–100.

78. St-Onge M, Mercier P, De Koninck J. Imagery rehearsal therapy for frequent nightmares in children. Behav Sleep Med 2009;7(2):81–98.

79. Gregory AM, Rijsdijk FV, Lau JY, et al. The direction of longitudinal associations between sleep problems and depression symptoms: a study of twins aged 8 and 10 years. Sleep 2009;32(2):189–99.

80. Owens JA, Spirito A, McGuinn M. The Children's Sleep Habits Questionnaire (CSHQ): psychometric properties of a survey instrument for school-aged children. Sleep 2000;23(8):1043–51.

81. Bruni O, Ottaviano S, Guidetti V, et al. The Sleep Disturbance Scale for Children (SDSC) construction and validation of an instrument to evaluate sleep disturbances in childhood and adolescence. J Sleep Res 1996;5(4):251–61.

82. Werner H, Lebourgeois MK, Geiger A, et al. Assessment of chronotype in four- to eleven-year-old children: reliability and validity of the Children's Chronotype Questionnaire (CCTQ). Chronobiol Int 2009;26(5):992–1014.

83. Belicki K. The relationship of nightmare frequency to nightmare suffering with implications for treatment and research. Dreaming 1992;2(3):143–8.

84. Krakow B, Melendrez D, Santana E, et al. Prevalence and timing of sleep disturbance in Cerro Grande Firestorm victims. Sleep 2001;24:A394–5.

# *Moving?*

## Make sure your subscription moves with you!

To notify us of your new address, find your **Clinics Account Number** (located on your mailing label above your name), and contact customer service at:

**Email: journalscustomerservice-usa@elsevier.com**

**800-654-2452** (subscribers in the U.S. & Canada)
**314-447-8871** (subscribers outside of the U.S. & Canada)

**Fax number: 314-447-8029**

**Elsevier Health Sciences Division**
**Subscription Customer Service**
**3251 Riverport Lane**
**Maryland Heights, MO 63043**

*To ensure uninterrupted delivery of your subscription, please notify us at least 4 weeks in advance of move.